Fetal Growth Restriction

Luciano Marcondes Machado Nardozza
Edward Araujo Júnior
Giuseppe Rizzo • Russell Lee Deter
Editors

Fetal Growth Restriction

Current Evidence and Clinical Practice

Springer

Editors
Luciano Marcondes Machado Nardozza
Paulista School of Medicine
Federal University of São Paulo
São Paulo, SP
Brazil

Edward Araujo Júnior
Paulista School of Medicine
Federal University of São Paulo
São Paulo, SP
Brazil

Giuseppe Rizzo
University of Rome Tor Vergata
Roma
Italy

Russell Lee Deter
Baylor College of Medicine
Houston, TX
USA

ISBN 978-3-030-00050-9 ISBN 978-3-030-00051-6 (eBook)
https://doi.org/10.1007/978-3-030-00051-6

Library of Congress Control Number: 2018963221

This Springer imprint is published by the registered company Springer Nature Switzerland AG
The registered company address is: Gewerbestrasse 11, 6330 Cham, Switzerland

Foreword

Fetal growth restriction remains as one of the most common pregnancy complications which can have devastating consequences for both mother and fetus or neonate. Growth restricted fetuses suffer increased risks for stillbirth, neonatal death, preterm birth, neonatal morbidity, and abnormal neurodevelopment. Long-term risks include adult chronic disorders such as obesity, diabetes, metabolic syndrome, and cardiovascular disease. One of the most recent fascinating observations is that the diagnosis of fetal growth restriction also carries a significant risk for the mother including recurrent ischemic placental disease: preeclampsia and placental abruption in the pregnancies to follow, and increased risk for ischemic cardiac disease and premature death following the birth of the growth restricted neonate.

Given the huge impact of fetal growth restriction on both maternal and fetal/neonatal health, this book is an extremely significant and timely contribution. The book is unique because of its international scope written by world-renowned experts that represent seven countries and span four continents! Given the short- and long-term health consequences for both mother and baby, it remains vital for the international community to be familiar with cutting-edge information regarding the prenatal and postnatal diagnosis of fetal growth restriction as well as its pathophysiology, management, prognosis, neurological sequalae, and maternal cardiovascular involvement. This book covers everything!

The book, "Fetal Growth Restriction: Current Evidence and Clinical Practice," is the result of a combined effort of four distinguished editors, Drs. Edward Araujo Júnior, Luciano Marcondes Machado Nardozza, Giuseppe Rizzo, and Russell Lee Deter. These individuals are well-recognized authorities who dedicated their careers to the field of fetal medicine and specifically in the area of fetal growth restriction. These editors have undertaken a successful task of recruiting individuals known for their innovative research and technologies to contribute to the various chapters of the book.

The book presents the most current thinking about fetal growth restriction including: the concept of fetal growth potential which is an individualized approach for each fetus to be used as its own control; the early detection of growth restriction and transition from adaption to fetal growth pathology; the pathophysiology and causes of fetal growth restriction; the genomic factors regulating the process of fetal-placental vasculogenesis; early and late onset fetal growth restriction; the value of current biochemical, biophysical, ultrasound, and Doppler markers in the prenatal diagnosis and prognosis; current and future treatment; obstetrical management and interventions; and evaluation, treatment, and follow-up after birth including neurodevelopmental complications. The book concludes with the maternal cardiovascular long-term consequences for the woman after the birth of a growth restricted infant.

In my view, this book, "Fetal Growth Restriction: Current Evidence and Clinical Practice," covers every aspect of the topic of fetal growth restriction and provides up-to-date information like no other text or monograph before. This book will serve as *the* source for valuable information for clinicians and investigators and also as the basis for future research. I remain confident that this comprehensive book will come to stay as a classic reference in the area of fetal growth restriction and I strongly recommend its reading by all those health-care providers who are involved in the care of pregnant women and their fetuses.

Anthony M. Vintzileos, MD
Deputy Editor for Obstetrics,
American Journal of Obstetrics and Gynecology
Mineola, NY, USA

Preface

Fetal Growth Restriction: Current Evidence and Clinical Practice was conceived as a means for keeping the health professional up to date on a subject of great relevance to Obstetrics. It was written in clear and objective language, reflecting the experience of the authors in their respective fields. The book addresses aspects of normal intrauterine growth, as well as placental function, etiopathogenesis, and pathophysiology of this disease process. Clinical evaluation of fetal growth restriction (FGR) is described through its classification, diagnosis, and management. Long-term consequences of growth restriction are considered from the neurological and cardiovascular points of view.

We address recent knowledge about the new definition and recent classification of FGR, merging with the still important clinical evaluation. The presented proposal of pathology management appears as a consensus in the world literature.

This is a book for all professionals involved in Perinatology. It is the result of teamwork between professionals from different countries. However, this is not an exhaustive presentation of the subject but rather an update of the most important aspects of this topic.

We would like to thank all the professionals and friends from different countries who participated in this important work, especially the group that studies restriction of fetal growth at the Federal University of São Paulo, which encouraged us to undertake this important project.

São Paulo, SP, Brazil — Edward Araujo Júnior
São Paulo, SP, Brazil — Luciano Marcondes Machado Nardozza
Rome, Italy — Giuseppe Rizzo
Houston, TX, USA — Russell Lee Deter

Acknowledgment

I dedicate this book to my group of the Fetal Medicine Discipline, Federal University of São Paulo, and to my mother Antonia and my wife Renata who are with me in all moments.

Edward Araujo Júnior

I would like to thank all my family, especially my wife, daughter, and son for their wonderful collaboration and for always being by my side.

Luciano Marcondes Machado Nardozza

I would like to dedicate this book to Wes Lee for his help and support over the last 20 years, to Roberto Romero for his critical thinking that significantly improved IGA, to Ivar Rossavik whose insight made IGA possible, and to my beautiful wife, Susan, who has always been the first to appreciate what I have done.

Russell Lee Deter

I dedicate this book to my research team.

Giuseppe Rizzo

Contents

Contributors

Matteo Andolfatto, MD Department of Woman and Child Health, Maternal Fetal Medicine Unit, University of Padua, Padua, Italy

Matteo Arata, MD Department of Woman and Child Health, Maternal Fetal Medicine Unit, University of Padua, Padua, Italy

Roland Axt-Fliedner Division of Prenatal Medicine and Fetal Therapy, Campus Gießen and Marburg, Justus-Liebig University Gießen, University Hospital Gießen and Marburg, Gießen, Germany

Maria Paola Bonasoni Fetal Pathology Section, Department of Human Pathology, Arcispedale "Santa Maria Nuova", AUSL Istituto di Ricerca a Carattere Clinico Scientifico (IRCCS) di Reggio Emilia, Reggio Emilia, Italy

Danilo Buca Department of Obstetrics and Gynaecology, University of Chieti, Chieti, Italy

Ana Carolina Rabachini Caetano, MD Discipline of Fetal Medicine, Department of Obstetrics, Paulista School of Medicine, Federal University of São Paulo (EPM-UNIFESP), São Paulo, SP, Brazil

Marilia Calanducci, MD Department of Woman and Child Health, Maternal Fetal Medicine Unit, University of Padua, Padua, Italy

Inma Castilla-Cortázar Tecnologico de Monterrey, Escuela de Medicina y Ciencias de la Salud, Monterrey, NL, Mexico

Fundacion de Investigacion HM Hospitales, Madrid, Spain

Erich Cosmi, MD, PhD University of Padua School of Medicine, Deparment of Woman and Child Health, Padua, Italy

Department of Woman and Child Health, Maternal Fetal Medicine Unit, University of Padua, Padua, Italy

Fabricio Da Silva Costa, MD, PhD Department of Obstetrics and Gynaecology, Monash University and Perinatal Services, Monash Medical Centre, Melbourne, VIC, Australia

Francesco D'Antonio, MD, PhD Department of Clinical Medicine, Faculty of Health Sciences, UiT – The Arctic University of Norway, Tromsø, Norway

Andrea Dall'Asta Department of Medicine and Surgery, Obstetrics and Gynecology Unit, University of Parma, Parma, Italy

Russell L. Deter, MD Department of Obstetrics and Gynecology, Baylor College of Medicine, Houston, TX, USA

Elisenda Eixarch Fetal i+D Fetal Medicine Research Center, BCNatal | Barcelona Center for Maternal Fetal and Neonatal Medicine - Hospital Clínic and Hospital Sant Joan de Déu, IDIBAPS, University of Barcelona and Centre for Biomedical Research on Rare Diseases (CIBER-ER), Barcelona, Spain

Francesc Figueras Fetal i+D Fetal Medicine Research Center, BCNatal | Barcelona Center for Maternal Fetal and Neonatal Medicine - Hospital Clínic and Hospital Sant Joan de Déu, IDIBAPS, University of Barcelona and Centre for Biomedical Research on Rare Diseases (CIBER-ER), Barcelona, Spain

Nicola Fratelli Department of Obstetrics and Gynaecology, ASST Spedali Civili di Brescia, University of Brescia, Brescia, Italy

Tiziana Frusca Department of Medicine and Surgery, Obstetrics and Gynecology Unit, University of Parma, Parma, Italy

Tullio Ghi Department of Medicine and Surgery, Obstetrics and Gynecology Unit, University of Parma, Parma, Italy

Eduard Gratacos Fetal i+D Fetal Medicine Research Center, BCNatal | Barcelona Center for Maternal Fetal and Neonatal Medicine - Hospital Clínic and Hospital Sant Joan de Déu, IDIBAPS, University of Barcelona and Centre for Biomedical Research on Rare Diseases (CIBER-ER), Barcelona, Spain

Talita Micheletti Helfer Fetal i+D Fetal Medicine Research Center, BCNatal | Barcelona Center for Maternal Fetal and Neonatal Medicine - Hospital Clínic and Hospital Sant Joan de Déu, IDIBAPS, University of Barcelona, Barcelona, Spain

Anna Iacoi Division of Prenatal Medicine and Fetal Therapy, Campus Gießen and Marburg, Justus-Liebig University Gießen, University Hospital Gießen and Marburg, Gießen, Germany

Edward Araujo Júnior Discipline of Fetal Medicine, Department of Obstetrics, Paulista School of Medicine, Federal University of São Paulo (EPM-UNIFESP), São Paulo, SP, Brazil

Jader de Jesus Cruz Fetal Medicine Unit, Maternidade Alfredo da Costa, Centro Hospitalar Lisboa Central, Lisbon, Portugal

Annie Kroushev Department of Obstetrics and Gynaecology, Monash University and Perinatal Services, Monash Medical Centre, Melbourne, VIC, Australia

Marco Liberati Women's Health and Perinatology Research Group, Department of Clinical Medicine, Faculty of Health Sciences, UiT – The Arctic University of Norway, Tromsø, Norway

Department of Obstetrics and Gynaecology, University Hospital of Northern Norway, Tromsø, Norway

Laudelino Marques Lopes Department of Obstetrics and Gynaecology, Schulich School of Medicine and Dentistry, University of Western Ontario, London, ON, Canada

Irene Martín-Estal Tecnologico de Monterrey, Escuela de Medicina y Ciencias de la Salud, Monterrey, NL, Mexico

Luciano Marcondes Machado Nardozza, PhD Discipline of Fetal Medicine, Department of Obstetrics, Paulista School of Medicine, Federal University of São Paulo (EPM-UNIFESP), São Paulo, SP, Brazil

Kirsten Palmer Department of Obstetrics and Gynaecology, Monash University and Perinatal Services, Monash Medical Centre, Melbourne, VIC, Australia

Alberto Borges Peixoto, MD Discipline of Fetal Medicine, Department of Obstetrics, Paulista School of Medicine, Federal University of São Paulo (EPM-UNIFESP), São Paulo, SP, Brazil

Discipline of Obstetrics and Gynecology, University of Uberaba (UNIUBE), Uberaba, MG, Brazil

Department of Obstetrics and Gynecology, Federal University of Triângulo Mineiro (UFTM), Uberaba, MG, Brazil

Federico Prefumo, MD, PhD Department of Obstetrics and Gynaecology, ASST Spedali Civili di Brescia, University of Brescia, Brescia, Italy

Maya Reddy, MBBS, BMed Sci Department of Obstetrics and Gynaecology, Monash University and Perinatal Services, Monash Medical Centre, Melbourne, VIC, Australia

Miguel Angel Rodriguez-Zambrano Fundacion de Investigacion HM Hospitales, Madrid, Spain

Daniel Rolnik Department of Obstetrics and Gynaecology, Monash University and Perinatal Services, Monash Medical Centre, Melbourne, VIC, Australia

Gabriele Tonni, PhD, MD Maternal-Fetal Medicine Section, Department of Obstetrics and Gynecology, AUSL Istituto di Ricerca a Carattere Clinico Scientifico (IRCCS) di Reggio Emilia, Reggio Emilia, Italy

Silvia Visentin, MD, PhD Department of Woman and Child Health, Maternal Fetal Medicine Unit, University of Padua, Padua, Italy

Ana Cristina Perez Zamarian, MD Discipline of Fetal Medicine, Department of Obstetrics, Paulista School of Medicine, Federal University of São Paulo (EPM-UNIFESP), São Paulo, SP, Brazil

Cristina Zanardini Department of Obstetrics and Gynaecology, ASST Spedali Civili di Brescia, University of Brescia, Brescia, Italy

Standards for Fetal Growth and Neonatal Growth Outcomes

1

Russell L. Deter

Introduction

While the focus of this book is on *fetal growth restriction*, this condition cannot be discussed without defining normal growth in more general terms. The purpose of this chapter is to review how growth in both the fetus and neonate is assessed, and it will examine various ways of defining what is normal. With normal growth defined, growth restriction can be identified.

Growth Assessment

There are several fundamental aspects of growth assessment that are common to all methods now in use.

Choice of Growth Parameters

Fetal growth and development is a process by which a single cell evolves into an organism with 7500 named structures of different sizes [1, 2]. However, before the advent of obstetrical ultrasonography, this process could only be monitored noninvasively by measuring birth weight [3]. With ultrasound, the main components of the fetus can be visualized and measured [4]. For historical reasons [5], considerable effort has also been made to estimate fetal weight, a parameter that cannot be directly measured with ultrasound [6].

R. L. Deter (✉)
Department of Obstetrics and Gynecology, Baylor College of Medicine, Houston, TX, USA
e-mail: russelld@bcm.edu

L. M. M. Nardozza et al. (eds.), *Fetal Growth Restriction*,
https://doi.org/10.1007/978-3-030-00051-6_1

Table 1.1 Prenatal and neonatal growth profiles

Prenatal growth profile	
Growth variable	*Measured parameter*
Head size	Head circumference (HC)
Trunk size	Abdominal circumference (AC)
Soft tissue	Partial thigh volume (TVol) [ThC included]
Length	Femur diaphysis length (FDL)
Weight	Estimated weight (EWT)
Neonatal growth profile	
Growth outcome variable	*Measured parameter*
Head size	Head circumference (HC)
Trunk size	Abdominal circumference (AC)
Soft tissue	Thigh circumference (THC), arm circumference (ArmC), percent body fat
Length	Crown-heel length
Weight	(WT)

This table presents the anatomical variables that provide a comprehensive evaluation of prenatal growth and neonatal growth outcomes

Studies of growth abnormalities in both fetuses and neonates suggest that a comprehensive assessment of growth is needed as these abnormalities manifest themselves in different anatomical parameters in individual fetuses/neonates [7–10]. These observations have led to the development of a prenatal growth profile and a neonatal growth profile (Table 1.1) [11]. The prenatal growth profile provides a comprehensive evaluation of the major anatomical components of the fetus and can detect most, but not all, growth abnormalities [8].

All components of the prenatal growth profile can be measured directly with ultrasound except weight. Fetal weight estimations are obtained from functions relating sets of measureable anatomical parameters [obtained within 1–3 days of delivery] to birth weight [12, 13]. The weight estimation functions are obtained by multiple regression analysis and may have increased systematic errors if not sample specific [14, 15].

Choice of Measurement Parameters

A quantitative description of anatomical parameter growth during pregnancy requires the use of dimensional measurements [length, surface area, volume]. Since assessment is primarily with ultrasound, direct measurements of length are used primarily. However, profile area [16, 17] and volumes [18, 19] can be measured. Weight is estimated from sets of length and volume measurements [14].

Selecting the appropriate measure for an anatomical parameter involves the use of latent and observable variables [20, 21], the former having multiple definitions while the latter precisely defined (Table 1.2). This process involves having a clear concept of the information needed and establishing (through a chain of latent variables) that the observable variable contains this information. The observable variable chosen for each anatomical parameter needs to be specifically justified.

Table 1.2 Procedure for selecting a fetal growth parameter

Selection of an observable variable (accessible to ultrasound measurement) that can be used to quantify fetal growth requires a logical process involving latent variables. Given below is an example of such a process:
Latent variable 1 (definition of "growth assessment"): size or change in size with change in age
Size: Change in size with age is more appropriate but cannot be carried out if only one measurement is available
Latent variable 2 (anatomical parameter): head, abdomen, thigh, or femur
Head: All would be more appropriate since they represent different aspects of fetal growth, but *head* was chosen to simplify this example
Latent variable 3 (measure of size): profile circumference, profile area, volume
Profile circumference: Head volume would be more appropriate as it is not affected by shape changes, but complex technology is required for measurement. A head profile with unique anatomy can be defined
Latent variable 4 (method of measurement): tracing of perimeter of head profile or use of elliptical tool
Elliptical tool: *It has been* shown to give similar results as tracing, is less operator dependent and much faster
Latent variable 5 (standard to which measurement is compared): reference range, local prescriptive standard, national prescriptive standard, or international prescriptive standard
The observable variable in this example is the HC measured on the BPD plane with the elliptical tool and compared to the appropriate prescriptive standard

This table gives an example of the procedure used for selecting a growth parameter based on latent variables. Such a procedure provides a well-defined observable variable with the characteristics needed for a specific evaluation of a growth process

Choice of Age Estimate

As standards are age-specific, it is essential that the chosen fetal age be biologically justifiable and be determined as accurately as possible.

Types of Age Estimates

Menstrual age (MA) is the most widely used age estimate. It is measured from the first day of the last menstrual cycle [22]. This age includes a 2-week (on average) period *before* there is a fertilized zygote [22].

Conceptual age (CA) is measured from the date of either ovulation or fertilization and is synonymous with biological age [22].

Gestational age (GA) is synonymous with menstrual age even though its name suggests conceptual age. Because of this name discrepancy, it is not recommended as an age designation even though widely used.

Determining Age Estimates

Menstrual age is primarily determined from the patient's history. Estimates can also be obtained by ultrasound [4]. The most accurate estimates are provided by crown-rump length [CRL] measurements, followed by sets of biometric measurements made in the early 2nd trimester [22].

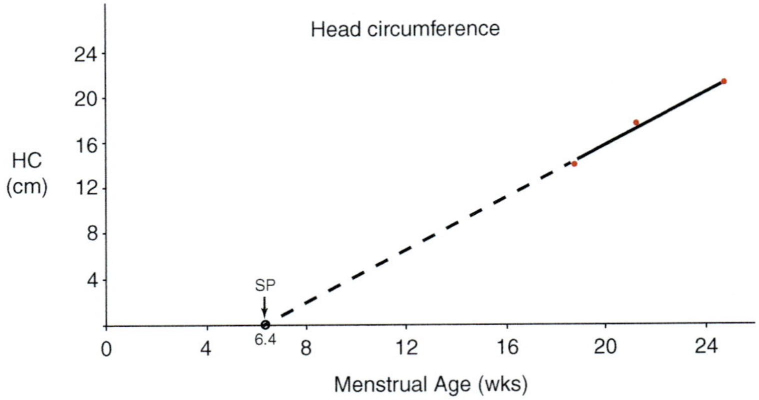

Fig. 1.1 Determination of start point. This figure gives an example of how the start point [SP] used to generate the time variable [t] of individualized growth assessment [IGA] is obtained [t = MA-SP]. A linear function [solid line] is fitted to three second trimester measurements of HC [red dots] and then extrapolated [broken line] back to where it crosses the menstrual age [MA] line. The crossing point [6.4 weeks in this example] is the start point for HC in this example. (HC head circumference)

Conceptional age can be determined by direct observation (IVF) and the LH surge or from basal body temperature and intercourse records [22].

Duration of growth {t} involves both menstrual age and a start point [t = MA − SP]. Start point values can be obtained by extrapolating a line fit to 2nd trimester measurements back to where it crosses the MA axis (Fig. 1.1) [10]. On average, SP values are in good agreement with the embryological appearance ages for various anatomical structures [10]. However, because of variation among individuals, better results are obtained when individual SP values are used [23].

Processing Fetal Measurements Related to Growth

Group Approach

Conventionally, the primary means for defining normal growth involves comparing an individual to the group to which he/she can reasonably be considered a member. Past studies have defined these groups on a local, regional, national, or international basis. The issue of which group should be used in these comparisons is currently a major topic of discussion among investigators [24–26], and no consensus has been reached.

Types of Reference Samples

Descriptive In past studies, biometric data has been collected on unselected samples from a given race, ethnic group, geographical location, or economic class [24–28]. Such samples provide a simple description of the distribution of measurements within the group. Adequate sample size to assure representativeness is the main requirement for such sampling.

Table 1.3 Criteria for selecting prescriptive samples

Criterion	Villar et al. [30]	Kiserud et al. [29]
Maternal age (years)	≥18 to ≤35	≥18 to ≤40
Maternal BMI (kg/m^2)	≥18.5 to ≤30	≥18 to ≤30
Maternal height (cm)	≥153	–
Singleton pregnancy	Yes	Yes
Fetal age	Known, normal MA	CRL confirmed MA
Type of pregnancy	Natural	Not stated
Medical history	No previous problems	No previous problems
Socioeconomic constraints	None	None
Tobacco/drug use	None in this pregnancy	None in this pregnancy
Alcohol use	<50 ml/week	Not stated
Recurrent miscarriage	None	None
Premature/LBW delivery	None	None
Congenital disease	None	Not in this pregnancy
Vascular disease of pregnancy	None	Not stated
Rh disease	None	Not stated
Urinalysis	Negative	Not stated
Blood pressure (mm Hg)	<140, <90	Not stated
Anemia	None	Not stated
Sexually transmitted disease	None	Not stated
Environment/physical work	Not adverse to pregnancy	Not adverse to pregnancy

This table lists the criteria used in two recent studies for selecting a patient sample which optimizes fetal growth and minimizes growth abnormalities

Prescriptive More recent studies have specified conditions that maximize normal growth and minimize factors causing growth pathology (Table 1.3) [29, 30]. Fetal growth in pregnancies meeting these criteria has been presented as how fetuses *should* grow. Results obtained using these samples have been proposed as international *standards* for normal growth since similar growth was found in different countries, at least for skeletal parameters [31].

A second type of prescriptive sample is chosen on the basis of a particular desirable neonatal characteristic [e.g., normal neonatal growth outcome as determined with the modified neonatal growth assessment score and a sample-specific reference range] [32]. Fetuses having this desired characteristic were assumed to have grown normally so were used to define size and growth reference ranges.

A third precriptive approach has been applied only to birth weight. The relationships between birth weight and known size determinants [maternal height, weight in early pregnancy, parity and ethnic group, as well as fetal sex] were established in a large, unselected sample using regression analysis [33, 34]. A function containing these variables was then used to determine the "term optimal weight" for any neonate at 280 days.

Classification of Size

With selection of a specific measurement, a fetal age parameter, and an appropriate sample, regression analysis is used to create cross-sectional, *population* size charts (Fig. 1.2) [29]. These charts usually present a set of continuous lines that represent *group percentile lines*. Comparison of individual biometric measurements to such a

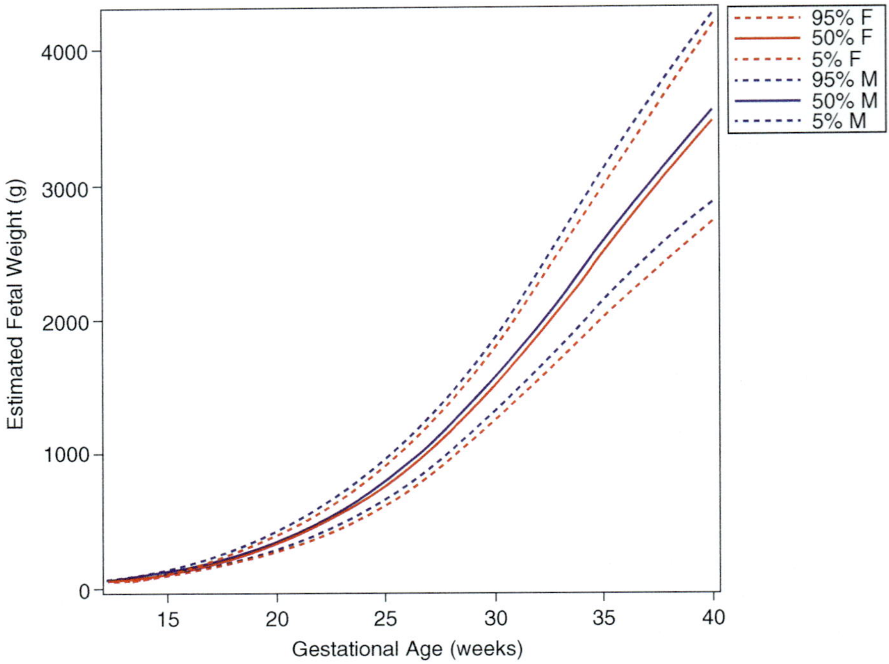

Fig. 1.2 Example of size standard for a specified group. This figure shows the conventional size [estimated weight] reference range used in comparing an individual measurement to the group. In this example, the 5th, 50th, and 95th percentile lines are plotted for both males (blue lines) and females (red lines). (These curves were obtained from the prescriptive sample of Kiserud T, et al. PLOS Med. 2017;14:1–36. [Figure used with permission])

group standard requires calculation of the appropriate *percentiles*. The percentile for a given measurement involves determining the number of standard deviation (SD) units between the measurement value and its expected, or 50th percentile, value in a normal distribution. The difference between the measurement and its expected value is calculated (deviation), and this difference is divided by the SD value (z-score [21]). The z-score value can be converted to a percentile, assuming a normal distribution, using a look-up table [35]. Obtaining expected and SD values for percentile calculation requires mathematical techniques found in the regression analysis literature and is age-specific [36].

Obtaining Expected and SD Values for Percentile Calculation

Cross-Sectional Data If all measurements are independent (one measurement per fetus), ordinary least squares regression analysis can be used to generate the expected value function with respect to fetal age and calculate the variability. If the variability is uniform with respect to age, a single SD value can be obtained and used at any age in the percentile calculation [37]. If there is a change in variability with respect to age, regression analysis has to be used to generate a function relating variability to age [38].

Longitudinal Data The use of longitudinal data to generate expected values and SDs is a relatively recent development but has the advantages of being more efficient and providing knowledge of growth outcomes which can be used to select a more appropriate reference sample. However, in addition to variability variation with age, the repeated measurements in each fetus are correlated with each other [autocorrelation] [39]. This results in biased estimates of the variability [40].

These statistical problems can be solved by using two-level, hierarchical linear modeling (first level, characteristics of the group; second level, characteristics of the individuals in the group) and generalized least squares regression analysis [41]. These procedures generate expected value and total variance functions that are age-dependent. With these functions, the expected value and SD at any age can be obtained.

Customized Percentiles In this procedure, the term optimal weight, based on known, physiological size determinants, is taken as the expected value at 40 weeks [33, 34]. The 40-week standard deviation of the birth weight sample used for specifying the term optimal weight function (expressed as a percent of the 40-week mean value) is taken as the variability parameter. These statistics are used to determine the percentile of the measured birth weight if delivery is at 40 weeks. In deliveries before 40 weeks, the term optimal weight is adjusted using a "proportionality curve" obtained by comparing 50th percentile *estimated weights* at ages before 40 weeks to the 50th percentile estimated weight value at 40 weeks [34]. The SD, as a proportion of the adjusted term optimal weight, is considered to be the same as that determined at term [34].

Distribution-Free Percentile Values A new technique, called *quantile regression*, is now available for obtaining age-specific percentile values directly from the data [42, 43]. This method makes no distributional assumptions and is more robust against the influence of outliers than conventional methods.

Criteria for Classifying Percentiles

The traditional, though still arbitrary, definition of a group of values is the 95% range because there are usually outliers due to errors of different kinds. This definition is independent of any distributional assumptions. For a normal distribution (usually assumed by most reference range studies), this is equivalent to the 2.5–97.5 percentile range. However, beginning in 1967 with birth weight [44], many clinical studies have used the <10th, 10–90th, and >90th percentiles to define abnormally low, normal, and abnormally high values for biometric parameters. More recently [45–47], below the 5th or the 3rd percentile has been used to define abnormally low values.

However, as pointed out by Deter and Harrist [11], what actually needs to be done is to find boundaries *empirically* that optimally separate normal and abnormal cases (Fig. 1.3). The objective of this approach is to choose a boundary that minimizes misclassification. However, this approach has the disadvantages of giving boundaries that change with different types of abnormalities and even with the same

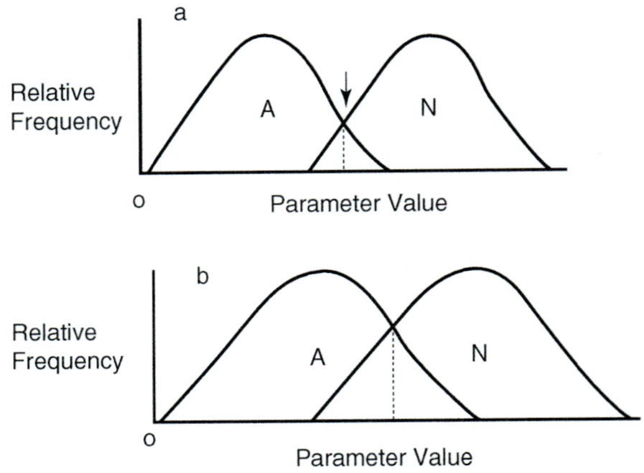

Fig. 1.3 Overlap of normal and abnormal size distributions. (**a**) shows an acceptable degree of overlap between the distributions of normal [N] and abnormal [A] values for a specific size parameter. This degree of overlap gives reasonable numbers for false positives and false negatives. (**b**) shows an unacceptable degree of overlap because the number of false positives and false negatives would be too high

abnormality, in different samples. Such boundaries are also subject to change with sample size until representativeness has been reached. However, such boundaries provide the most definitive information on the quality of the separation boundary in any given sample.

Finally, it must be pointed out that most symmetric distributions have theoretical limits of plus and minus infinity, so no matter what boundary is chosen, there will be some normal values below the boundary and some abnormal values above the boundary. The best that can be done is to minimize misclassification.

Problems with Conventional Classification

Descriptive Reference Ranges Reference ranges from unselected samples may contain individuals with growth abnormalities since growth outcome is not evaluated. They also may or may not be representative, and as they do not take differences in growth potential into account, this source of variation is included in the "normal variability." Group percentile lines cannot be considered individualized size trajectories [5].

Prescriptive Standards Because of the strict and comprehensive inclusion criteria, growth abnormalities are likely to be rare but still possible unless sample selection includes neonatal growth outcome information. Differences in growth potential are not taken into account so are again part of "normal variability." Again, group percentile lines cannot be considered individualized size trajectories [5].

There is also controversy over which biometric parameters to include in international standards [24–26]. Only skeletal parameters [more invariant between countries] have been proposed by one group [31], while other groups also include soft tissue measures and estimated weight (more sensitive to socioeconomic factors [31]) [28, 29]. This difference in approach appears to be due to what the standards are designed to do. The former would provide a means for evaluating overall obstetrical performance of different *groups* [e.g., countries]. The latter would be most useful in determining the growth status of *individuals* in different groups.

Customized Percentiles These percentiles are limited by their availability only for birth weight. Previous studies have shown that birth weight may not be affected in neonates with clear evidence of growth restriction [9, 47, 48]. The demographic parameters in the "term optimal weight" function only account for <10% of the birth weight variability [49–51], and including sex and birth age increases the percentage to around 25% [49, 50]. Adding pathological variables [50] or using a more comprehensive set of size determinants [52] increased the percentage to no more than 36% of the variability. These results indicate that the "term optimal weight" is being derived from only a fraction of the birth weight determinants and thus is very unlikely to be "optimal."

The "proportionality curve" used to adjust for delivery before 40 weeks may or may not be valid as it is based on weight *estimates*, not actual weight measurements, that are derived from a parameter set that does not include a measure of fat/muscle [12]. Its use also assumes that *group percentile lines* are the actual growth trajectories of individual fetuses. This assumption has been tested against individualized growth trajectories generated from empirical estimates of individual growth potential in fetuses with normal neonatal growth outcomes [53]. The use of percentile lines as individual trajectories resulted in significantly larger systematic and random prediction errors, indicating that an *individual*'s growth does not follow *group* percentile lines.

Individualized Approach

An alternative to the group approach described above is called individualized growth assessment [IGA] [10]. This procedure uses each fetus as its own control, generating individual- and parameter-specific size trajectories and predicted birth characteristics from empirical estimates of growth potential. A detailed presentation of IGA and its implementation (individualized growth assessment program [iGAP]) has recently been published [5].

Estimating Growth Potential and Start Points

Growth in the 2nd trimester has been shown to be quite linear in fetuses with normal growth outcomes and those with growth restriction for one-dimensional measurements [54]. This has also been found for two-dimensional and three-dimensional parameters after linearization with the appropriate mathematical manipulation [2D, square root;

3D, cube root] [10]. Linear functions fit to 2nd trimester measurements can be used for two purposes: estimating growth potential and determining start points for all anatomical parameters in each fetus.

Start Points [SP] Fetal age is customarily determined from the first day of the last menstrual period [menstrual age {MA}] [22]. However, this is, on average, 2 weeks *before* there is a fertilized zygote and over a month before embryological development has produced the first structure [head] that will be measured as part of the prenatal growth profile [1, 22]. Since it is not logical to talk about the growth of an anatomical structure before it exists (at least microscopically), an estimate of the *start point* [5, 10] for each measured anatomical parameter is needed for all fetuses. Start point values can be obtained by extrapolating the line fit to 2nd trimester measurements back to where it crosses the MA axis (Fig. 1.1). On average, SP values are in good agreement with the embryological appearance ages for various anatomical structures [10]. The availability of SP values allows definition of a new time variable for IGA, the *duration of growth* [t = MA − SP] [5, 10].

Growth Potential Linear growth in the 2nd trimester implies that the nutritional requirements of these very small fetuses are easily satisfied in normal pregnancies and even those with future growth restriction [54]. Under these circumstances, growth of the fetus is being determined by other growth controllers, both known and unknown [5, 54]. This is one of the several characteristic of 2nd trimester growth velocities (Table 1.4) that has led to these empirical measurements being proposed as estimators of growth potentials [each biometric parameter has its own growth potential] [54]. Second trimester growth velocities can be calculated directly if only two measurements are available. With three or more, regression analysis can be used to fit a linear function. The slope of this linear function is

Table 1.4 Second trimester growth velocity estimates of fetal growth potentials

Characteristics of second trimester growth velocities
Measures of change in size with age, not size alone, so most appropriate *growth* measurements
Empirical measures reflecting the effects of both known and unknown growth determinants
Measured during pregnancy when fetal nutritional requirements are low, thus primarily reflecting intrinsic determinants of growth
Remain constant during the second trimester, consistent with intrinsic control of growth and adequate nutritional supply
Specify Rossavik size models that accurately predict third trimester size trajectories and birth characteristics in fetuses with normal neonatal growth outcomes
Similar second trimester growth in fetuses with normal growth, growth restriction, and macrosomia

This table gives the characteristics of second trimester growth velocities that support their use as estimators of the growth potential of different anatomical parameters

taken as an estimate of the growth potential for that parameter in the fetus being studied. At least two sets of measurements (anatomical measurement and menstrual age measurement) separated by 2–3 weeks must be available between 14 and 26–28 weeks, MA [5].

Rossavik Size Model Specification

Rossavik Model IGA utilizes the Rossavik size model [55, 56] to generate 3rd trimester size trajectories and predict anatomical birth characteristics:

$$P = c(t)^{k+st}$$

1. $P \equiv$ anatomical parameter value
2. $t \equiv$ time variable [$t = \text{MA}-\text{SP}$]
3. $c, k, s \equiv$ model coefficients

A Rossavik size model is completely specified when values for the start point and for coefficients *c*, *k*, and *s* are known. The method for determining SP values is given in Fig. 1.1. Values for coefficients *c*, *k*, and *s* have been determined for nine anatomical parameters [BPD, HC, AC, FDL, ThC, HDL, ArmC, AVol, and TVol] by regression analysis in 118 fetuses with normal neonatal growth outcomes [32]. Coefficient *k* was found to represent the anatomical characteristics of the measured parameters (Table 1.5). Since coefficient *k* reflects anatomical characteristics that do not change, it is held constant at its mean values (Table 1.5). Repeated regression analysis with a fixed *k* gave new sets of coefficients *c* and *s* [c^*, s^*], c^* being linearly related to growth velocity (Fig. 1.4) and s^* being linearly related to

Table 1.5 Coefficient *k* values for different anatomical parameters

Head measurements	Abdominal measurements
HC: 1.405 BPD, 1.367	AC: 1.043
HA: 2.624	AA: 2.180
HV: 4.056	AV: 5.206
Upper arm measurements	Thigh measurements
HDL: 1.355	FDL: 1.258
ArmC: 0.844	ThC: 0.878
AVol: 2.927	TVol: 3.030

This table presents the empirically determined mean values for the coefficient *k* of the Rossavik size model, obtained from fetal samples with normal neonatal growth outcomes. They illustrate how this coefficient is related to the anatomy of what is being measured

Deter et al. [32, 56]

HC head circumference, *HA* head profile area, *HV* head volume, *BPD* biparietal diameter, *AC* abdominal circumference, *AA* abdominal profile area, *AV* abdominal volume, *HDL* humerus diaphysis length, *ArmC* arm circumference, *AVol* partial arm volume, *FDL* femur diaphysis length, *ThC* thigh circumference, *TVol* partial thigh volume

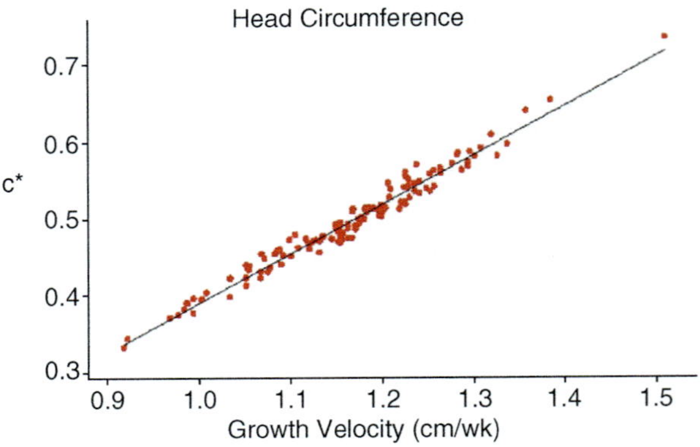

Fig. 1.4 Relationship of coefficient c^* to second trimester growth velocity. This figure demonstrates the strong linear relationship between coefficient c^* and the second trimester growth velocity of the head circumference in a sample of 119 fetuses with normal neonatal growth outcomes. The R^2 for this linear regression was 97.2% (see Table 1.6)

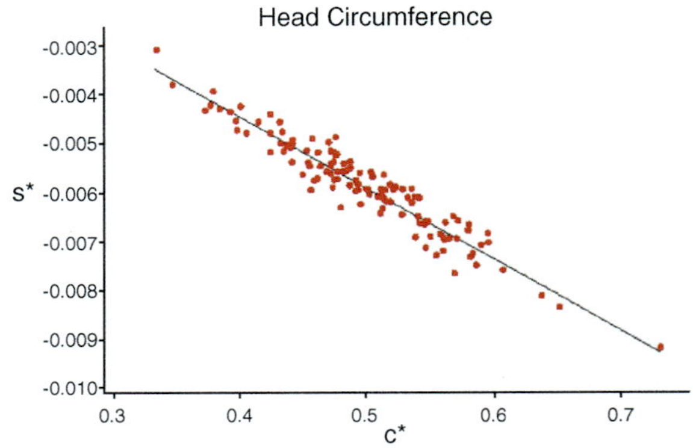

Fig. 1.5 Relationship of coefficient s^* to coefficient c^*. This figure demonstrates the strong linear relationship between coefficient s^* and c^* of the head circumference in a sample of 119 fetuses with normal neonatal growth outcomes. The R^2 for this linear regression was 91.3% (see Table 1.6)

Table 1.6 Mathematical functions used to obtain estimates of Rossavik size model coefficients

		$\log_e(c^*) = b_0 + b_1 \log_e(\text{slope})$			$s^* = c_0 - c_1(c^*)$		
Measurement	k	b_0	b_1	R^2	c_0	c_1	R^2
HC	1.405	−0.9326	1.4979	97.2	0.0013	0.0144	91.3
AC	1.043	−0.1306	1.3381	97.1	0.0060	0.0064	83.1
FDL	1.258	−0.0223	1.3665	97.7	0.0026	0.0448	88.7
HDL	1.355	−0.0196	1.4766	98.4	0.0016	0.0664	94.7
ThC	0.878	0.2952	1.1340	96.2	0.0076	0.0070	53.9
ArmC	0.844	0.4627	1.1779	96.2	0.0073	0.0084	53.9
AVol	2.927	2.0079	3.8187	97.1	0.0071	4.5928	75.3
TVol	3.036	1.2257	3.6705	97.5	0.0047	1.8970	69.5
BPD	1.367	−0.2207	1.4880	97.9	0.0016	0.0464	90.5

This table provides the functions needed to calculate estimates of the coefficient c^* from the slope of the linear function fit to second trimester measurements (growth velocity). It also gives the functions used to calculate estimates of coefficient s^* from coefficient c^*. Values for the coefficients k, c^*, and s^* specify a Rossavik size model in the second trimester

Deter et al. [32]

Note: *HC* head circumference, *AC* abdominal circumference, *FDL* femoral diaphysis length, *HDL* humeral diaphysis length, *ArmC* mid-arm circumference, *ThC* thigh circumference at level of mid-femoral diaphysis, *Hcube* head cube, *Acube* abdominal cube, *AVol* and *TVol* fractional arm and thigh volume, *BPD* biparietal diameter. HC and AC determined from short- and long-axis diameters

coefficient c^* (Fig. 1.5) {now known as coefficient predicted s^*}. Estimates of c^* and predicted s^* can be obtained for any growth velocity measurements using the functions shown in Table 1.6. This approach is able to specify models for two-dimensional parameters (e.g., head profile area, abdominal profile area [16, 17]) and three-dimensional parameters (e.g., head volume, abdominal volume, head cube, abdominal cube, partial thigh and arm volumes [10, 32, 56]).

Third Trimester Size Trajectories, Percent Deviations, and Pathological Percent Deviations

Third Trimester Size Trajectories Using models specified from 2nd trimester growth velocities [growth potential estimates], predicted anatomical measurements at various times in the 3rd trimester can be calculated. These predicted values form the predicted size trajectory for each anatomical parameter in any specified fetus (Fig. 1.6) [5, 32]. Such trajectories represent *individualized size standards* against which subsequent anatomical measurements can be compared.

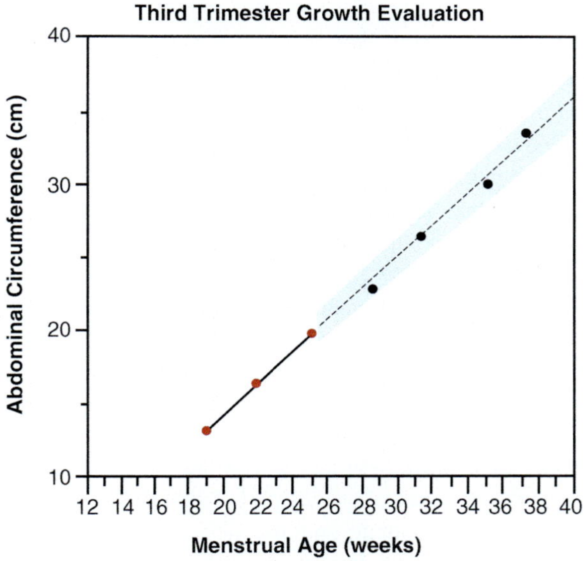

Fig. 1.6 Predicted size trajectory generated by IGA. Individualized growth assessment [IGA] provides third trimester size standards for each fetus as shown for the abdominal circumference [AC] in this figure. A linear function [solid line] was fitted to second trimester measurements [red dots], providing the growth velocity measurement [slope] needed for Rossavik size model specification. This model was then used to generate the expected size trajectory [broken line], which is the individualized size standard for this fetus. Subsequently, actual AC measurements at different time points [black dots] were placed on this graph to show how well actual growth followed the predicted trajectory. The blue area represents normal variation determined in fetuses with normal neonatal growth outcomes. (Deter et al. [5], figure used with permission)

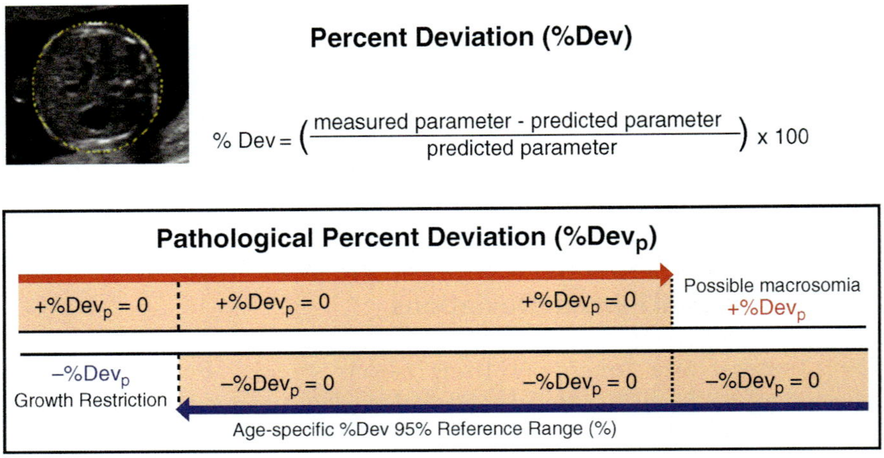

Fig. 1.7 Percent deviation and pathological percent deviation. In IGA, percent deviations [%Dev] are used to compare actual measurements to predicted measurements. This figure shows how this parameter is calculated. However, percent deviations are composed of random variations and potentially the effects of growth pathology. The growth pathology can be quantified using the pathological percent deviation [$\%Dev_p$]. This figure shows how both positive and negative $\%Dev_p$ values are determined by calculating the differences between the %Dev's and the appropriate upper or lower boundary of the age-specific 95% reference range. (Deter et al. [5], figure used with permission)

Percent Deviation Third trimester measurements are not compared to those of a *group* but to what the measurements *should have been* if growth continued as described in the 2nd trimester. The statistic carrying the information about such comparisons is called the *percent deviation* (%Dev, Fig. 1.7) [5, 47]. Percent deviations in normally growing fetuses reflect the effects of random variables such as measurement errors, modeling errors, and intrinsic biological control variability. They are independent of differences in growth potential and trajectory shape. Reference ranges for the percent deviations of ten anatomical parameters have been determined in fetuses with normal neonatal growth outcomes [32]. It has been shown that %Dev values are proportional to the difference between observed and expected average third trimester growth velocities so are measures of growth, not size [10].

Pathological Percent Deviation Percent deviations outside the appropriate reference range indicate the presence of growth pathology. The magnitude of this pathology can be determined by calculating the difference between the appropriate reference range boundary [upper boundary, accelerated growth; lower boundary, decelerated growth] and the percent deviation value, as shown in Fig. 1.7 [5, 47]. These differences are called *pathological percent deviations* [$\%Dev_p$] and can be either positive [comparisons with the upper boundary] or negative [comparison with the lower boundary]. Differences not giving information about the pathology being evaluated are assigned a value of zero (see Fig. 1.7) [5, 47].

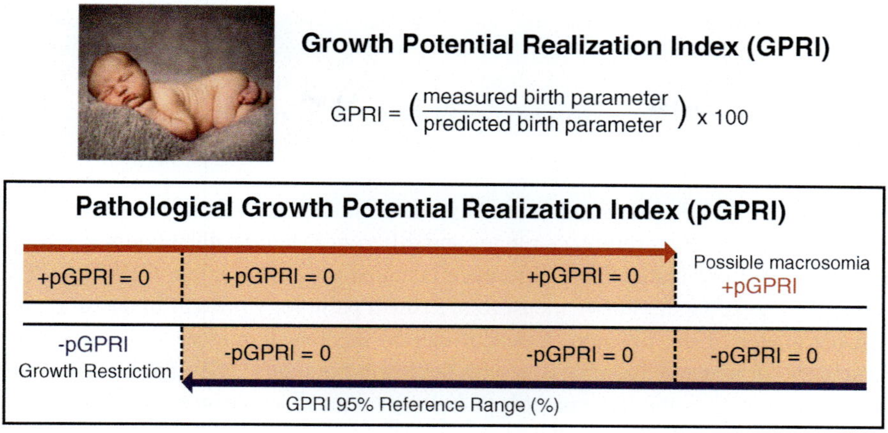

Fig. 1.8 Growth potential realization index and pathological growth potential realization index. In IGA, growth potential realization index [GPRI] values are used to compare actual neonatal measurements to predicted neonatal measurements. This figure shows how the GPRI is calculated. However, GPRI values are composed of random variation and potentially the effects of growth pathology. The growth pathology can be quantified using the pathological GPRI [pGPRI]. This figure shows how both positive and negative pGPRI values are determined by calculating the difference between the GPRI value and the appropriate upper or lower boundary of the 95% reference range. (Deter et al. [5], figure used with permission)

Growth Potential Realization Index [GPRI], Pathological Growth Potential Realization Index, and Modified Neonatal Growth Assessment Score

Evaluation of growth outcome in the neonate follows a similar pattern to evaluation of fetal growth except there is only one time of measurement. Previous studies [57] of late fetal growth have shown continued growth up to 38 weeks, MA. Beyond that point, very little growth is seen in fetuses with normal neonatal growth outcomes. For this reason, 38 weeks is considered the growth cessation age [57].

GPRI As with fetal growth, neonatal growth outcome assessment is based on comparisons of measured and predicted birth characteristics [WT, HC, AC, ThC, CHL, ArmC]. Direct measurements at birth provide the sizes of anatomical structures, while Rossavik size models are used to obtain predicted values, at birth age up to 38 weeks and at 38 weeks if delivery occurs later. For some parameters, systematic prediction errors have been observed due to differences in prenatal and postnatal measurement procedures [58]. These can be eliminated using appropriate correction factors [57]. The statistic containing the information about comparisons of measured and predicted birth characteristics is the *growth potential realization index* (GPRI, Fig. 1.8) [5, 47]. This parameter is the ratio of the measured value to the predicted value multiplied by 100 [ideal GPRI value = 100%]. The GPRI is independent of differences in growth potential, age at delivery, growth cessation, and systematic measurement errors. GPRI reference ranges have been established in pregnancies with normal neonatal growth outcomes [5, 10]. The GPRI has been shown to be proportional to the difference in measured and predicted average, 3rd trimester growth velocities so is a measure of growth, not size [10].

Pathological GPRI As with percent deviations, GPRI values can be compared to the boundaries of their reference ranges and differences between the boundary value and the GPRI calculated. This difference is called the *pathological GPRI* (pGPRI, Fig. 1.8) and is a quantitative measure of growth pathology present in the anatomical parameter of the neonate. Again, it can be positive [comparison to the upper boundary] or negative [comparison with the lower boundary]. GPRI values containing no information about the pathology being evaluated are assigned a pGPRI value of zero (see Fig. 1.8) [5, 47].

mNGAS Finally, the ultimate parameter for determining neonatal growth outcome is the modified neonatal growth assessment score [mNGAS] [9]:

$$m_3NGAS_{5.1} = 0.660(GPRI_{WT}) + 0.602\ (GPRI_{ThC}) + 0.394\ (GPRI_{AC}) + 0.159\ (GPRI_{CHL}) + 0.146\ (GPRI_{HC}).$$

This comprehensive, composite parameter utilizes multiple GPRI values (with all their advantages) and weighs them according to their importance to the mNGAS. The mNGAS has separated growth restricted, normal, and macrosomic neonates with accuracy of 96.9% in a previous study [9].

Prenatal-Postnatal Growth Assessment Concordance

As indicated above, IGA provides evaluations of 3rd trimester fetal growth and neonatal growth outcomes. These evaluations are independent of each other [i.e., information about 3rd trimester fetal growth is not needed to assess neonatal growth outcomes and vice versa] [5]. Agreement between these two assessments provides definitive information on growth status. This is because the alternative interpretation, that the different prenatal and postnatal sources of error cancel each other out to give the *same wrong answer*, is extremely improbable. Concordance can be considered the most definitive determinant of growth status.

Summary

Group standards are needed for assessments of single measurements or growth velocities calculated from two sets of measurements. With three or more sets of measurements, if obtained early in pregnancy, individualized standards based on growth potential estimates can be used. IGA evaluations of growth provide a wealth of information not available in the "snapshots" provided by the cross-sectional approach. A web-based computer program (individualized growth assessment program {iGAP} [5]) for implementing IGA is freely available at https://igap.reseach.bcm.edu. Particularly in high-risk pregnancies, this new information may prove useful in improving management and outcomes in these difficult cases.

Acknowledgment The author would like to thank Ms. Rajshi Gandhi for her help in the preparation of this chapter.

References

1. Blechschmidt E. The beginnings of human life. New York: Springer; 1977.
2. Dorland W. Dorland's medical dictionary for health consumers. New York: Saunders, an imprint of Elsevier; 2007.
3. Steckel RH. Birth weights and stillbirths in historical perspective. Eur J Clin Nutr. 1998;52:S16–20.
4. Callen PW. Ultrasonography in obstetrics and gynecology. 4th ed. Philadelphia: W.B. Saunders Company; 2000.
5. Deter RL, Lee W, Yeo L, Erez O, Ramamurthy U, Naik M, et al. Individualized growth assessment: conceptual framework and practical implementation for the evaluation of fetal growth and neonatal growth outcome. Am J Obstet Gynecol. 2018;218:S656–78.
6. Salomon LJ, Alfirevic Z, Berghella V, Bilardo C, Hernandez-Andrade E, Johnsen SL, et al. Practice guidelines for performance of the routine midtrimester fetal ultrasound scan. Ultrasound Obstet Gynecol. 2011;37:116–26.
7. Deter RL, Stefos T, Harrist RB, Hill RM. Detection of intrauterine growth retardation in twins using individualized growth assessment. II. Evaluation of third-trimester growth and prediction of growth outcome at birth. J Clin Ultrasound. 1992;20:579–85.
8. Deter RL, Xu B, Milner LL. Prenatal prediction of neonatal growth status in twins using individualized growth assessment. J Clin Ultrasound. 1996;24:53–9.
9. Deter RL, Spence LR. Identification of macrosomic, normal and intrauterine growth retarded neonates using the modified neonatal growth assessment score. Fetal Diagn Ther. 2004;19:58–67.
10. Deter RL. Individualized growth assessment: evaluation of growth using each fetus as its own control. Semin Perinatol. 2004;28:23–32.
11. Deter RL, Harrist RB. Assessment of normal fetal growth. In: Chervenak FA, Isaacson G, Campbell S, editors. Ultrasound in obstetrics and gynecology. Boston: Little, Brown and Co; 1993. p. 361–85.
12. Hadlock FP, Harrist RB, Deter RL, Park SK. Estimation of fetal weight using head, body and femur measurements – a prospective study. Am J Obstet Gynecol. 1985;151:333–7.
13. Melamed N, Yogev Y, Meizner I, Mashiach R, Bardin R, Ben-Haroush A. Sonographic fetal weight estimation: which model should be used? J Ultrasound Med. 2009;28:617–29.
14. Lee W, Balasubramaniam M, Deter RL, Yeo L, Hassan SS, Gotsch F, et al. New fetal weight estimation models using fractional limb volume. Ultrasound Obstet Gynecol. 2009;34:556–65.
15. Faschingbauer F, Dammer U, Raabe E, Kehl S, Schmid M, Schild RL, et al. A new sonographic weight estimation formula for small-for-gestational-age fetuses. J Ultrasound Med. 2016;35:1713–24.
16. Rossavik IK, Deter RL, Hadlock FP. Mathematical modeling of fetal growth: III. Evaluation of head growth using the head profile area. J Clin Ultrasound. 1987;15:23–30.

17. Rossavik IK, Deter RL, Hadlock FP. Mathematical modeling of fetal growth: IV. Evaluation of trunk growth using the abdominal profile area. J Clin Ultrasound. 1987;15:31–5.
18. Lee W, Deter RL, McNie B, Gonçalves LF, Espinoza J, Chaiworapongsa T, et al. Individualized growth assessment of fetal soft tissue using fractional thigh volume. Ultrasound Obstet Gynecol. 2004;24:766–74.
19. Lee W, Deter RL, McNie B, Gonçalves LF, Espinoza J, Chaiworapongsa T, et al. The fetal arm: individualized growth assessment in normal pregnancies. J Ultrasound Med. 2005;24:817–28.
20. Harris RJ. A primer of multivariate statistics. Orlando: Academic Press; 1985.
21. Salomon LJ, Deter RL, Alfirevic Z. How to improve on the analysis and presentation of research data submitted to our journal. Ultrasound Obstet Gynecol. 2008;32:721–7.
22. Deter RL. Fetal age determination and growth assessment: their roles in prenatal diagnosis. In: Evans MI, Johnson MP, Yaron Y, Drugan A, editors. Prenatal diagnosis. New York: McGraw-Hill; 2006. p. 387–405.
23. Deter RL, Rossavik IK, Cortissoz C, Hill RM, Hadlock FP. Longitudinal studies of thigh circumference growth in normal fetuses. J Clin Ultrasound. 1987;15:388–93.
24. Papageorghiou AT, Kennedy SH, Salomon LJ, Altman DG, Ohuma EO, Stones W, et al. The INTERGROWTH-21 fetal growth standards: toward the global integration of pregnancy pediatric care. Am J Obstet Gynecol. 2018;218:S630–40.
25. Kiserud T, Benach A, Perez RG HK, Carvalho J, Piaggio G, et al. The World Health Organization fetal growth charts: concept, findings, interpretation and application. Am J Obstet Gynecol. 2018;218:S619–29.
26. Gardosi J, Francis A, Turner S, Williams M. Customized growth charts: rationale, validation and clinical benefits. Am J Obstet Gynecol. 2018;218:S609–18.
27. Deter RL, Harrist RB, Birnholz JC, Hadlock FP. Quantitative obstetrical ultrasonography. New York: Wiley; 1986.
28. Buck Louis GM, Grewal J, Albert PS, Sciscione A, Wing DA, Grobman WA, et al. Racial/ethnic standards for fetal growth: the NICHD Fetal Growth Studies. Am J Obstet Gynecol. 2015;213:449.e1–449.e41.
29. Kiserud T, Piaggio G, Carroli G, Widmer M, Carvalho J, Neerup Jensen L, et al. The World Health Organization fetal growth charts: a multinational longitudinal study of ultrasound biometric measurements and estimated fetal weight. PLoS Med. 2017;14:e1002220.
30. Villar J, Altman DG, Purwar M, Noble JA, Knight HE, Ruyan P, et al. The objectives and implementation of the INTERGROWTH-21st project. BJOG. 2013;120(Suppl 2):9–26.
31. Papageorghiou AT, Ohuma EO, Altman DG, Todros T, Cheikh Ismail L, Lambert A, et al. International standards for fetal growth based on serial ultrasound measurements: the Fetal Growth Longitudinal Study of the INTERGROWTH-21st Project. Lancet. 2014;384:869–79.
32. Deter RL, Lee W, Sangi-Haghpeykar H, Tarca AL, Yeo L, Romero R. Individualized fetal growth assessment: critical evaluation of key concepts in the specification of third trimester size trajectories. J Matern Fetal Neonatal Med. 2014;27:543–51.
33. Gardosi J, Chang A, Kalyan B, Sahota D, Symonds EM. Customised antenatal growth charts. Lancet. 1992;339:283–7.
34. Gardosi J. Customized fetal growth standards: rationale and clinical application. Semin Perinatol. 2004;28:33–40.
35. Stell RGD, Torrie JH, Dickey DA. Principles and procedures of statistics a biometrical approach. New York: McGraw-Hill; 1997.
36. Altman DG, Chitty LS. Design and analysis of studies to derive charts of fetal size. Ultrasound Obstet Gynecol. 1993;3:378–84.
37. Draper NR, Smith H. Applied regression analysis. 2nd ed. New York: Wiley; 1981.
38. Altman DG, Chitty LS. Charts of fetal size: 1. Methodology. Br J Obstet Gynaecol. 1994;101:29–34.
39. Diggle PJ, Liang K-Y, Zeger SL. Analysis of longitudinal data. Oxford: Clarendon Press; 1994.
40. Elston RC, Grizzle JE. Estimation of time-response curves and their confidence bands. Biometrics. 1962;18:148–59.

41. Bryk AS, Raudenbush SW. Hierarchical linear models. Newbury Park: Sage; 1992.
42. Wei Y, Pere A, Koenker R, He X. Quantile regression methods for reference growth charts. Stat Med. 2006;25:1369–82.
43. Daniel-Spiegel E, Weiner E, Yarom I, et al. Establishment of fetal biometric charts using quantile regression analysis. J Ultrasound Med. 2013;32:23–33.
44. Battaglia FC, Lubchenco LO. A practical classification of newborn infants by weight and gestational age. J Pediatr. 1967;71:159–63.
45. Mlynarczyk M, Chauhan SP, Baydoun HA, Wilkes CM, Earhart KR, Zhao Y, et al. The clinical significance of an estimated fetal weight below the 10th percentile: a comparison of outcomes of <5th vs 5th–9th percentile. Am J Obstet Gynecol. 2017;217:198.e1–198.e11.
46. Poljak B, Agarwal U, Jackson R, Alfirevic Z, Sharp A. Diagnostic accuracy of individual antenatal tools for prediction of small-for-gestational age at birth. Ultrasound Obstet Gynecol. 2017;49:493–9.
47. Deter RL, Lee W, JCP K, Romero R. Fetal growth pathology score: a novel ultrasound parameter for individualized assessment of third trimester growth abnormalities. J Matern Fetal Neonatal Med. 2018;31:866–76.
48. Xu B, Deter RL, Milner LL, Hill RM. Evaluation of twin growth status at birth using individualized growth assessment: comparison with conventional methods. J Clin Ultrasound. 1995;23:277–86.
49. Hutcheon JA, Zhang X, Crattingius S, Kramer MS, Platt RW. Customized birthweight percentiles: does adjusting for maternal characteristic matter? BJOG. 2008;115:1397–404.
50. Anderson NH, Sadler LC, Stewart AW, LM MC. Maternal and pathological pregnancy characteristics in customised birthweight centiles and identification of at-risk small-for-gestational age infants: a retrospective cohort study. BJOG. 2012;119:848–56.
51. Sovio U, Smith GC. The effect of customization and use of a fetal growth standard on the association between birthweight percentile and adverse perinatal outcome. Am J Obstet Gynecol. 2018;218:S738–44.
52. Bukowksi R, Uchida T, Smith GC, Malone FD, Ball RH, Nyberg DA, et al. Individualized norms of optimal fetal growth. Obstet Gynecol. 2008;111:1065–76.
53. Deter RL, Lee W, Sangi-Haghpeykar H, Tarca AL, Li J, Yeo L, et al. Personalized third trimester fetal growth evaluation: comparisons of individualized growth assessment, percentile line and conditional probability methods. J Matern Fetal Neonatal Med. 2016;29:177–85.
54. Deter RL, Lee W, Kingdom J, Romero R. Second trimester growth velocities: assessment of fetal growth potential in SGA singletons. J Matern Fetal Neonatal Med. 2017 Nov;7:1–8. https://doi.org/10.1080/14767058.2017.1395849.
55. Rossavik IK, Deter RL. Mathematical modeling of fetal growth I. Basic principles. J Clin Ultrasound. 1984;12:529–33.
56. Deter RL, Rossavik IK, Harrist RB, Hadlock FP. Mathematical modeling of fetal growth: development of individual growth curve standards. Obstet Gynecol. 1986;68:156–61.
57. Deter RL, Lee W, Sangi-Haghpeykar H, Tarca AL, Yeo L, Romero R. Fetal growth cessation in late pregnancy: its impact on predicted size parameters used to classify small for gestational age neonates. J Matern Fetal Neonatal Med. 2015;28:755–65.
58. Hata T, Deter RL, Hill RM. Individual growth curve standards in triplets: prediction of third trimester growth and birth characteristics. Obstet Gynecol. 1991;78:379–84.

Small for Gestational Age Versus Fetal Growth Restriction

2

Russell L. Deter

Introduction

A discussion of this topic has to begin by pointing out that small for gestational age (SGA) is a neonatal growth outcome classification based on birth weight [1], while fetal growth restriction (FGR) is a process by which the fetus tries to adapt to in utero malnutrition [2]. It is often assumed that the latter results in the former, but as this chapter will show, that is frequently not true if proper growth assessment methods are used [3–5]. However, both terms can signify the presence of a growth abnormality, which can increase the risk for perinatal complications [6]. The etiology of these growth abnormalities will be discussed in another chapter (Chap. 3). This chapter will deal with how to correctly identify growth restriction in both the fetus and neonate.

Evolutionary Perspective

In order to detect and evaluate a fetal growth abnormality, it is important to consider the evolutionary aspects of human pregnancy. Recent paleoanthropology studies of *Homo sapiens* remains [7] indicate that humans have been procreating for at least 250,000–300,000 years, long before recorded history (10,000–15,000 BCE) or "modern times" (after 1400 CE). Therefore, the current reproductive system is primarily designed for "cave women and cave fetuses." As with all systems resulting from "survival of the fittest" evolution, its primary objective is to perpetuate the parents' DNA in the next generation. This requires survival of the fetus in utero and

R. L. Deter (✉)
Department of Obstetrics and Gynecology, Baylor College of Medicine, Houston, TX, USA
e-mail: russelld@bcm.edu

L. M. M. Nardozza et al. (eds.), *Fetal Growth Restriction*,
https://doi.org/10.1007/978-3-030-00051-6_2

the neonate during the first month after delivery in a hostile environment where his/her caretakers know very little about the survival requirements. In essence, given this level of ignorance, the system had to perform *automatically* almost all the time or none of us would be here!

Beginning around 28 weeks, menstrual age (MA) (after which postnatal survival of "cave" babies might even be possible [8]), the fetus starts to deposit muscle and fat on the limbs [9, 10] to provide stores of energy for use postnatally. Only after 38 weeks, MA, does normal growth stop [3], most likely to shift energy to those processes preparing the fetus for extrauterine life in the "cave." If the nutrient supply supporting the growth process is compromised (for whatever reason), adaption must occur or the "cave fetus" would die since there was no understanding of the situation and technical help was not available. If the fetus died, without antibiotics and operative delivery, the "cave mother" would also die and her genetic line would be gone.

Fetal Adaption to Compromised Nutrient Supply

Modern scientific studies of malnourished primate and human fetuses have shown various adaptions to growth restriction including (1) increased red cell production during hypoxia [2], (2) metabolic downregulation of growth processes [11] and blood redistribution to vital organs [12]. Various regulatory systems are involved [2], and differential vasoconstriction/vasodilatation produce blood flow changes [12]. Since quantification and characterization of growth restriction evolution has only recently been possible [5, 13], it is not known how these adaptive processes are related to the severity and progression of different types of growth restriction. However, it would be logical to speculate that if growth restriction developed slowly and was not too severe, metabolic downregulation would predominate and only at the latter stages (provided the abnormality was severe enough) would vascular changes be seen. If severe and rapidly developing, vascular changes would be expected to predominate since they maximize protection of the brain [12].

Small for Gestational Age (SGA)

Definition

In the early 1800s, birth weights became the first measurement to reflect fetal growth in utero [14], even though it is a measure of *size* not *growth* [15]. By the 1960s, it was recognized that neonates with small birth weights had higher incidences of perinatal complications and death [16, 17]. This resulted in a number of studies concerned with outcomes in low birth weight (LBW, <2500 g) infants [17]. Later, however, it was recognized that a neonate could be LBW because it was growth restricted, premature, or both [17]. To eliminate this confounding, Battaglia and Lubchenco published their now classic paper [1] which considered both age and weight in classifying neonatal birth weights. This system, still in use today, subdivides neonates into three groups, small for gestational age {SGA} (less than the 10th percentile for birth age), appropriate for gestational age {AGA} (between the 10th and 90th percentiles for birth age), and large for gestational age {LGA} (above the 90th percentile for birth age). The only justification given for these boundaries was that the 10th percentile values in various studies of birth weight were similar [1]. This is a classification of *size* (not growth) with respect to the *group* (not the individual). However, the SGA-AGA-LGA system did provide a means for relating size and prematurity to neonatal mortality [18].

For many years following publication of the Battaglia-Lubchenco system, SGA neonates were considered growth restricted and the designation used to identify fetuses with this growth abnormality [19]. With the advent of obstetrical ultrasound in the late 1970s, direct studies of fetal growth became possible. Given the history with birth weight, investigators focused on developing ways to estimate fetal weight (EFW) [20–22] since this is a parameter that cannot be measured directly with ultrasound. As a result, some obstetrical organizations have defined *fetal growth restriction* as an *estimated weight* below the 10th percentile for age [23]. Considerable effort has been made to use EFW to predict birth weight categories so that the relationships between birth weight and perinatal complication/developmental abnormalities could be used in risk assessment. However, recent studies have concluded that such predictions are not accurate enough for clinical use [24, 25].

Fetal Growth Restriction (FGR)

Even if EFW or some other prenatal measurement could predict SGA status accurately, there is another major problem. A birth weight categorization of SGA does not necessarily mean that the fetus was growth restricted. This categorization is based on comparison of the individual to a *group* and does not take into account the growth potential of the individual [26]. Normally growing, genetically small fetuses would also be classified as SGA, and genetically larger fetuses with growth restriction would be classified as AGA. Therefore a different approach to identifying growth-restricted fetuses and neonates is needed.

Definition of FGR in Individual Fetuses

The most logical definition of *growth restriction* is failure to achieve growth potential [15]. However, this definition requires a definition of *growth potential* to be meaningful. Deter et al. [26–28] have proposed the use of the second trimester growth velocity as an empirically determined parameter that can be used to estimate growth potential. As can be seen in Table 2.1, these velocities have properties that make them appropriate estimators of the latent variable, *growth potential* [28]. However, use of this definition results in multiple growth potentials, one for each anatomical parameter measured. Therefore, there are multiple *growth restrictions*,

Table 2.1 Specific fetal growth pathology parameters

Trimester	Parameter name	Abbreviation	Description and use
Second	Abnormal Growth Velocity Score	AGVS	Difference between the reference range boundary and the measurement; classifies growth velocities as abnormally high or low and gives abnormality magnitudes. This score can be used to detect growth abnormalities beginning in either the first or second trimester
Third	Pathological Percent Deviation	$\%Dev_p$	Difference between the reference range boundary and the measurement (Fig. 1.7, Chap 1). This parameter provides a measure of growth pathology for individual anatomical parameters at specified time points
	Anatomical Parameter Prenatal Growth Assessment Score	apPGAS	Average pathological percent deviation for a single anatomical parameter during the third trimester. This score provides a measure of growth pathology during the third trimester for individual anatomical parameters
	Individual Composite Prenatal Growth Assessment Score	icPGAS	Average pathological percent deviation for a set of anatomical parameters at a specific time point. This score provides a way to evaluate growth abnormalities that manifest themselves differently among fetuses (Fig. 2.1)
	Fetal Growth Pathology Score	FGPS	Average pathological percent deviation for all available anatomical measurements at specific time points in the third trimester (Fig. 2.2). The FGPS measures growth pathology found in the third trimester using all anatomical parameters and time points

This table presents the five parameters utilized by individualized growth assessment [IGA] to detect and quantify growth pathology in the second [AGVS] and third [%Devp, apPGAS, icPGAS, FGPS] trimesters. On the right-hand side are the descriptions and uses of these growth pathology parameters Deter et al. [15], table used with permission

one for each anatomical parameter, or set of parameters, regardless of how they may be defined at different times in pregnancy. What is not clear is how *clinically significant* growth restriction should be defined.

Second Trimester FGR

Previous studies [29] have shown that a small percentage (>10%) of fetal growth restriction can be caused by abnormalities in the first trimester (e.g., genetic problems, congenital infections, exposure to toxins, etc.). These cases may be detected in the early second trimester using growth velocity measurements. Velocities measured later in the second trimester might identify early growth restriction due to other causes (e.g., smoking).

In a previous publication [27], Deter et al. presented second trimester growth velocity reference ranges for nine anatomical parameters (BPD, HC, AC, FDL, ThC, HDL, ArmC, AVol, and TVol) in pregnancies with normal neonatal growth outcomes. Comparison of growth velocity measurements made in the second trimester to these reference ranges can be used to detect very early growth restriction. For individual anatomical parameters, the growth restriction is quantified by calculation of the Abnormal Growth Velocity Score (AGVS) [28]. This Score sets all growth velocities above the lower reference range boundary equal to zero. It uses the difference between the boundary and the actual velocity as the measure of growth pathology magnitude. The AGVS is one of several IGA parameters that can quantify growth pathology.

Single Anatomical Parameter Third Trimester FGR

In certain fetuses, growth restriction can be limited to a single anatomical parameter (head [4], soft tissue [30]). As this condition cannot be detected at every third trimester time point, more consistent results can be obtained by using the modified anatomical parameter Prenatal Growth Assessment Score (apPGAS, Fig. 2.1) [31]. The apPGAS (e.g., hcPGAS, thcPGAS) is the average of the negative, pathological percent deviations ($-\%Dev_p$; see Chap. 1) obtained for the studied parameter during the third trimester. Reference ranges for these parameters, determined in fetuses with normal neonatal growth outcomes, are found in Ref. [31]. Since apPGAS values are derived from $-\%Dev_p$ values, they quantify the growth pathology (Table 2.1) [15].

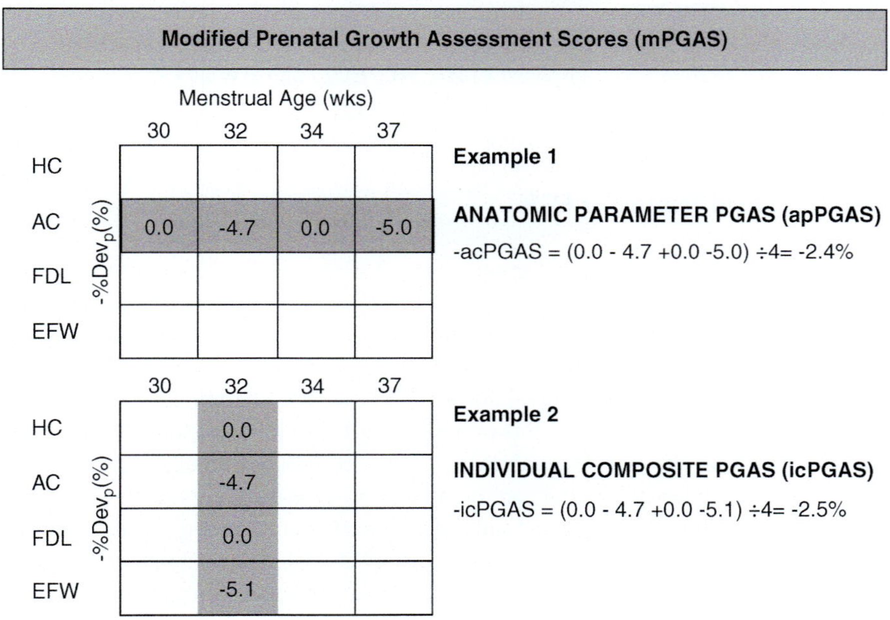

Fig. 2.1 Modified Prenatal Growth Assessment Scores. This figure presents the calculation of an anatomical parameter Prenatal Growth Assessment Score [apPGAS]. This IGA parameter provides a means for summarizing growth pathology for a single anatomical parameter during the third trimester [see Table 2.1]. Also presented is the calculation of an individual composite Prenatal Growth Assessment Score [icPGAS]. This IGA parameter provides a summary of growth pathology at a single time point (see Table 2.1). (HC head circumference, AC abdominal circumference, FDL femur diaphysis length, EFW estimated fetal weight. Deter et al. [15], figure used with permission)

Single Time Point Third Trimester FGR

In many longitudinal studies of fetal growth, serial ultrasound scans are complemented by intermittent scans using other imaging modalities (e.g., MRI), physiological assessments (e.g., Doppler evaluations of blood velocity; see Chap. 10), or measurement of biochemical parameters (e.g., placental biomarkers; see Chap. 7). In these situations, fetal growth status at the same time points where additional information was acquired is needed for making comparisons. These assessments are more consistent between fetuses if a set of anatomical parameters is used since different fetuses manifest growth restriction in different ways [15, 26]. EFW has been used for this purpose by many investigators, but it has a number of significant problems: (1) it is estimated, not measured [32]; (2) the accuracy of estimates in the second trimester may not be well defined because the number of birth weights available for comparison within 3 days of the scan is often small [32]; (3) normal variability is large (12–20% [20–22]); (4) estimation coefficients are related to birth weight, which may produce errors since all growth-restricted fetuses do not have abnormal birth weights [33]; (5) estimation coefficients often need to be sample-specific [34, 35].

An alternative to EFW is the individual composite Prenatal Growth Assessment Score (icPGAS, Fig. 2.1) [31]. The icPGAS is the average of the -%Dev values obtained for each of a set of growth measures at a specific time point. As the set can be defined in different ways, a number of different icPGASs can be specified. The only one used to date was composed of HC, AC, FDL, and EWT [13]. The icPGAS is also a quantifier of growth pathology (Table 2.1) [15].

General Third Trimester FGR

In ongoing as well as completed pregnancies, it is frequently important to have an overall view of growth restriction in the third trimester. With IGA, the quantitative measures of growth restriction, $-\%\mathrm{Dev}_\mathrm{p}$ values, are being collected for a set of anatomical parameters sequentially at each time point studied. These data can be used to calculate the desired general measure of growth restriction, the Fetal Growth Pathology Score (FGPS) [5]. As shown in Fig. 2.2, the FGPS is the cumulative moving average of all the $-\%\mathrm{Dev}_\mathrm{p}$ values collected up through the current scan. This method of calculation retains the history of the growth restriction process and allows for variations in the parameter and time of occurrence of pathological findings frequently observed in growth restriction processes [15, 26]. As an average of all available $-\%\mathrm{Dev}_\mathrm{p}$ values, it is the best general statistic for representing third trimester growth restriction in any given fetus. Any number of FGPSs can be defined, depending on the composition of the anatomical parameter set; so many types of growth restriction can be investigated. However, only one (FGPS1) has been used to date. Its set includes the conventional biometric parameters HC, AC, FDL, and EWT [5,

a

Fetal Growth Pathology Score (FGPS1)

Menstrual age (weeks)	30	32	34	37
	Negative Pathological Percent Deviation (-%Dev $_p$)			
HC	0.0	0.0	0.0	0.0
AC	0.0	-4.7	0.0	-5.0
FDL	0.0	0.0	0.0	0.0
EWT	0.0	-5.1	-0.4	-8.8
FGPS1$_{At1}$ = 0.0%				
HC	0.0	0.0	0.0	0.0
AC	0.0	-4.7	0.0	-5.0
FDL	0.0	0.0	0.0	0.0
EWT	0.0	-5.1	-0.4	-8.8
FGPS1$_{At2}$ = -1.23%				
HC	0.0	0.0	0.0	0.0
AC	0.0	-4.7	0.0	-5.0
FDL	0.0	0.0	0.0	0.0
EWT	0.0	-5.1	-0.4	-8.8
FGPS1$_{At3}$ = -0.85%				
HC	0.0	0.0	0.0	0.0
AC	0.0	-4.7	0.0	-5.0
FDL	0.0	0.0	0.0	0.0
EWT	0.0	-5.1	-0.4	-8.8
FGPS1$_{At4}$ = -1.53%				

b

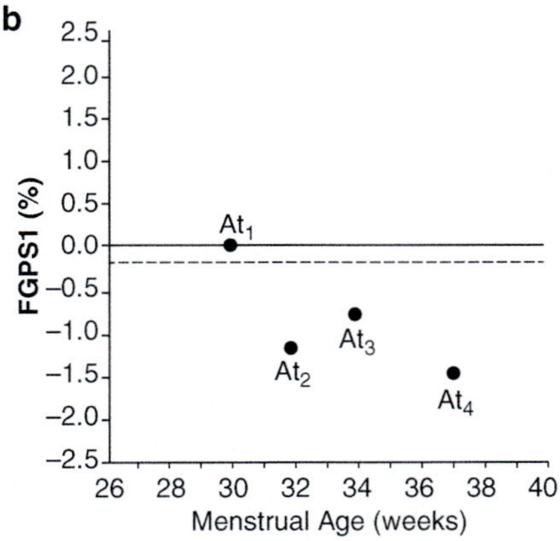

Fig. 2.2 Fetal Growth Pathology Score. (**a**) presents the serial calculation of a Fetal Growth Pathology Score [FGPS1] at each fetal age when the anatomical parameters were measured. This Score is the cumulative moving average of all %Dev$_p$ values available up through the current scan. The shaded areas indicate which -%Dev$_p$ were used in the FGPS1 calculation at a particular age. The non-zero -%Dev$_p$ values are indicated in red. The FGPS1 values at each time point are given in the purple shaded areas. (**b**) is a plot of the FGPS1 values obtained in this example. After the first scan, growth restriction was indicated by the negative value. There was some improvement between the second and third time points, but further progression was seen between the third and fourth time points. (HC head circumference, AC abdominal circumference, FDL femur diaphysis length, EFW estimated fetal weight. Deter et al. [15], figure used with permission)

13]. In a retrospective study (no control of the number of scans, the fetal age at the time of scan, or the composition of the neonatal growth assessment set) of SGA singletons, concordance between fetal and neonatal growth assessments was nearly 70%, with 42% of these confirmed cases showing normal growth [5].

An unexpected benefit of using the FGPS to characterize growth restriction in this SGA sample is shown in Fig. 2.3 [13]. Plotting of FGPS1 values after each scan in the 73 fetuses with confirmed growth restriction gave five patterns in 70/73 (95.9%) of these cases [13]. These patterns represent different evolutions of growth restriction during the third trimester: Pattern 1, continuously getting worse; Pattern 2, abnormality only at the last scan (70% were within 2 weeks of delivery); Pattern 3, initial significant abnormality that was relatively constant afterward; Pattern 4, initial abnormality followed by partial recovery and then further worsening; and Pattern 5, initial abnormality followed by a progressive recovery back toward normal. These patterns are distinct, few in number, repeated in different fetuses and have reasonable biological interpretations. Such characteristics suggest that they are not due to random processes but their exact significance is currently unknown. However, they strongly suggest that fetal growth restriction in the third trimester is NOT a single biological process!

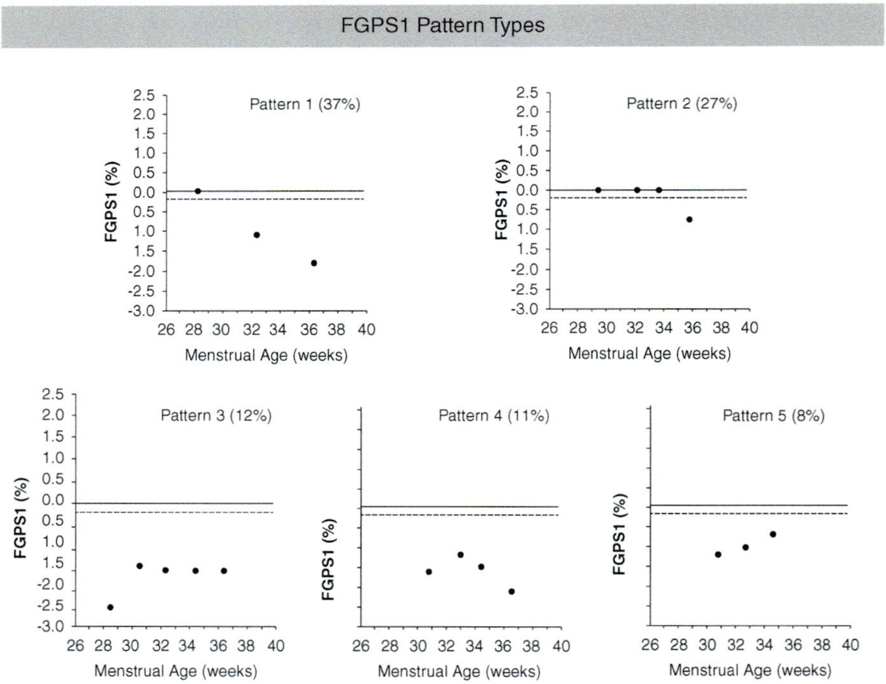

Fig. 2.3 Patterns of growth restriction found in the third trimester. This figure presents the five FGPS1 patterns found in 70/73 SGA singletons with fetal growth restriction, confirmed by neonatal growth outcome. Pattern 1 was most frequent [37%] followed by Pattern 2 [27%]. This latter pattern was found within two weeks of delivery in 70% of the cases. The significance of these patterns is not known but they are few in number, distinctly different, occur repeatedly in other fetuses and have plausible biology interpretations. (Deter et al. [15], figure used with permission)

Neonatal Growth Restriction (NGR)

As discussed in Chap. 1, fetal and neonatal growth assessments are made independently with IGA. Therefore, the strongest evidence for the presence or absence of growth pathology is concordance between fetal and neonatal evaluations [15]. This necessitates a comprehensive approach to neonatal growth assessments (Neonatal Growth Profile; see Chap. 1) rather than the limited evaluation used by conventional methods (weight, length, head circumference). However, such assessments are rarely done [3, 27, 30, 36] even in prospective research studies.

Single Anatomical Parameter NGR

Any anatomical parameter can be evaluated using the Growth Potential Realization Index (GPRI; see Chap. 1) if it can be measured prenatally and postnatally (e.g., HC, AC) or prenatal measurements can be used to estimate postnatal measurements (e.g., EWT parameter set for predicted WT; FDL for predicted CHL) [4]. To identify and quantify the presence of NGR in individual anatomical parameters, GPRI values are compared to their reference ranges [3] and pathological GPRIs calculated (see Chap. 1). These pGPRI values are specific neonatal growth abnormality parameters which quantify the growth pathology of individual anatomical parameters (see Table 2.2).

An unpublished study [5] of 112 cases in neonates with normal growth outcomes has shown that -$pGPRI_{WT}$, -$pGPRI_{HC}$, -$pGPRI_{CHL}$, -$pGPRI_{AC}$, and -$pGPRI_{ThC}$ values were primarily zero (545/560 {97.3%}), indicating normal growth. However, 1–5 values (depending on anatomical parameter) were non-zero. This is probably due to the use of GPRI 95% reference ranges in -pGPRI calculations. Such ranges classify 2.5% of normal values as being outside the normal range. Since only 1–2 -pGPRI values for any of anatomical parameter were more negative than −2.0%, we consider those less negative than −2.0% to be abnormal but potentially normal.

Table 2.2 Specific neonatal growth pathology parameters

Parameter name	Abbreviation	Description and use
Pathological Growth Potential Realization Index	pGPRI	Difference between the reference range boundary and the measurement for a *single anatomical parameter* (Fig. 1.8, Chap 1). This outcome parameter can be used to detect abnormal growth outcomes that express themselves differently in different individuals
Average Pathological Growth Potential Realization Index	av. pGPRI	Average pGPRI value for a *set of anatomical parameters*. This composite parameter provides a comprehensive measure of neonatal growth pathology
Pathological Modified Neonatal Growth Assessment Score	pNGAS	Difference between the reference range boundary and the mNGAS measurement. The pNGAS provides a comprehensive assessment of neonatal growth outcome based on multiple anatomical parameters weighted for their importance in detecting abnormal growth outcomes

This table presents the three parameters utilized by individualized growth assessment [IGA] to detect and quantify growth pathology at birth [pGPRI, av pGPRI, pNGAS]. On the right-hand side are the descriptions and uses of these growth pathology parameters Deter et al. [15], table used with permission

General NGR

Due to the differences in NGR in individual neonates [30], there is a need for composite parameters that can identify and quantify this condition in groups of neonates. There are two such composite parameters, the average, negative, pathological GPRI (av. –pGPRI) and the modified Neonatal Growth Assessment Score (mNGAS) {Table 2.2} [5, 15]. The former is simpler and easier to use since no special anatomical parameters or mathematical procedures are required. However, all parameters are given equal weight even though it is known that some are more important than others in detecting NGR [33, 37]. The unpublished study of Deter et al. [5] cited above found that the 95% reference range for the five members (WT, HC, AC, ThC, CHL) av. –pGPRI was 0.0 to −0.72% in neonates with normal growth outcomes. For the three members (WT, HC, CHL) av. –pGPRI, it was 0.0 to −0.40%. Since these ranges were obtained in neonates with normal growth outcomes, those with av. –pGPRIs outside these ranges are considered to have NGR. These statistics are corrected for most confounding variables (differences in growth potential, birth age, growth cessation age, systematic measurement error, normal variation) so are much less subject to error than conventional standards.

The principal confounding variable not corrected for in the av. –pGPRI are differences in the sensitivity of values for any of the anatomical paramters for detecting growth abnormalities. Previous studies [33, 37] have shown that ThC and WT are the most important variables in NGR identification; AC has an intermediate importance, while CHL and HC are of minor importance. These results indicate that anatomical parameters used to detect and quantify NGR should be weighted, and this can be done using GPRI values in a principal component analysis (PCA) [38]. The optimal function obtained for separating normal and growth-restricted neonates is:

$$\begin{aligned} m_1NGAS_{51} = {} & 0.685\ (GPRI_{ThC}) + 0.600\ (GPRI_{WT}) \\ & + 0.349\ (GPRI_{AC}) + 0.169\ (GPRI_{CHL}) + 0.142\ (GPRI_{HC}). \end{aligned}$$

This function correctly classified 97.3% of cases. Despite this (and other [3]) evidence for the importance of neonatal ThC measurements in detecting NGR, ThC is rarely measured prenatally or postnatally. Previous studies of the mNGAS have shown detection of NGR with the m_1NGAS_{51} dropped from 98.6% to 86.5% when ThC was omitted [37]. This lack of adequate postnatal measurements was found to be a major cause of discordance between prenatal and postnatal growth assessments using the -FGPS and av. –pGPRI in SGA singletons [5]. Without appropriate measurements (ThC prenatally; ThC and AC postnatally), the use of this powerful tool for detecting NGR is greatly restricted.

Special Uses of IGA

Although definitive interpretations of IGA cannot be made until they are compared to physiological parameters, perinatal complications, and long-term neurobehavioral outcomes [15], current observations allow some comments to be made.

More accurate assessment of growth status: As IGA evaluations are based on empirical estimates of growth potential [28], utilize sets of anatomical parameters instead of single parameters [5, 31], and quantify growth pathology [15], they provide a more complete and accurate assessment of fetal/neonatal growth status. This information can be obtained for singletons, twins, and triplets [36]. Use of the Fetal Growth Pathology Score [5] has, for the first time, revealed differences in the evolution of growth restriction [13]. This allows more precise classification of the growth restriction processes, which may have different outcomes.

Improved detection of early FGR: As expected by eliminating the differences in growth potential, IGA is more sensitive to growth abnormalities since the normal reference ranges are smaller. For example, the conventional 2SD reference range value for HC at 30 weeks [39], expressed as a percent deviation from the 50th percentile (mean) value, is 7.8%. The similar IGA value is 5.3% [27], a 32% decrease. This indicates that IGA is very likely to detect growth abnormalities earlier in pregnancy. This has been demonstrated in 73 fetuses with proven FGR [5]. In 46/73 (63%) cases, there was clear evidence of FGR before 34 weeks. In 15/46 (33%), FGR was seen before 30 weeks. With conventional methods, early FGR has an incidence of only 20–30% [40]. These results suggest that IGA can improve the detection of early FGR.

Separation of normal and growth-restricted small fetuses/neonates: The vexing problem of which small fetus is truly growth restricted has been resolved using IGA [5]. Based on standards derived from estimates of individual growth potential [30] and using composite growth parameters [5], it has been possible to conclusively separate 69% of 184 SGA singletons into normally growing or growth-restricted categories (in this retrospective study, most of those misclassifications were due to lack of appropriate scans or inadequate neonatal growth assessment methods) [5]. Of the 126 cases with prenatal-postnatal concordance, 42% showed normal prenatal growth. Smaller studies using more complete neonatal growth assessment [3] or inclusion of placental evaluation [4] confirm these findings. During pregnancy, plots of the Fetal Growth Pathology Score clearly show differences that can be used to identify these two subgroups [15].

Identification of end of adaption process: As described above (Fetal Adaption to Compromised Nutrient Supply), the early response to an inadequate nutrient supply could be an adaption process in the "cave fetus" to enhance survival. However, when the magnitude of the pathological process reaches a certain level, physiological changes within the fetus become necessary to protect vital organs. As IGA provides quantitative assessments of growth pathology [15], it might be possible to determine the point where this change becomes likely. In a small, preliminary study (unpublished) of fetuses with progressive FGR (Pattern 1), FGPS1 and middle cerebral artery pulsatility index (MCA PI) values were compared. In subgroups with [17] and without [10] decreased MCA PI values (1–5 tests/fetus), mean FGPS1 values were −4.12% and −2.29%, respectively. This difference was statistically significant. Although these sample sizes are small, it may be possible to find a FGPS1 value beyond which changes in fetal physiology begin to occur.

Summary

Although conventional comparisons of the individual to the *group* provide the only means for detecting FGR through the first two scans, they are far from ideal. Beginning with the third scan, such evaluations can shift to *individualized* methods (each fetus is its own control) based on empirical estimates of growth potential (IGA). Subsequent longitudinal studies (through delivery) can be carried out which provide new and more comprehensive information about both normal and abnormal growth. IGA utilizes parameters based on differences in growth velocities and provides both qualitative and quantitative information about the growth process and any abnormalities. This approach can be used with multiple anatomical parameters (which are in a form allowing formation of composite parameters), thus significantly reducing the problems associated with growth abnormalities manifesting themselves differently in different fetuses. NGR can be detected and quantified using these methods. Since fetal and neonatal growth assessments are independent of each other, their concordance can be used to definitively establish growth status. The way is now prepared for making new comparisons of growth with physiological/biochemical changes, perinatal/long-term complications, and new methods of managing growth abnormalities.

Acknowledgment The author would like to thank Ms. Rajshi Gandhi for her help in the preparation of this chapter.

References

1. Battaglia FC, Lubchenco LO. A practical classification of newborn infants by weight and gestational age. J Pediatr. 1967;71:159–63.
2. Neerhof MG, Thaete LG. The fetal response to chronic placental insufficiency. Semin Perinatol. 2008;32:201–5.
3. Deter RL, Lee W, Sangi-Haghpeykar H, Tarca AL, Yeo L, Romero R. Fetal growth cessation in late pregnancy: its impact on predicted size parameters used to classify small for gestational age neonates. J Matern Fetal Neonatal Med. 2015;28:755–65.
4. Deter RL, Levytska K, Lee W, Melamed N, Kingdom JCP. Classifying neonatal growth outcomes: use of birth weight, placental evaluation and individualized growth assessment. J Matern Fetal Neonatal Med. 2016;29:3939–49.
5. Deter RL, Lee W, Kingdom JCP, Romero R. Fetal growth pathology score: a novel ultrasound parameter for individualized assessment of third trimester growth abnormalities. J Matern Fetal Neonatal Med. 2018;31:866–76.
6. McIntire DD, Bloom SL, Casey BM, Leveno KJ. Birth weight in relation to morbidity and mortality among newborn infants. N Engl J Med. 1999;340:1234–8.
7. Hershkovitz I, Weber GVV, Quam R, Duval M, Grün R, Kinsley L, Ayalon A, et al. The earliest modern humans outside of Africa. Science. 2018;359:456–9.
8. Pritchard JA, Macdonald PC. Williams obstetrics. 15th ed. New York: Appleton-Century-Crofts; 1976.
9. Lee W, Deter RL, McNie B, Gonçalves LF, Espinoza J, Chaiworapongsa T, et al. Individualized growth assessment of fetal soft tissue using fractional thigh volume. Ultrasound Obstet Gynecol. 2004;24:766–74.

10. Lee W, Deter RL, McNie B, Goncalves LF, Espinoza J, Chaiworapongsa T, et al. The fetal arm: individualized growth assessment in normal pregnancies. J Ultrasound Med. 2005;24:817–28.
11. Antonow-Schlorke I, Schwab M, Cox LA, Stuchlik K, Witte OW, Nathanielsz PW, et al. Vulnerability of the fetal primate brain to moderate reduction in maternal global nutrient availability. Proc Natl Acad Sci U S A. 2011;108:3011–6.
12. Nardozza LM, Caetano AC, Zamarian AC, Mazzola JB, Silva CP, Marçal VM, et al. Fetal growth restriction: current knowledge. Arch Gynecol Obstet. 2017;295:1061–77.
13. Deter RL, Lee W, Kingdom J, Sangi-Haghpeykar H, Romero R. Third trimester growth restriction patterns: individualized assessment using a fetal growth pathology score. J Matern Fetal Neonatal Med. 2018;31:2155–63.
14. Steckel RH. Birth weights and stillbirths in historical perspective. Eur J Clin Nutr. 1998;52:S16–20.
15. Deter RL, Lee W, Yeo L, Erez O, Ramamurthy U, Naik M, et al. Individualized growth assessment: conceptual framework and practical implementation for the evaluation of fetal growth and neonatal growth outcome. Am J Obstet Gynecol. 2018;218:S656–78.
16. Nelson WE, Vaighan VC. Textbook of pediatrics. 9th ed. Philadelphia: W B Saunders Co.; 1969.
17. Cassady G. The small-for date infant. In: Avery GB, editor. Neonatology, pathophysiology and management of the newborn. 2nd ed. Philadelphia: J B Lippincott Co.; 1981. p. 262.
18. Lubchenco LO, Searls DT, Brazie JV. Neonatal mortality rate: relationship to birth weight and gestational age. J Pediatr. 1972;81:814–22.
19. Nyberg DA, Abuhamad A, Ville Y. Ultrasound assessment of abnormal fetal growth. Semin Perinatol. 2004;28:3–22.
20. Deter R, Harrist R. Assessment of normal fetal growth. In: Chervenak FA, Isaacson GC, Campbell S, editors. Ultrasound in obstetrics and gynecology. Boston: Little, Brown & Co.; 1993. p. 361–85.
21. Dudley NJ. A systematic review of the ultrasound estimation of fetal weight. Ultrasound Obstet Gynecol. 2005;25:80–9.
22. Melamed N, Yogev Y, Meizner I, Mashiach R, Bardin R, Ben-Haroush A. Sonographic fetal weight estimation: which model should be used? J Ultrasound Med. 2009;28:617–29.
23. RCoOa G. Small-for-gestational-age fetus, investigation and management, Green-top guideline, vol. 31. London: Royal College of Obstetricians and Gynecologists; 2014.
24. Monier I, Blondel B, Ego A, Kaminiski M, Goffinet F, Zeitlin J. Poor effectiveness of antenatal detection of fetal growth restriction and consequences for obstetric management and neonatal outcomes: a French national study. BJOG. 2015;122:518–27.
25. Poljak B, Agarwal U, Jackson R, Alfirevic Z, Sharp A. Diagnostic accuracy of individual antenatal tools for prediction of small-for-gestational age at birth. Ultrasound Obstet Gynecol. 2017;49:493–9.
26. Deter RL. Individualized growth assessment: evaluation of growth using each fetus as its own control. Semin Perinatol. 2004;28:23–32.
27. Deter RL, Lee W, Sangi-Haghpeykar H, Tarca AL, Yeo L, Romero R. Individualized fetal growth assessment: critical evaluation of key concepts in the specification of third trimester growth trajectories. J Matern Fetal Neonatal Med. 2014;27:537–42.
28. Deter RL, Lee W, Kingdom J, Romero R. Second trimester growth velocities: assessment of fetal growth potential in SGA singletons. J Matern Fetal Neonatal Med. 2017:1–8. https://doi.org/10.1080/14767058.2017.1395849.
29. Smith GC. First trimester origins of fetal growth impairment. Semin Perinatol. 2004;28:41–50.
30. Deter RL, Xu B, Milner LL. Prenatal prediction of neonatal growth status in twins using individualized growth assessment. J Clin Ultrasound. 1996;24:53–9.
31. Deter RL, Lee W, Sangi-Haghpeykar H, Tarca AL, Yeo L, Romero R. A modified prenatal growth assessment score for the evaluation of fetal growth in the third trimester using single and composite biometric parameters. J Maternal Fetal Neonatal Med. 2015;28:745–54.
32. Hadlock FP, Harrist RB, Deter RL, Park SK. Estimation of fetal weight using head, body and femur measurements – a prospective study. Am J Obstet Gynecol. 1985;151:333–7.

33. Deter RL, Spence L. Identification of macrosomic, normal and intrauterine growth retarded neonates using the modified Neonatal Growth Assessment Score. Fetal Diagn Ther. 2004;19:58–67.
34. Lee W, Balasubramaniam M, Deter RL, Yeo L, Hassan SS, Gotsch F, et al. New fetal weight estimation models using fractional limb volume. Ultrasound Obstet Gynecol. 2009;34:556–65.
35. Faschingbauer F, Dammer U, Raabe E, Kehl S, Schmid M, Schild RL, et al. A new sonographic weight estimation formula for Small-for-Gestational-Age fetuses. J Ultrasound Med. 2016;35:1713–24.
36. Hata T, Deter RL, Hill RM. Individual growth curve standards in triplets: prediction of third trimester growth and birth characteristics. Obstet Gynecol. 1991;78:379–84.
37. Deter RL, Nazar R, Milner LL. Modified neonatal growth assessment score: a multivariate approach to the detection of intrauterine growth retardation in the neonate. Ultrasound Obstet Gynecol. 1995;6:400–10.
38. Harris RJA. Primer of multivariate statistics. Orlando: Academic Press; 1985.
39. Kiserud T, Piaggio G, Carroli G, Widmer M, Carvalho J, Neerup Jensen L, et al. The World Health Organization fetal growth charts: a multinational longitudinal study of ultrasound biometric measurements and estimated fetal weight. PLoS Med. 2017;14:e1002284.
40. Dall'Asta A, Brunelli V, Prefumo F, Frusca T, Lees CC. Early onset fetal growth restriction. Mater Health Neonatol Perinatol. 2017;3:2.

Etiopathogeny

3

Anna Iacoi and Roland Axt-Fliedner

Introduction

Fetal growth restriction (FGR) refers to a poor growth of the fetus while inside the mother's womb during gestation and is to be distinguished from *small for gestational age* (SGA) fetuses. FGR is defined as a birth weight less than the 10th percentile [1]: the fetus has not reached its genetic determined growth potential at a given gestational age due to one or more causative factors. In contrast to this, the SGA fetus has reached its growth potential, and there is no pathology causing the poor growth. This fetus grows with a constant velocity, parallel to a specific percentile through the pregnancy. A normal postnatal outcome is to be expected. Differentiation can be very difficult, and umbilical artery Doppler can be useful to differentiate the constitutionally small fetus from the pathologically small fetus [2–6].

Since birth weight is a strong predictor of pregnancy outcomes, it is important to identify the causes of FGR, which can be divided into fetal, maternal, and placental causes. Regulation of fetal growth is multifactorial and complex. It is known that fetal weight is directly associated with placental size. Placental insufficiency is associated with most cases of FGR. There are many causes not primarily caused by placental insufficiency but indirectly leading to it [7]. So placental and maternal causes for FGR have a common final pathway of decreased placental perfusion and transfer of nutrients to the fetus. Fetal-induced FGR is caused secondarily through genetic or infectious diseases.

Until 20 weeks of gestational age, fetal growth is characterized by hyperplasia, which means through growth of the number of cells. Later on, fetal growth is primarily characterized by hypertrophy, the growth of existing cells [4]. FGR in the first half of pregnancy is caused especially by intrinsic factors like chromosomal

A. Iacoi · R. Axt-Fliedner (✉)
Division of Prenatal Medicine and Fetal Therapy, Campus Gießen and Marburg, Justus-Liebig University Gießen, University Hospital Gießen and Marburg, Gießen, Germany
e-mail: Roland.Axt-Fliedner@gyn.med.uni-giessen.de

L. M. M. Nardozza et al. (eds.), *Fetal Growth Restriction*,
https://doi.org/10.1007/978-3-030-00051-6_3

aberration or infections, whereas FGR in the second half of pregnancy is primarily caused by extrinsic factors that lead to placental insufficiency. If FGR is caused by intrinsic factors, FGR is symmetric. Extrinsic factors cause asymmetric FGR. In these cases, there is an increase in the head circumference to the abdominal circumferences, the so-called brain sparing.

Fetal Causes

Fetal causes are numerous and range from genetic and structural malformations to infective diseases. Genetic diseases lead to 5–20% of causes of FGR [7]. Trisomies are often associated with fetal growth restriction, which is more severe with trisomy 18 than trisomies 13 and 21 [5, 6]. FGR is also associated with trisomy 16 as well as with Wolf-Hirschhorn syndrome (4q deletion) and Cri du chat syndrome (5q deletion). Also to be taken into consideration is monosomy X, also known as Turner syndrome. Triploidy and an extra set of chromosomes are also highly linked to fetal growth restriction. Since incidence of FGR is high in fetuses with genetic abnormalities, an amniocentesis or placental biopsy should be considered in cases of unexplained and early occurring FGR.

Congenital malformations without genetic cause are responsible for 1–2% of FGR. This includes malformations like congenital heart disease, diaphragmatic hernia, omphalocele, gastroschisis, and anencephaly [6, 8].

Infections during gestation are important to mention when talking about causes for FGR. In fact they make up to 10% of the cases. The TORCH (toxoplasmosis, other (syphilis), rubella, cytomegalovirus, and HIV) organisms are considered the leading organisms causing FGR. In developed countries toxoplasmosis and cytomegalovirus are considered the most important infections and should be therefore tested in pregnancy in order to control costs [9]. There is no evidence for testing all TORCH organisms also considering rising costs. However it should be taken into consideration that malaria is the most common cause of FGR worldwide [10, 11]. Single umbilical artery is also considered as a cause for FGR.

Multiple gestations are also associated with FGR and make 3% of the cases. Twin pregnancies should be under constant control. After 28 weeks of gestation, growth rate decreases. FGR of one fetus could indicate genetic abnormalities or infections of the fetus or be a hint for twin-to-twin transfusion syndrome [12, 13].

Maternal Causes

Size at birth depends on numerous factors including race, sex, parity, maternal weight, and height [14, 15]. Fetal nutrition depends on the ability of the mother to provide oxygenated blood. Maternal causes of FGR are usually related to placental insufficiency, the main reason for FGR that can concern up to 3% of all pregnancies. Pathogenesis is not totally clear yet, but it seems that defects in placental circulation and transport affect nutrient transport to the fetus and therefore lead to FGR.

Placental insufficiency and FGR are risk factors for stillbirth. In fact up to 43% of stillborn are FGR fetuses [16]. Placental insufficiency is not a specific placental disease, in fact there a numerous factors leading to it. Abnormal fetal genome as well as chronic infection and many maternal diseases can affect placental tissue and therefore cause FGR. To conclude decreased uteroplacental blood flow, reduced blood volume, and reduced oxygen transport capacity are responsible for placental insufficiency [17].

Decreasing fetal perfusion leads to hypoxia and therefore to FGR. Chronic hypertension, preeclampsia, pregestational diabetes, chronic renal insufficiency, systemic lupus erythematodes, and antiphospholipid syndrome affect fetal microcirculation. This causes decreasing fetal perfusion. Chronic hypertension, whether isolated or in the form of preeclampsia, is the most important maternal factor influencing fetal growth: severe, pregnancy-induced hypertension reduces birth weight by approximately 10%. A history of prior low-birth-weight infants is responsible for the same amount of reduction in birth weight. Interestingly, a preexisting, uncomplicated maternal hypertension does not reduce fetal growth.

In addition to maternal disorders, also poor nutrition status, substance abuse, and pharmacotherapy affect fetal growth and can lead to FGR. Women with lower socioeconomic status as well as women living in developing countries are at higher risk of a poor nutrition status but also of maternal anemia, poor prenatal care, and substance abuse problems. Smoking during gestation, especially smoking of more than 15 cigarettes per day, is highly associated with a lower birth weight and associated with reduced oxygen transport capacity. Important to mention is that especially smoking in the third trimester of the pregnancy leads to FGR [18, 19]. If pregnant women quit smoking until 16 weeks of gestation, birth weight does not differ from women who never smoked before [20]. Therefore women should be motivated to quit smoking in early pregnancy. Women living in high altitudes are also at risk of FGR, also because of reduced oxygen transport capacity.

Placental Causes

Placental causes for IUGR are placental abruption, maternal floor infarct, placental mosaicism, velamentous cord insertion, as well as placenta accreta [7, 17, 21]. Genetic and environmental factors can influence early placental development including poor placental growth, inadequate trophoblast invasion, and altered immuno-regulatory environment. These processes in turn can trigger altered nutrient delivery, hypoxic response, and/or a variety of inflammatory responses that are linked to adverse perinatal outcomes.

Placental-Mediated Complications

There are multiple obstetrical concerns for which placental biomarkers can have beneficial clinical applications. Early prediction of poor fetal growth, premature delivery, and maternal preeclampsia (PE) is important, as careful monitoring and interventions can improve outcomes and save the lives of babies and mothers. However, these are heterogeneous conditions for which a variety of genetic and environmental influences (e.g., maternal obesity, diabetes, low socioeconomic status, and poor nutrition) can contribute to risk. Defining abnormal placental health is also challenging as, even in normal pregnancies, there is extensive within and between placenta variation in terms of gross pathology and molecular changes [22]. Recently, protein and nucleic acid biomarkers have been identified by modern genomic technologies which have been discussed to be related to placental and fetal health outcomes. In the future it is expected that incorporation of a combination of biomarkers along with clinical maternal and fetal parameters will serve to a better understanding of placental pathology and would optimize risk assessment.

Conclusion

The ethiopathogeny of intrauterine growth restriction is diverse. Besides well-established maternal, extrinsic, and intrinsic causes, recent improvements in genomic technologies and increase in knowledge have directed the interest toward biomarkers in investigating placental and fetal status. A combination of clinical data along with new results from biomarkers is probably the way to go forward in diagnosing and surveilling the fetus at risk for fetal growth restriction in the future.

References

1. American College of Obstetricians and Gynecologists. Intrauterine growth restriction. Practice Bulletin no. 12, 2000, Washington, DC.
2. Gagnon R, Van de Hof M. The use of fetal Doppler in obstetrics. J Obstet Gynecol Can. 2003;25:601–7.
3. ACOG committee opinion. Utility of antepartum umbilical artery Doppler velocimetry in intrauterine growth restriction. Number 188, October 1997 (replaces no. 116, November 1992). Committee on Obstetric Practice. American College of Obstetricians and Gynecologists. Int J Gynaecol Obstet. 1997;59:269–70.
4. Winick M. Fetal malnutrition. Clin Obstet Gynecol. 1970;13:526–41.
5. Viora E, Zamboni C, Mortara G, Stillavato S, Bastonero S, Errante G, et al. Trisomy 18: fetal ultrasound findings at different gestational ages. Am J Med Genet A. 2007;143A:553–7.
6. Khoury J, Erickson D, Cordero J, McCarthy BJ. Congenital malformations and intrauterine growth retardation: a population study. Pediatrics. 1988;82:83–90.
7. Hendrix N, Berghella V. Non-placental causes of intrauterine growth restriction. Semin Perinatol. 2008;32:161–5.
8. Lin CC, Santolaya-Forgas J. Current concepts of fetal growth restriction: part I. Causes, classification, and pathophysiology. Obstet Gynecol. 1998;92:1044–55.
9. Khan NA, Kazzi SN. Yield and costs of screening growth-retarded infants for TORCH infections. Am J Perinatol. 2000;17:131–5.
10. Wendel GD. Cytomegalovirus, genital herpes, rubella, syphilis and toxoplasmosis. In: Queenan JT, Hobbins JC, Spong CY, editors. Protocols for high-risk pregnancies: an evidence-based approach. 5th ed. Oxford: Wiley-Blackwell; 2010.

11. Adanu RM. Malaria in pregnancy. In: Queenan JT, Hobbins JC, Spong CY, editors. Protocols for high-risk pregnancies: an evidence-based approach. 5th ed. Oxford: Wiley-Blackwell; 2010.
12. Divon MY, Weiner Z. Ultrasound in twin pregnancy. Semin Perinatol. 1995;19:404–12.
13. D'Alton ME, Simpson LL. Syndromes in twins. Semin Perinatol. 1995;19:375–86.
14. Strobino DM, Ensminger ME, Kim YJ, Nanda J. Mechanisms for maternal age differences in birth weight. Am J Epidemiol. 1995;142:504–14.
15. Wen SW, Goldenberg RL, Cutter GR, et al. Intrauterine growth retardation and preterm delivery: prenatal risk factors in an indigent population. Am J Obstet Gynecol. 1990;162:213–8.
16. Reddy UM. Prediction and prevention of recurrent stillbirth. Obstet Gynecol. 2007;110:1151–64.
17. Divon MY, Ferber A. Overview of causes and risk factors for fetal growth restriction. In: Lockwood CJ, Barss VA, editors. UpToDate. http://www.uptodate.com. Accessed 28 Dec 2014.
18. Lieberman E, Gremy I, Lang JM, Cohen AP. Low birth weight at term and the timing of fetal exposure to maternal smoking. Am J Public Health. 1994;84:1127–31.
19. Shu XO, Hatch MC, Mills J, Clemens J, Susser M. Maternal smoking, alcohol drinking, caffeine consumption, and fetal growth: results from a prospective study. Epidemiology. 1995;6:115–20.
20. MacArthur C, Knox EG. Smoking in pregnancy: effects of stopping at different stages. Br J Obstet Gynaecol. 1988;95:551–5.
21. Wilkins-Haug L, Roberts DJ, Morton CC. Confined placental mosaicism and intrauterine growth retardation: a case control analysis of placentas at delivery. Am J Obstet Gynecol. 1995;172:44e50.
22. Manokhina I, Wilson SL, Robinson WP. Noninvasive nucleic acid–based approaches to monitor placental health and predict pregnancy-related complications. Obstet Gynecol. 2015;213:S197–206.

4 Physiopathology

Gabriele Tonni, Edward Araujo Júnior, and Maria Paola Bonasoni

The Role of Abnormal Trophoblastic Invasion

Trophoblast cells derive from the trophectoderm of the developing blastocyst. They differentiate into main lineages: syncytiotrophoblasts and invasive trophoblasts. Syncytiotrophoblasts are the outer component of the chorionic villi and are involved in nutrient and gas exchange. Invasive trophoblasts, on the other hand, originate from the cytotrophoblast columns and can be interstitial or endovascular. Interstitial invasive trophoblasts invade the uterine tissues, assuring placental anchorage, whereas endovascular invasive trophoblasts migrate to the uterine spiral arteries, replacing endothelial cells and promoting degeneration of the parietal smooth muscle cells. This process, called conversion, allows the uterine spiral arteries to become vessels with low resistance and high capacitance, promoting adequate blood flow and feto-maternal exchange. Defective placentation, such as trophoblast failure in the conversion of spiral arteries, underlies many diseases in pregnancy, especially fetal growth restriction (FGR) and preeclampsia (PE) [1].

The conversion of decidual arteries is indirectly modulated by intravascular trophoblasts that prompt endothelial cells to secrete chemokines. These molecules attract natural killer cells (NK) and macrophages, which in turn induce vascular

G. Tonni (✉)
Maternal-Fetal Medicine Section, Department of Obstetrics and Gynecology, AUSL Istituto di Ricerca a Carattere Clinico Scientifico (IRCCS) di Reggio Emilia, Reggio Emilia, Italy
e-mail: tonnig@ausl.re.it

E. Araujo Júnior
Discipline of Fetal Medicine, Department of Obstetrics, Paulista School of Medicine, Federal University of São Paulo (EPM-UNIFESP), São Paulo, SP, Brazil

M. P. Bonasoni
Fetal Pathology Section, Department of Human Pathology, Arcispedale "Santa Maria Nuova", AUSL Istituto di Ricerca a Carattere Clinico Scientifico (IRCCS) di Reggio Emilia, Reggio Emilia, Italy

L. M. M. Nardozza et al. (eds.), *Fetal Growth Restriction*,
https://doi.org/10.1007/978-3-030-00051-6_4

smooth muscle cell apoptosis, likely via the Fas/FasL system. In FGR, the number of trophoblast cells within the spiral arteries is reduced, a condition associated with increased apoptosis and a narrow vascular lumen. Impaired trophoblast invasion is associated with high-pressure placental blood flow, which indirectly damages the developing villous tree. This leads to hypoxia and impaired blood flow, as observed by aberrant Doppler ultrasound waveforms in FGR [2]. Impaired decidual artery remodeling can have different causes other than increased apoptosis within the placental bed. In FGR, trophoblast invasion is normal or even increased, but the cells fail to migrate into the vascular wall. This is probably due to anomalous interactions with maternal natural killer cells, which determine inhibitory reduction of protease secretion.

Improperly converted spiral arteries have negative consequences for placental blood flow. In this condition, maternal blood flow into the intervillous space maintains high velocity and pulsatility, leading to mechanical damage to the villous tree. Furthermore, the presence of arterial smooth muscle cells in the spiral arteries promotes vasoconstriction and intermittent placental perfusion, inducing recurrent ischemia- or reperfusion-type injuries. Furthermore, deficient arterial remodeling is the main cause of changes due to acute atherosis, with macrophage recruitment and luminal narrowing. This effect further impairs uteroplacental blood flow, exposing the placenta to oxidative stress. Excessive levels of reactive oxygen species (ROS) are caused by an overpowering of the cellular detoxification system. As a consequence, DNA and other biomolecules, such as proteins and lipids, can be randomly damaged, leading to abnormal cellular functionality or even death. ROS production particularly increases during hypoxia and ischemia-reperfusion injuries when the placenta is exposed to intermittent cycles of hypoxia and reoxygenation. ROS production within the mitochondria may influence endoplasmic reticulum (ER) protein synthesis via direct calcium signaling. In particular, as misfolded proteins are toxic for the cell, ER in the presence of oxidative stress activates the evolutionarily conserved signaling pathways, known as the unfolded protein response (UPR). This regulatory mechanism is incredibly quick and prevents unnecessary protein synthesis, thus sparing cellular reserves. This is enabled by phosphorylation of the alpha subunit of eukaryotic initiation factor 2 (eIF2alpha), which reduces the assemblage of ribosomal complexes on the messenger RNA (mRNA). Therefore, the UPR pathway is a conservative homeostatic mechanism essential to balancing feto-placental growth to oxygen levels [3]. In an *in vitro* experimental study, pleckstrin homology-like domain, family A, member 2 (PHLDA2), a maternally expressed imprinted gene, was tested on cell lines. The results showed that PHLDA2 overexpression inhibited cell proliferation, promoting apoptosis via the mitochondrial pathway and accumulation of ROS. In particular, PHLDA2 promoted cytochrome *c* releasing, loss of mitochondrial membrane potential, and ROS buildup in trophoblasts [4].

Hypoxia determines shallow extravillous trophoblast (EVT) invasion, inducing the expression of E3 ubiquitin ligase, Mcl-1 ubiquitin ligase E3 (MULE), through factor 1-alpha (HIF-1α). Elevated levels of HIF-1α further increase MULE expression, promoting trophoblast apoptosis by targeting Mcl-1, a pro-survival

Bcl-2 family member. Moreover, during hypoxia, the vascular endothelial growth factor (VEGF) family of growth factors and receptors is activated, as they regulate angiogenesis through endothelial cell proliferation, migration, and new vessel formation. In fact, hypoxia indirectly enhances VEGF-A gene expression. Soluble fms-like tyrosine kinase-1 (sFlt-1), a soluble truncated variant of the type 1 VEGF receptor (Flt-1), produced and secreted from the placenta, binds to pro-angiogenic factors VEGF and PlGF, reducing their levels. For example, in women with pre-eclampsia, high amounts of sFlt-1 and a high sFlt-1/PlGF ratio have been detected, indicating disequilibrium in angiogenetic factors. In FGR, endocrine gland-derived vascular endothelial growth factor (EG-VEGF) levels are elevated in the placenta and in the maternal circulation. In fact, hypoxia induces EG-VEGF, which interacts with the prokineticin receptor (PROKR1), and their deregulation is considered a cause of FGR.

Anomalous maternal inflammatory response is also responsible for failure in trophoblast migration and spiral artery transformation. In FGR, pro-inflammatory cytokines interleukin-8 (IL-8), interferon gamma (IFN-γ), and tumor necrosis factor-alpha (TNF-α) are elevated, whereas anti-inflammatory cytokines IL-13 and IL-10 are reduced. In addition, complement activation induces dysregulation of angiogenic factors. *In vitro* studies have demonstrated that complement activation induces sFlt1 secretion in human monocytes. In a mouse model, neutrophil infiltration in the placenta and TNF-α release determined excessive C3 deposition and reduced levels of VEGF. EVT invasion is also regulated by decidua basalis and its microenvironment, composed of leukocytes, natural killer cells, macrophages, and T lymphocytes. During physiological conditions, developing fetal tissue is protected by maternal inflammatory response in different ways. For example, EVT invasion could transform CD4+ T cells to resting regulatory T cells expressing CD4+, CD25HIFOXP3+, and CD45RA+. NK cells interact with EVTs, regulating their migration and spiral artery remodeling through natural killer cell receptors (NKR) and major histocompatibility complex (MHC). EVTs express human leukocyte antigen class I ligands (HLA-E, HLA-G, and HLA-C), recognized on NK receptors CD94/NKG2, LILR, and KIR. The binding frequency of KIR to HLA-C2 leads to decreased or increased secretion of cytokines, regulating angiogenesis and EVT invasion. Decidual NK cells express sphingosine-1-phosphate receptor-5 (S1PR5). Specific inhibition of this pathway decreases VEGF levels, and trophoblast migration is impaired. Moreover, in FGR, decidual NK cells not only are reduced, but they express by activating KIR2DL/S1PR5 and LILRB1 receptors. HLA-C and HLA-G receptors on EVTs in decidual tissue are significantly reduced. NK cells with decreased LILRB1 binding capacity show higher expression of TNF-α and lower expression of CXCL10. On the whole, this reflects a pro-inflammatory feature of FGR placenta dysregulated by NK release of cytokines [5].

As mentioned above, macrophages are important cells involved in the regulation of trophoblast invasion. Physiologically, they secrete IL-10, prostaglandin E2 (PGE2), TGF-β, IL-1b, TNF-α, IFN-γ, and indolamine 2,3-dioxygenase (IDO). They also have low-level expression of CD80 and CD86, preventing maternal T lymphocyte activation. Macrophages are also able to phagocytize apoptotic cells and debris, especially apoptotic EVTs. In FGR, macrophages are aberrantly activated, secreting TNF-α, nitric oxide (NO), and TGF-β. TNF-α can induce apoptosis in trophoblast cells. On the contrary, *in vitro* studies have shown that macrophage-derived NO reduces trophoblast migration associated with decreased levels of urokinase plasminogen activator receptor (uPAR) on the surface of trophoblast cells. TGF-β enhances trophoblast expression of plasminogen activator inhibitor 1 (PAI-1), which inhibits trophoblast invasion. Moreover, TNF-α and IFN-γ promote trophoblast apoptosis, increasing the expression of the pro-apoptotic factor XAF1 via the caspase-dependent death pathway [6].

EVT migration is also influenced by microRNAs (miRNAs), which are small noncoding, single-stranded RNAs (made up of 22 nucleotides) that silence genes by targeting mRNAs at the posttranscriptional level. miRNAs are first transcribed by RNA polymerase II. Two enzymes, DROSHA and DICER, process pri-miRNA to pre-miRNA and pre-miRNA to mature miRNA in the nucleus and cytoplasm, respectively. Mature miRNAs are then transferred to a multiprotein complex, which contains the RNA-induced silencing complex (RISC), involved in silencing specific genes. In human placenta, most miRNAs originate from two miRNA clusters, the chromosome 14-miRNA cluster (C14MC) and the chromosome 19-miRNA cluster (C19MC). *In vitro* studies have shown that C19MC miRNAs reduce EVT migration, as they specifically target genes associated with invasion, such as CXCL6, NR4A2, and FOXL2. However, miRNA dysregulation may partially explain FGR, as miRNAs are involved in trophoblast cell invasion. For example, miR-125b-1-3p targets S1PR1, whereas miR-210 acts through extracellular signal-regulated kinase (ERK) signaling. miRNA-144 inhibits titin and then reduces the expression of ERK1/2 and the activity of MMP2/9. miR-29b inhibits its target genes, myeloid cell leukemia sequence 1 (*MCL1*), *MMP2*, *VEGF-A*, and *ITGB1* (integrin β1). miRNA-424, a hypoxia-related miRNA, is highly expressed, reducing mRNAs and proteins of mitogen-activated protein kinase 1 (MEK1) and fibroblast growth factor receptor 1 (FGFR1) genes. FGFR1 is associated with the functions of VEGF; therefore increased miRNA-424 may affect placental vascularity. Moreover, enhanced levels of miRNA-141 downregulate E2F3 and PLAG1 target genes, reducing corresponding miRNAs and protein levels of PLAG1 [5]. miR-346 and miR-582-3p target and bind EG-VEGF, suppressing its expression. This results in matrix metalloproteinase (MMP 2 and MMP 9) downregulation, which affects trophoblast invasion [7].

Under normal conditions, the H19 gene promotes EVT migration and invasion by inhibiting microRNA let-7. The H19 gene encodes a polyadenylated, long noncoding RNA (lncRNA) of 2600 nucleotides mainly located in the cytoplasm but with a minor fraction in the nucleus. H19 is predominantly expressed during fetal life and downregulated after birth in adult tissues. In mice, H19 lncRNA recruits nuclear repressive histone markers to differentially methylated regions of imprinted network genes, preventing their transcription and indirectly regulating embryo growth and development. Nuclear H19 serves as precursor for microRNA miR-675 that inhibits placental growth in late pregnancy. In the cytoplasm, H19 binds microRNA let-7, reducing its bioavailability and consequently preventing its action on repressing target gene expression at the posttranscriptional level. In a recent *in vitro* study, impaired trophoblast invasion was demonstrated by H19 knockdown, which decreased type 3 TGF-β receptor (TGF-β) signaling via the Par6/Smurf1/RhoA pathway activated by TβR3 [8]. In another study, TGF-β signaling was altered via the canonical SMAD pathway, leading to an elevated sphingosine/ceramide ratio, which was responsible for increased trophoblast cell death [9].

Many other molecular events are involved in abnormal trophoblast migration and invasion. Connective tissue growth factor (CTGF), also known as CCN2, is a matricellular protein highly expressed in FGR placentas. In a human trophoblast cell line, HTR-8/SVneo, TGF-β1 treatment upregulates CTGF expression, preventing trophoblast cell invasion, via the SMAD2/3 signaling pathway [10]. Rac1, Cdc42, and ROCK via prostaglandin E2 induce trophoblast cell migration, which is inhibited by RhoGDI2 suppressing Rac1 activity. Decreased Rac1 levels are reported in PE, and genetic knockout of mouse ROCK2 determines placental dysfunction and FGR [11–16]. Table 4.1 summarizes regulatory agents, localization, and mechanisms of trophoblastic cell invasion.

The expression of the transcription factor glial cell missing 1 (GCM1) is decreased in PE and FGR. GCM1 targets the synapse defective 1 (SYDE1) gene, which encodes a RhoGAP that promotes cytoskeletal reshaping and cellular movement. In a mouse model experiment, SYDE1 knockout resulted in FGR and abnormal placental vascularization. The results also showed altered expression of renin-1, angiotensin I-converting enzyme 2, angiotensin II type 1a receptor, and membrane metalloendopeptidase of the renin-angiotensin system [17].

The Role of Fetal-Placental Angiogenesis

Fetal growth restriction (FGR) involves multifactorial causes affecting the normal development potential of the fetus. FGR may be harmful not only for the fetus itself but is also associated with a series of diseases that may appear later in childhood or in adulthood, such as cardiovascular disease and diabetes [18], intellectual impairment, and psychiatric disorders [19, 20].

Reduced activity of the placenta may involve altered cytotrophoblastic invasion of the maternal uterine arteries as well as thrombotic lesions to the villous tree or placental maldevelopment [21–23]. A prevalence of thrombotic activity may be related to a decrease in the expression of placental dermatan sulfate [24], a biglycan that is highly concentrated in the placenta [25, 26], as well as a decrease in decorin (DCN) expression, especially in idiopathic FGR [27]. Glycosaminoglycans are the major component of the extracellular matrix and play an important role in the control of collagen fibrillogenesis and matrix remodeling [28, 29], modulating cell adhesion [24] by binding TGF-β [30].

The reduced expression of dermatan sulfate and decorin may reduce thrombin inhibition at the endothelial level of the fetal circulation, predisposing to thrombosis of the vascular bed [31–33]. Although thrombin concentration during pregnancy is largely due to placental production, the true mechanism by which this mechanism

Table 4.1 Regulatory agents and mechanisms of trophoblastic cell invasion

Regulatory agents	Localization/action site	Biological effects
Chemokines	Decidual arteries Attract natural killer cells and macrophages through the Fas/FasL system	Induce vascular smooth muscle cell apoptosis
PHLDA2	Placenta; reduced thrombin inhibition at the endothelial level	Prevalence of thrombotic activities
HIF-1α	↑ Levels of HIF-1α ↑ MULE expression	↑ MULE expression favors trophoblast apoptosis by targeting Mcl-1, a pro-survival Bcl-2 family member
EG-VEGF	Placenta and maternal circulation Binds to VEGFR-1/flt-1 and KDR/flk1	VEGF interacts with PROKR1: a deregulation is considered a cause of FGR
IL-8, TNF, IFN-γ	Maternal inflammatory response ↑ IL-8, TNF, IFN-γ in FGR	Failure in trophoblast migration and spiral artery transformation
C3	C3 induces sFlt1 secretion in human monocytes	C3 activation favors dysregulation of angiogenic factors; neutrophil infiltration in the placenta and TNF-α release determined excessive C3 deposition and reduced levels of VEGF
NK	Decidua basalis Regulates extravillous trophoblast and spiral artery remodeling	NK receptors regulates ↑ or ↓ secretion of cytokines, regulating angiogenesis and invasion of EVT Decidual NK cells express S1PR5: inhibition of this pathway decreases VEGF levels with impaired trophoblast migration
H19 gene	Encodes a lncRNA	Nuclear H19 serves as precursor for microRNA miR-675 that inhibits placental growth in late pregnancy H19 gene favors EVT migration and invasion
TGF-β	Regulates SMAD pathway	↑ Sphingosine/ceramide ratio, responsible for increased trophoblast cell death TGF-β1 upregulates CTGF expression preventing trophoblast cell invasion, via SMAD signaling pathway
RAC1, CDC42, ROCK1	Prostaglandin E2	Induces trophoblast cell migration

EG-VGEF, endocrine gland-derived vascular endothelial growth factor; EVT, extravillous trophoblast; C3, complement; CDC42, cell division cycle 42; CTGF, connective tissue growth factor; HIF-1α, factor 1-α; IL-8, interleukin-8; IFN-γ, interferon gamma; lncRNA, long noncoding RNA; MULE, Mcl-1 ubiquitin ligase E3; NK, natural killer cells; PHLA2, pleckstrin homology-like domain, family A, member 2; ROCK1, Rho-associated coiled-coil-containing protein kinase 1; S1PR5, sphingosine-1-phosphate receptor-5; SMAD, Specific E3 ubiquitin protein ligase 1; TGF-β, tumor growth factor-β; TNF, tumor necrosis factor

acts is yet to be completely elucidated [34]. Murthi et al. have demonstrated that reduced expression of decorin (DCN) may contribute to the pathogenesis of idiopathic FGR; idiopathic FGR accounts for 70% of all cases of uteroplacental insufficiency [34]. The cellular mechanism by which DCN exerts its action may be related to its binding to heparin cofactor II (HCII) [35] and regulation of angiogenic growth factors such as epidermal growth factor (EGF) and vascular growth factor (VGFA) [30]. Chui et al. [34] demonstrated that fibroblast growth factor 17 (FGF17), interleukin-18 (IL18), and myostatin (MSTN) represent targeted genes of DCN on primary placental microvascular endothelial cells (PLECs). The downstream regulation by DCN on these targeted genes and a reduction of DCN gene expression imply a decrease in human microvascular endothelial cell (HMVEC) type proliferation in FGR-affected placentas [27, 34] and decreased expression of VEGA, IGFR1 (insulin growth factor 1), and PLGF (placental growth factor) [34]. As a final consequence, the reduced expression of DCN in HMVECs promotes increased thrombin generation in the microvascular system [25].

More recently, Murthi et al. [24] demonstrated that DCN mRNA was significantly decreased in first-trimester placental tissue by analyzing 15 chorionic villus samplings of FGR pregnancies over 50 normal controls ($p < 0.03$). The remodeling of the spiral arterioles by extravillous cytotrophoblasts (EVCTs) [36], which replace the maternal endothelium, is essential in the process of normal placental development [37], and a reduction in DCN expression may disrupt trophoblast proliferation and migration [38, 39]. It has been postulated that DCN may have gestation-dependent effects: early in pregnancy, DCN regulates cytotrophoblast proliferation, migration, and syncytium formation and interacts with the critical growth factor signaling pathway. As demonstrated, decreased DCN expression during the first trimester is associated with small for gestational age (SGA) fetuses late in pregnancy [40], since DCN also interacts with IGFR1 [41].

The process of fetal-placental vessel formation derives from vasculogenesis, a process that takes place very early in pregnancy and soon after implantation (from day 21 postconception to day 32). In order to occur, vasculogenesis requires endothelial progenitor cells (EPCs), extracellular matrix (ECM) components, and a series of soluble molecules [42, 43]. From day 32 until approximately 24 weeks of gestation, the process of vasculogenesis will end in the formation of 10–16 generations of stem villi [44, 45] (Fig. 4.1). Abnormal villous vasculogenesis may further lead to pregnancy complications such as PE with superimposed FGR [46, 47] (Fig. 4.2).

The fetal-placental vessels are composed of different cells, such as mesenchymal stem cells, fibroblasts, and tissue macrophages [48]. An important role in angiogenesis is played by M2 macrophages activated by IL4/IL13 to promote ECM construction and cell proliferation, called Hofbauer cells, which are numerous in the villous stroma [49–51]. Characteristically, Hofbauer cells produce vascular endothelium growth factor (VEGF), participating in the process of vasculogenesis of fetal-placental vessels [52–54]. Loegl et al. demonstrated that Hofbauer cells promote *in vitro*

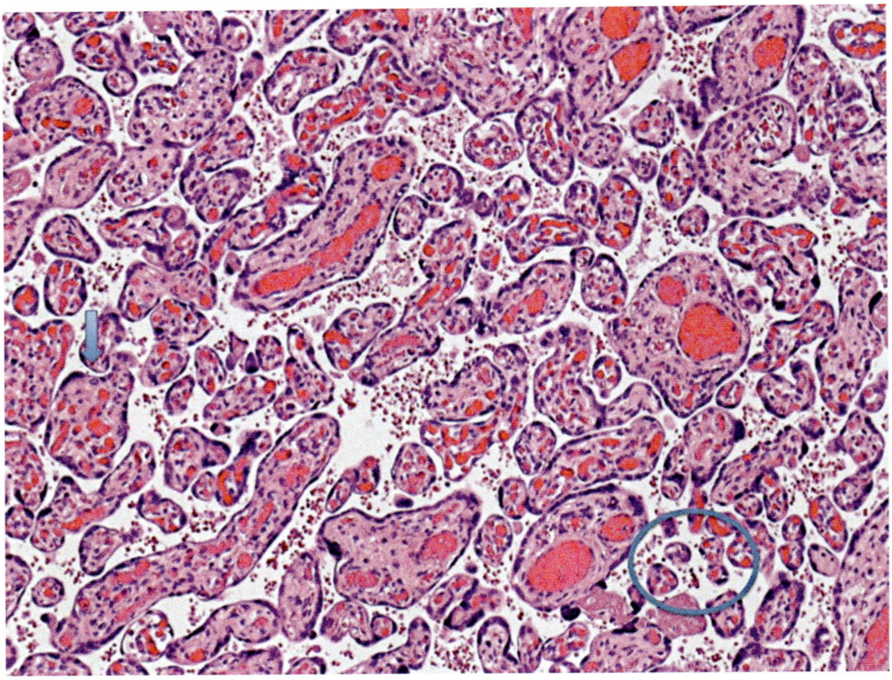

Fig. 4.1 Term placenta: the image shows mature intermediate villi (blue arrow) and terminal villi (circle). The first type of villi has abundant cellular stroma, and capillaries are less than 50%. Terminal villi are small, mainly composed of capillaries and scant stromal tissue (hematoxylin and eosin 4HPF)

angiogenesis of feto-placental endothelial cells (fpEcs) [55]. The process of fetal-placental vasculogenesis is very complex at the cellular level and is regulated by a large number of growth factors with their pathways, mainly represented by VEGF with its binding protein and placental growth factor (PlGF). VEGF and PIGF exert their biological effects by binding to their fms-like tyrosine kinase (Flt-1) receptors, namely, VEGFR-1/flt-1 and kinase insert domain-containing region (KDR)/flk1 (VEGFR2), respectively, whereas PlGF acts by binding to VEGFR2 [56]. The activation of VEGFR receptors is dependent upon partial oxygen pressure (p02) induced by hypoxic-ischemic changes occurring to the placenta, where VEGFR receptors are activated by a low p02 and PlGF by an elevated p02 [57, 58]. During hypoxic-ischemic insults to the placenta, VEGF and KDR concentrations are increased by paracrine secretion, whereas PlGF and flt-1 are enhanced in villous trophoblasts by autocrine regulation [59, 60]. Moreover, VEGF-C increases vascular permeability and stimulates endothelial cell proliferation and migration, and reduced VEGF-C and the protein expression of its receptors VEGFR-3 (localized on trophoblasts) have been documented in the placenta of severe cases of FGR [58]. The lack of PlGF and VEGFR-2 observed in placentas from pregnancies with FGR may predispose to the development of FGR and might explain the loss of normal vascular branching and villous trees in such complications [61]. VEGF is the most effective angiogenetic

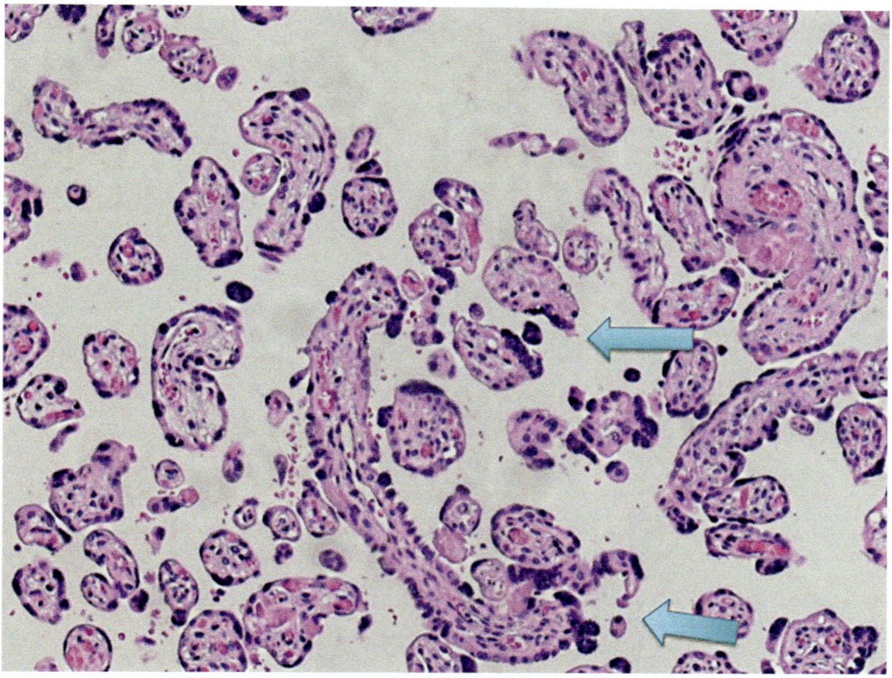

Fig. 4.2 Placenta at 28 weeks of gestational age with FGR (fetal growth restriction) and preeclampsia (PE): there is accelerated villous maturation with small villi and increased syncytial knots (blue arrows)

molecule, and its biological effects are partly regulated by PlGF and its receptors [62]. Interestingly in PE, there are an overproduction of VEGFR1 that inhibits VEGFR and PlGF and a downregulation of the membrane-bound form (VEGFR-1) in the placental bed that may contribute to causing abnormal placental development [63], which may be an antecedent of PE [64–67] (Figs. 4.3 and 4.4).

In addition, women who develop PE have a higher concentration than controls of soluble endoglin (sEnd) as well as soluble VEGFR-1 [68, 69]. sEnd is a glycoprotein and functional co-receptor for transforming growth factors (TGF)-β1 and TGF-β3 [70, 71] that display its antiangiogenic effects by inhibiting endothelial function *in vitro*, and endoglin mRNA is upregulated in women with PE and localized to the syncytiotrophoblast [68]. Chaiworapongsa et al. [72] demonstrated that the maternal plasma concentrations of sVEGFR1 increase 5–10 weeks prior to the development of PE and that increased concentration of sEnd and decreased concentration of PlGF are antecedents of delivering a small for gestational age (SGA) neonate [73]. On the contrary, while confirming that the concentration of PlGF is lower and the concentration of sFlt-1 is increased in women who later develop PE, no alterations could be found regarding angiogenic factor concentrations in women giving birth to SGA neonates in a case-control study of 12 mothers who developed PE, compared to 104 randomly selected controls [74]. Using a logistic model, Bakalis et al. [75] demonstrated that the best model for predicting, at a 10% false-positive rate (FPR),

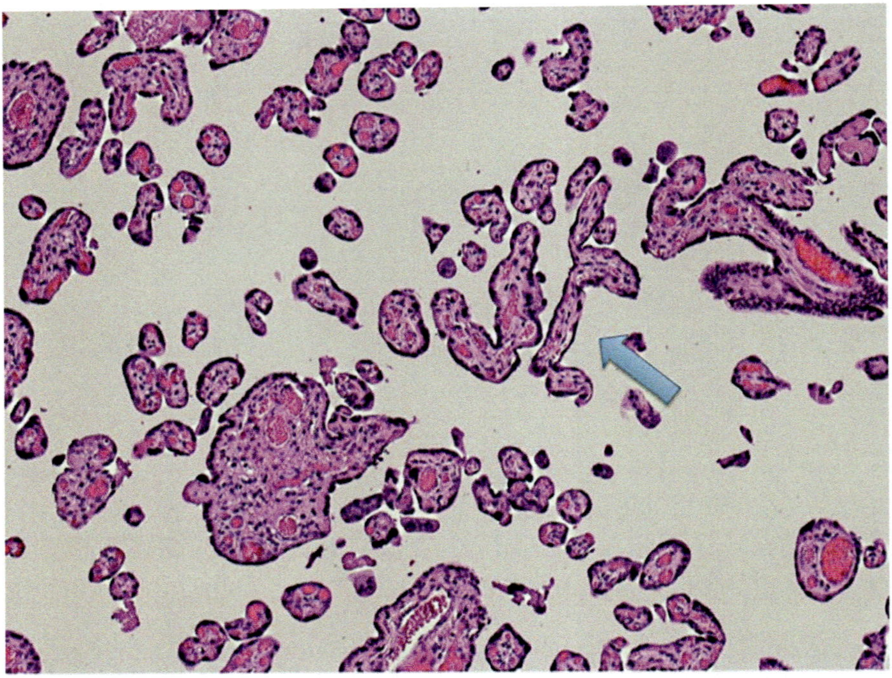

Fig. 4.3 Placenta at 28 weeks of gestational age with FGR and PE: there is distal villous hypoplasia with small and slender shaped villi (blue arrow)

89% of the deliveries of neonates with a birth weight <10 percentile was based on a combination of maternal risk factors, estimated fetal weight (EFW), uterine artery pulsatility index (Ut-A-PI), mean arterial pressure (MAP), and PlGF but no sFlt-1.

Angiopoietin 1 (Ang-1) and angiopoietin 2 (Ang 2) are another interesting recently discovered group of molecules acting as angiogenic factors by binding to their endothelium-specific receptor tyrosine kinase-2 [76]. Ang-1 and its antagonist Ang-2 act on the endothelial cell Tie-2 receptor to regulate vascular integrity, and fetal-placental artery remodeling and angiopoietin mRNA levels are a process dependent on placental oxygen tension [77]. Trophoblast outgrowth is regulated by Ang-1 and Ang-2 via stimulation of the Tie-2 receptor, promoting trophoblast proliferation and migration [78]. The angiogenic effect of Ang-1 and the angiopoietin/Tie2 signal is involved in the survival and migration of endothelial cells, which are important in maintaining the vascular integrity of newly formed blood vessels by binding to its angiopoietin-like proteins (Angptls) [79], whereas Ang-2 seems to have a destabilizing effect [80, 81].

Endothelin-1 is released from the maternal endothelium and is one of the most potent vasoconstrictors known. It has been demonstrated that maternal concentration of endothelin-1 is increased, while placental endothelin-1 synthesis is reduced in PE as a possible adaptive mechanism due to reduced blood flow to the placenta in PE placentas [82]. Moreover, it has been suggested that early and late PE might

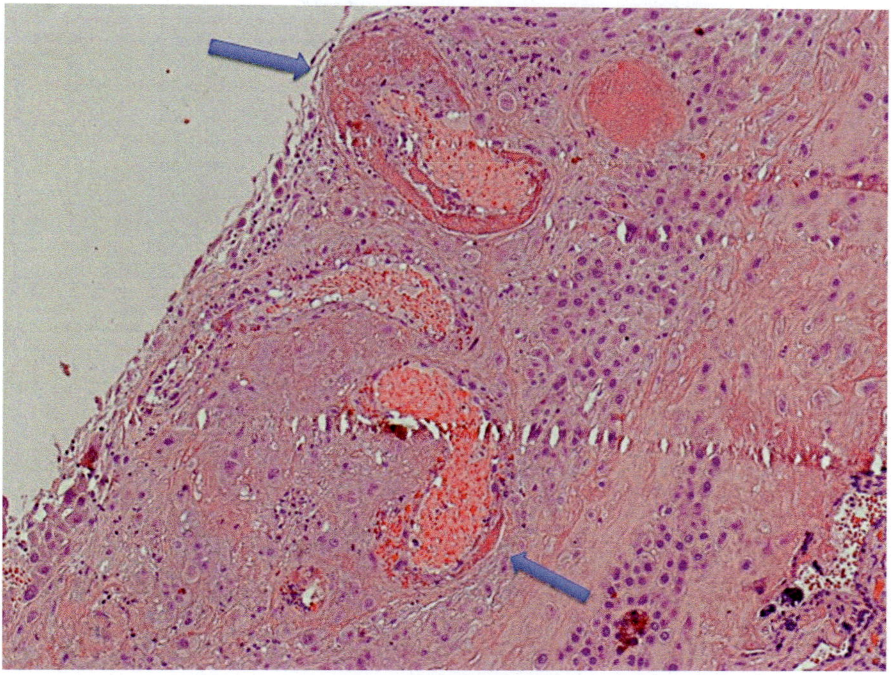

Fig. 4.4 Placenta at 28 weeks of gestational age with FGR and PE: decidual arteries show fibrinoid necrosis and lack of physiological conversion with persistence of smooth muscle in the wall (blue arrows)

be two distinct diseases, as early PE (<34 weeks) with or without FGR is associated with an increased expression of the endothelin-1-endothelin receptor (ET/ETR) system, whereas late PE is associated with an opposite effect [83]. Interestingly, in women developing FGR, the concentration of endothelin-1 is also increased in the amniotic fluid [84]. In the animal model, endothelin-1 has been shown to regulate placental perfusion, as ET-1 is upregulated in the setting of nitric oxide synthase (NOS) inhibition and NOS inhibition results in hypoxia-mediated FGR [85, 86]. ET-1 also counteracts the effect of leptin in pregnancy with FGR, where an increased fetal concentration of ET-1 and a decreased concentration of fetal leptin are observed [87]. In order to reduce the vasoconstrictor effect of ET-1 inducing hypoxia-FGR, a potential adaptive effect may be the reduced localization of ET-1 on placental tissue (capillary endothelial cells of villi, endothelial, decidual, and trophoblastic cells of the basal plate of the placenta) in pregnancies associated with FGR [88]. Table 4.2 summarizes the biologic effects of the major fetal-placental angiogenetic factors.

Severe FGR-complicated PE may also be associated with a tumor necrosis factor (TNF)-alpha G-308A single nucleotide polymorphism (SNP), as one study demonstrated that this mutant allele was statistically significantly higher among preeclamptic mothers with FGR compared with controls [89].

Table 4.2 Fetal-placental vasculo-angiogenetic factors and biological effects

Angiogenic factor	Localization/action site	Biological effect
Decorin (DCN)	Extracellular matrix: modulates cells adhesion by binding TGF-β and binding HCII; regulation of EGF and VGFA DCN regulates cytotrophoblastic proliferation, migration, and syncytium formation FGF17, IL18, and MSTN are targeted genes of DCN on primary PLECs Reduced thrombin inhibition at the endothelial level	Collagen fibrillogenesis and matrix remodeling Prevalence of thrombotic activity (↓ decorin expression in idiopathic type of FGR) Decrease in HMVECs in FGR-affected placentae and a decreased expression of VEGF, IGFR1, and PLGF Increased thrombin generation in the microvascular system
↓ Dermatan sulfate expression	Placenta; reduced thrombin inhibition at the endothelial level	Prevalence of thrombotic activities
Hofbauer cells (M2 macrophages)	Produce VEGF in the villous stroma	Promote *in vitro* angiogenesis of fpEcs VEGF interacts with PROKR1: a deregulation is considered a cause of FGR
VEGF	Binds to VEGFR-1/flt-1 and KDR/flk1	Increases vascular permeability, stimulates endothelial cell proliferation and migration
PlGF	Binds to VEGFR2 and regulates VEGF expression	↓ PlGF causes loss of normal vascular branching and villous trees
S-End	Co-receptor for TGF-β1 and TGF-β3	Inhibition of endothelial function in vitro
Ang-1	Inhibition of endothelial function *in vitro*; endothelial cell Tie-2 receptor	Regulates vascular integrity and fetal-placental arteries remodeling by binding to its Angptls; promotes trophoblast proliferation and migration
End-1	Maternal endothelium Regulates placental perfusion	ET-1 is upregulated in the setting of NOS inhibition and NOS inhibition results in hypoxia-mediated FGR ET-1 counteracts the effect of leptin in pregnancy with FGR (↑ ET-1 fetal concentration and ↓ leptin fetal concentration)

Ang-1, angiopoietin-1; Angptls, angiopoieting-like protein; DCN, decorin; EGF, epidermal growth factor; ET-1, endothelin-1; FGR, fetal growth restriction; FGF17, fibroblast growth factor 17; Flt-1, fms-like tyrosine kinase (VEGFR-1/flt-1); fpEcs, feto-placental endothelial cells; HCII, heparin cofactor II; HMVECs, human microvascular endothelial cells type proliferation; IGFR1, insulin growth factor, IL18, interleukin; KDR, kinase insert domain-containing region; NOS, nitric oxide synthase; PROKR1, prokineticin receptor; PLECs, primary microvascular endothelial cells; MSTN, myostatin; PlGF, placental growth factor; TGF, tumor growth factor; VGFA, vascular growth factor A; VEGF, vascular endothelial growth factor

The Role of Spiral Artery Remodeling

Spiral artery remodeling in the fetus is one of the most critical events that takes place in order to modify the maternal vascular bed and plays an essential role in preventing the development of PE, a disease affecting 4–6% of overall pregnancies [90] and capable of causing FGR. An abnormal impairment of this process, along with reduced extravillous cytotrophoblast invasion, is an important mechanism in the development of PE [91]. Altered spiral artery remodeling during pregnancy may be facilitated by different pathologic mechanisms involving the cytotrophoblast, such as inhibited proliferation [92], antiangiogenesis [93], and decreased migration and invasion of the decidual stroma of the maternal spiral arteries [94]. The underlying genetic mechanism predisposing to abnormal uteroplacental artery remodeling and consequent PE may be the deregulation of noncoding RNAs (IncRNAs) [95–97]. Interestingly, it has also been demonstrated that upregulation of IncRNA SPRY4-IT in the nucleus modulates apoptosis and suppresses cytotrophoblast migration into uteroplacental vessels in PE [98]. In addition, downregulation of IncRNA MEG3 in PE also promotes trophoblast apoptosis and impaired trophoblast invasion as well as IncRNA MVIH (microvascular invasion in hepatocellular carcinoma) [98, 99]. Zou et al. [100] have very recently demonstrated that IncRNA MVIH is downregulated in the placental tissue of PE and that MVIH acts synergically with the Jun-B protein. Jun-B is an endonuclease of 299 amino acids that along with other proteins constitutes the activator protein 1 [101], which regulates the proliferation and migration of trophoblast cells [100] and tumor angiogenesis [102]. Embryologically, the process of spiral artery remodeling starts very early in gestation, approximately 5 days postfertilization, when the trophoblast cells that form the outer layer of the blastocyst start to migrate [103]. This process occurs under hypoxic conditions, and the placental oxygen gradient regulates whether some types of trophoblast cells will migrate or proliferate [104–106]. The cytotrophoblast cells are considered stem-like, and column trophoblasts facilitate the passage of extravillous trophoblasts (EVTs) through the maternal decidua, a process called migration. The interstitial trophoblasts will then destroy the arterial media (invasion), and the endothelial trophoblasts will replace endothelial cells that have undergone apoptosis [107].

EVTs act in a manner that resembles that of cancer cells as regards their capacity for proliferation, migration, and invasion [108], and it is likely that EVT invasions are also promoted by elastin-derived peptides (EDPs) that are released during elastolysis early in pregnancy when the arterial wall of the uterine spiral arteries are transformed into dilated, high-flow and low-resistance vessels [109]. SPRY4-IT1 inhibits trophoblast cell migration and invasion by regulating the epithelial-to-mesenchymal transition (EMT) process via the Wnt/β-catenin pathway [110, 111], resulting in abnormal spiral artery remodeling. Furthermore, SPRY4-IT1 is overexpressed, and the Wnt/β-catenin pathway is activated in PE placentas [112].

Ephrin B2, which belongs to the largest family of receptor tyrosine kinases [113], participates in the process of uteroplacental artery remodeling [114], as it regulates embryonic vascular development and postnatal angiogenesis [115]. The Notch pathway is a regulator of ephrin B2 expression and could potentially interact with ephrin B2 in their role in migration and invasion and could promote angiogenesis repair in women with PE [114, 116, 117]. Furthermore, the Notch pathway is implicated in trophoblast function and differentiation [118–121], and Notch1 has been detected *in vivo* in extravillous trophoblast progenitors and clusters of villous trophoblasts initiating the invasive differentiation program [122].

In addition, endothelial progenitor cells (EPCs) and MMP-14 and MMP-15 also appear to play an important role in uteroplacental artery remodeling [123, 124], as well as the absence of decidual mesenchymal stem cells (DMSCs) in the vascular niche surrounding fully transformed spiral arterioles, implying that DMSCs are involved in replacement or destruction by extravillous trophoblast cells [125]. In PE, a reduction in the number of EPCs has been documented [107, 126].

The leucocyte population in the uterine decidua is another important mechanism involved in the local cytokine balance that may affect trophoblast invasion and spiral artery remodeling, as demonstrated by reduced CD56+ uNK (uterine natural killer) cells from FGR decidua [127, 128]. Nonetheless, decidual natural killer cells (dNKs) regulate vascular stability, contributing to uteroplacental artery remodeling [129].

Epigenetics

It is well known that maternal factors influence fetal growth more than paternal factors. However, increased paternal age does not seem to affect fetal growth or poor perinatal outcomes [130]. Genomic influences on FGR have been scantily investigated in the medical literature compared to placental and fetal factors, even though it has been reported that genomic mechanisms may be responsible for 40–80% of fetal growth development [131]. Genomic imprinting and DNA methylation play a critical role [132, 133]. Different methylated positions of DNA involved in gene regulation and transcription pathways related to organ development and metabolic function can be found in placentas and cord blood from fetuses and neonates affected by *in utero* FGR [134].

DNA methylation is an epigenetic mechanism which involves the addition of a methyl group to a cytosine base in the DNA, forming a methylated cytosine-phosphate-guanine (CpG) dinucleotide which is known to silence gene expression. One of the major fetal somatotrophic regulators of fetal growth is represented by the insulin growth factor (IGF) system. Insulin-like growth factors 1 and 2 (IGF1, IGF2) are expressed in the placenta and contribute to the regulation of fetal growth [135]. The biological expression of IGF is regulated by its seven binding proteins (IGFBP), of which IGFBP1 appears to play a major role in fetal growth [136]. The IGF1 gene is underexpressed, and IGFBP1, IGFBP2, IGFBP3, IGFBP4, and IGFBP7 are overexpressed in the placenta of SGA neonates [137].

Stewart et al. were the first to demonstrate that high methylation of HSB11B2, a key gene involved in glucocorticoid metabolism in the human placenta, is associated with FGR [138–140]. Epigenetic or genetic defects affecting specific imprinted genes, such as those involving the 11p15 region, may produce significant effects on fetal and postnatal growth. Imprinted genes are highly expressed in the placenta and play a key role in placental morphology and function [141, 142]. IGF2, which is imprinted in tandem with H19, is the most intensively studied imprinted gene. It has been demonstrated that the critical 11p15 region encoded for IGF2/H19 and mutations at this level, as well as on chromosomes 7 and 14, have been documented in cases of Silver-Russell syndrome (SRS) or Beckwith-Wiedemann syndrome (BWS), which represent two opposite phenotypes of fetal growth [143]. SRS and BWS are useful clinical models for fetal growth disturbances and are caused by a loss of paternal and maternal methylation of the imprinted control region (ICR1) at the IGF-2/H19 domain and of the imprinted control region (ICR2) at the KCNQ1/CDKN1C domain, respectively [144, 145].

In addition, mutations involving transcriptional insulators such as CTCF and OCT-binding sequences are involved in the fetal growth mechanism [146, 147]. Very recently, it was discovered that mutation of the oncogenic HMGA2-PLAG1-IGF2 pathway is involved in the pathogenetic mechanism of SRS [148]. Methylation of the IGF axis may contribute to FGR, as the expression of mRNA and protein levels of IGF1 were found to be lower in the placenta of SGA newborns, while IGFBPs were higher compared to AGA neonates [137]. Furthermore, high WNT2 promoter methylation (WNT2ProMe) in human placentas, an epigenetic variant of the WNT family of genes located in the 7q31.2 region, has been shown to be associated with FGR [149].

Nonetheless, DNA methylation and gene expression of WNT2, IGF2/H19, SERPINA3, HERVWE1, and PPARG have not shown to be altered in first-trimester placental samples from pregnancies with SGA newborns, indicating that the clinical effects of the downregulation of such genes are visible only at a later stage of fetal development [150]. Tabano et al. have demonstrated that ICR1 methylation status is a necessary and sufficient condition to drive the imprinting of IGF2 and H19 present in embryonic as well as in extraembryonic tissues and that hypomethylation of H19 promoter and DMR2 does not influence the expression pattern of IGF2 and H19 [151]. Interestingly, reduced methylation of ICR1 is associated with normotensive FGR, but not FGR associated with PE, suggesting a different etiology of FGR in this subgroup [152].

Decreased synapse defective gene 1 (SYDE1) expression has been seen in cases of preterm or term FGR. SYDE1 promotes cytoskeletal remodeling and cell migration and invasion and is a target gene of transcriptional factor glial cell missing 1 (GCM1) that regulates trophoblast differentiation and function during placentation and is implicated in the pathogenesis of PE [17]. A case-control study on 250 pregnancies with FGR reported that rs6046 polymorphism of the FVII gene is associated with the development of FGR, confirming the role of thrombophilia as one of several pathogenetic mechanisms [153].

The upregulation of maternal PHLDA2 and IGF2R expression in FGR infants supports the "parental conflict hypothesis" [154]. PHLDA2 might be influenced by environmental factors, and its use as a placental marker of FGR should be encouraged [155]. It is known that maternal inheritance of a promoter variant in the imprinted PHLDA2 gene increases birth weight [156]. Pleckstrin homology-like domain, family A, member 2 (PHLDA2), located on 11p15.4, is close to the 11p15.5, a 1 Mb region that contains several genes, such as H19, IGF2, and CDKN1C, involved in Beckwith-Wiedemann syndrome.

Conclusion

Maternal, placental, and fetal factors interact to promote embryo and fetal growth. Trophoblastic invasion with uterine spiral arteries remodeling is a key-point event occurring at endothelial level and is critical for physiologic development of the embryo and fetus. The process of fetal-placental vasculogenesis is regulated by genomic factors and by multiple regulatory molecules and interactive pathway mechanisms. An altered expression of this process at different levels may cause defective intervillous perfusion, leading to preeclampsia and fetal growth restriction.

References

1. Goldman-Wohl D, Yagel S. Regulation of trophoblast invasion: from normal implantation to pre-eclampsia. Mol Cell Endocrinol. 2002;187:233–8.
2. Sharp AN, Heazell AE, Crocker IP, Mor G. Placental apoptosis in health and disease. Am J Reprod Immunol. 2010;64:159–69.
3. Burton GJ, Jauniaux E. Pathophysiology of placental-derived fetal growth restriction. Am J Obstet Gynecol. 2018;218:S745–S61.
4. Jin F, Qiao C, Luan N, Li H. Lentivirus-mediated PHLDA2 overexpression inhibits trophoblast proliferation, migration and invasion, and induces apoptosis. Int J Mol Med. 2016;37:949–57.
5. Tang L, He G, Liu X, Xu W. Progress in the understanding of the etiology and predictability of fetal growth restriction. Reproduction. 2017;153:R227–40.
6. Ning F, Liu H, Lash GE. The role of decidual macrophages during normal and pathological pregnancy. Am J Reprod Immunol. 2016;75:298–309.
7. Su MT, Tsai PY, Tsai HL, Chen YC, Kuo PL. miR-346 and miR-582-3p-regulated EG-VEGF expression and trophoblast invasion via matrix metalloproteinases 2 and 9. Biofactors. 2017;43:210–9.
8. Zuckerwise L, Li J, Lu L, Men Y, Geng T, Buhimschi CS, et al. H19 long noncoding RNA alters trophoblast cell migration and invasion by regulating TβR3 in placentae with fetal growth restriction. Oncotarget. 2016;7:38398–407.
9. Chauvin S, Yinon Y, Xu J, Ermini L, Sallais J, Tagliaferro A, et al. Aberrant TGFβ signalling contributes to dysregulation of sphingolipid metabolism in intrauterine growth restriction. J Clin Endocrinol Metab. 2015;100:E986–96.
10. Cheng JC, Chang HM, Leung PCK. TGF-β1 inhibits human trophoblast cell invasion by upregulating connective tissue growth factor expression. Endocrinology. 2017;158:3620–8.
11. Nicola C, Lala PK, Chakraborty C. Prostaglandin E2-mediated migration of human trophoblast requires RAC1 and CDC42. Biol Reprod. 2008;78:976–82.

12. Nicola C, Chirpac A, Lala PK, Chakraborty C. Roles of Rho guanosine 5′-triphosphatase A, Rho kinases, and extracellular signal regulated kinase (1/2) in prostaglandin E2-mediated migration of first-trimester human extravillous trophoblast. Endocrinology. 2008;149:1243–51.
13. Liu S, Cui H, Li Q, Zhang L, Na Q, Liu C. RhoGDI2 is expressed in human trophoblasts and involved in their migration by inhibiting the activation of RAC1. Biol Reprod. 2014;90:88.
14. Fan M, Xu Y, Hong F, Gao X, Xin G, Hong H, et al. Rac1/beta-catenin signalling pathway contributes to trophoblast cell invasion by targeting Snail and MMP9. Cell Physiol Biochem. 2016;38:1319–32.
15. Hannke-Lohmann A, Pildner von Steinburg S, Dehne K, Benard V, Kolben M, Schmitt M, et al. Downregulation of a mitogen-activated protein kinase signaling pathway in the placentas of women with preeclampsia. Obstet Gynecol. 2000;96:582–7.
16. Thumkeo D, Keel J, Ishizaki T, Hirose M, Nonomura K, Oshima H, et al. Targeted disruption of the mouse rho-associated kinase 2 gene results in intrauterine growth retardation and fetal death. Mol Cell Biol. 2003;23:5043–55.
17. Lo HF, Tsai CY, Chen CP, Wang LJ, Lee YS, Chen CY, et al. Association of dysfunctional synapse defective 1 (SYDE1) with restricted fetal growth – SYDE1 regulates placental cell migration and invasion. J Pathol. 2017;241:324–36.
18. Godfrey KM, Barker DJ. Fetal nutrition and adult disease. Am J Clin Nutr. 2002;71:13445–525.
19. Rosso IM, Cannon TD, Huttunen T, Huttunen MO, Lonnqvist J, Gasperoni TL. Obstetric risk factors for early-onset schizophrenia in a Finnish birth cohort. Am J Psychiatry. 2000;157:801–7.
20. Gale CR, Martyn CN. Birth weight and later risk of depression in a national birth cohort. Br J Psychiatry. 2004;184:28–33.
21. Gagnon R. Placental insufficiency and its consequences. Eur J Obstet Gynecol Reprod Biol. 2003;110:S99–S107.
22. Kingdom J, Huppertz B, Seaward G, Kaufmann P. Development of the placental villous tree and its consequences for fetal growth. Eur J Obstet Gynecol Reprod Biol. 2000;92:35–43.
23. Salafia CM, Silberman L, Herrera NE, Mahoney MJ. Placental pathology at term associated with elevated midtrimester maternal serum alpha-fetoprotein concentration. Am J Obstet Gynecol. 1988;158:1064–6.
24. Murthi P, Faisal FA, Rajaraman G, Stevenson J, Ignjatovic V, Monagle PT, et al. Placental biglycan expression is decreased in human idiopathic fetal growth restriction. Placenta. 2010;31:712–7.
25. Delorme MA, Xu L, Berry L, Mitchell L, Andrew M. Anticoagulant dermatan sulfate proteoglycan (decorin) in the term human placenta. Thromb Res. 1998;90:147–53.
26. Giri TK, Tollefsen DM. Placental dermatan sulfate: isolation, anticoagulant activity, and association with heparin cofactor II. Blood. 2006;107:2753–8.
27. Swan B, Murthi P, Rajaraman G, Pathirage NA, Said JM, Ignjatovic V, et al. Decorin expression is decreased in human idiopathic fetal growth restriction. Reprod Fertil Dev. 2010;22:949–55.
28. San Martin S, Zorn TM. The small proteoglycan biglycan is associated with thick collagen fibrils in the mouse decidua. Cell Mol Biol. 2003;49:673–8.
29. Douglas T, Heinemann S, Bierbaum S, Scharnweber D, Worch H. Fibrillogenesis of collagen types I, II, and III with small leucine-rich proteoglycans decorin and biglycan. Biomacromolecules. 2006;7:2388–93.
30. Reinboth B, Thomas J, Hanssen E, Gibson MA. Beta ig-h3 interacts directly with biglycan and decorin, promotes collagen VI aggregation, and participates in ternary complexing with these macromolecules. J Biol Chem. 2006;281:7816–24.
31. Klaritsch P, Haeusler M, Karpf E, Schlembach D, Lang U. Spontaneous intrauterine umbilical artery thrombosis leading to severe fetal growth restriction. Placenta. 2008;29:374–7.
32. Wilkins-Haug L, Quade B, Morton CC. Confined placental mosaicism as a risk factor among newborns with fetal growth restriction. Prenat Diagn. 2006;26:428–32.
33. Tovar AM, de Mattos DA, Stelling MP, Sarcinelli-Luz BS, Nazareth RA, Mourão PA. Dermatan sulfate is the predominant antithrombotic glycosaminoglycan in vessel walls: implications for a possible physiological function of heparin cofactor II. Biochim Biophys Acta. 1740;2005:45–53.

34. Chui A, Murthi P, Gunatillake T, Brennecke SP, Ignjatovic V, Monagle PT, et al. Altered decorin leads to disrupted endothelial cell function: a possible mechanism in the pathogenesis of fetal growth restriction? Placenta. 2014;35:596–605.
35. Chen J, Liu J. Characterization of the structure of antithrombin-binding heparan sulfate generated by heparan sulfate 3-O-sulfotransferase 5. Biochim Biophys Acta. 1725;2005:190–200.
36. Lyall F, Bulmer JN, Kelly H, Duffie E, Robson SC. Human trophoblast invasion and spiral artery transformation: the role of nitric oxide. Am J Pathol. 1999;154:1105–14.
37. McFadyen IR, Price AB, Geirsson RT. The relation of birthweight to histological appearances in vessels of the placental bed. Br J Obstet Gynaecol. 1986;93:476–81.
38. Iacob D, Cai J, Tsonis M, Babwah A, Chakraborty C, Bhattacharjee RN, et al. Decorin-mediated inhibition of proliferation and migration of the human trophoblast via different tyrosine kinase receptors. Endocrinology. 2008;149:6187–97.
39. Xu G, Guimond MJ, Chakraborty C, Lala PK. Control of proliferation, migration, and invasiveness of human extravillous trophoblast by decorin, a decidual product. Biol Reprod. 2002;67:681–9.
40. Murthi P, van Zanten DE, Eijsink JJ, Borg AJ, Stevenson JL, Kalionis B, et al. Decorin expression is decreased in first trimester placental tissue from pregnancies with small for gestation age infants at birth. Placenta. 2016;45:58–62.
41. Schonherr E, Sunderkötter C, Iozzo RV, Schaefer L. Decorin, a novel player in the insulin-like growth factor system. J Biol Chem. 2005;280:15767–72.
42. Adams RH, Alitalo K. Molecular regulation of angiogenesis and lymphangiogenesis. Nat Rev Mol Cell Biol. 2007;8:464–78.
43. Carmeliet P. Mechanisms of angiogenesis and arteriogenesis. Nat Med. 2000;6:389–95.
44. Charnock-Jones DS, Kaufmann P, Mayhew TM. Aspects of human fetoplacental vasculogenesis and angiogenesis. I. Molecular regulation. Placenta. 2004;25:103–13.
45. Kaufmann P, Mayhew TM, Charnock-Jones DS. Aspects of human fetoplacental vasculogenesis and angiogenesis. II. Changes during normal pregnancy. Placenta. 2004;25:114–26.
46. Maulik D, Evansa JF, Ragolia L. Fetal growth restriction: pathogenetic mechanisms. Curr Obstet Gynecol. 2006;2:219–27.
47. Krebs C, Macara LM, Leiser R, Bowman AW, Greer IA, Kingdom JC. Intrauterine growth restriction with absent end-diastolic flow velocity in the umbilical artery is associated with maldevelopment of the placental terminal villous tree. Am J Obstet Gynecol. 1996;175:1534–42.
48. Abumaree MH, Al Jumah MA, Kalionis B, Jawdat D, Al Khaldi A, AlTalabani AA, et al. Phenotypic and functional characterization of mesenchymal stem cells from chorionic villi of human term placenta. Stem Cell Rev. 2013;9:16–31.
49. Tang Z, Tadesse S, Norwitz E, Mor G, Abrahams VM, Guller S. Isolation of hofbauer cells from human term placentas with high yield and purity. Am J Reprod Immunol. 2011;66:336–48.
50. Jetten N, Verbruggen S, Gijbels MJ, Post MJ, De Winther M, Donners MM. Anti-inflammatory M2, but not pro-inflammatory M1 macrophages promote angiogenesis in vivo. Angiogenesis. 2014;17:109–18.
51. Martinez FO, Gordon S. The M1 and M2 paradigm of macrophage activation: time for reassessment. F1000Prime Rep. 2014;6:13.
52. Seval Y, Korgun ET, Demir R. Hofbauer cells in early human placenta: possible implications in vasculogenesis and angiogenesis. Placenta. 2007;28:841–5.
53. Cooper JC, Sharkey AM, McLaren J, Charnock-Jones DS, Smith SK. Localization of vascular endothelial growth factor and its receptor, flt, in human placenta and decidua by immunohistochemistry. J Reprod Fertil. 1995;105:205–13.
54. Khan S, Katabuchi H, Araki M, Nishimura R, Okamura H. Human villous macrophage-conditioned media enhance human trophoblast growth and differentiation in vitro. Biol Reprod. 2000;62:1075–83.
55. Loegl J, Hiden U, Nussbaumer E, Schliefsteiner C, Cvitic S, Lang I, et al. Hofbauer cells of M2a, M2b and M2c polarization may regulate feto-placental angiogenesis. Reproduction. 2016;152:447–55.

56. Hiratsuka S, Maru Y, Okada A, Seiki M, Noda T, Shibuya M. Involvement of Flt-1 tyrosine kinase (vascular endothelial growth factor receptor-1) in pathological angiogenesis. Cancer Res. 2001;61:1207–13.
57. Regnault TR, de Vrijer B, Galan HL, Davidsen ML, Trembler KA, Battaglia FC, et al. The relationship between transplacental O2 diffusion and placental expression of PlGF, VEGF and their receptors in a placental insufficiency model of fetal growth restriction. J Physiol. 2003;550:641–56.
58. Dunk C, Ahmed A. Expression of VEGF-C and activation of its receptors VEGFR-2 and VEGFR-3 in trophoblast. Histol Histopathol. 2001;16:359–75.
59. Khaliq A, Dunk C, Jiang J, Shams M, Li XF, Acevedo C, et al. Hypoxia down-regulates placenta growth factor, whereas fetal growth restriction up-regulates placenta growth factor expression: molecular evidence for "placental hyperoxia" in intrauterine growth restriction. Lab Investig. 1999;79:151–70.
60. Ahmed A, Dunk C, Ahmad S, Khaliq A. Regulation of placental vascular endothelial growth factor (VEGF) and placenta growth factor (PIGF) and soluble Flt-1 by oxygen – a review. Placenta. 2000;21(Suppl A):S16–24.
61. Alahakoon TI, Zhang W, Arbuckle S, Zhang K, Lee V. Reduced angiogenic factor expression in intrauterine fetal growth restriction using semiquantitative immunohistochemistry and digital image analysis. J Obstet Gynaecol Res. 2018;44:861. https://doi.org/10.1111/jog.13592.
62. Vrachnis N, Kalampokas E, Sifakis S, Vitoratos N, Kalampokas T, Botsis D, et al. Placental growth factor (PlGF): a key to optimizing fetal growth. J Matern Fetal Neonatal Med. 2013;26:995–1002.
63. Tsatsaris V, Goffin F, Munaut C, Brichant JF, Pignon MR, Noel A, et al. Overexpression of the soluble vascular endothelial growth factor receptor in preeclamptic patients: pathophysiological consequences. J Clin Endocrinol Metab. 2003;88:5555–63.
64. Maynard SE, Min JY, Merchan J, Lim KH, Li J, Mondal S, et al. Excess placental soluble fms-like tyrosine kinase 1 (sFlt1) may contribute to endothelial dysfunction, hypertension, and proteinuria in preeclampsia. J Clin Invest. 2003;111:649–58.
65. Levine RJ, Maynard SE, Qian C, Lim KH, England LJ, Yu KF, et al. Circulating angiogenic factors and the risk of preeclampsia. N Engl J Med. 2004;350:672–83.
66. Torry DS, Wang HS, Wang TH, Caudle MR, Torry RJ. Preeclampsia is associated with reduced serum levels of placenta growth factor. Am J Obstet Gynecol. 1998;179:1539–44.
67. Tidwell SC, Ho HN, Chiu WH, Torry RJ, Torry DS. Low maternal serum levels of placenta growth factor as an antecedent of clinical preeclampsia. Am J Obstet Gynecol. 2001;184:1267–72.
68. Venkatesha S, Toporsian M, Lam C, Hanai J, Mammoto T, Kim YM, et al. Soluble endoglin contributes to the pathogenesis of preeclampsia. Nat Med. 2006;12:642–9.
69. Levine RJ, Lam C, Qian C, Yu KF, Maynard SE, Sachs BP, et al. Soluble endoglin and other circulating antiangiogenic factors in preeclampsia. N Engl J Med. 2006;355:992–1005.
70. Barbara NP, Wrana JL, Letarte M. Endoglin is an accessory protein that interacts with the signaling receptor complex of multiple members of the transforming growth factor-beta superfamily. J Biol Chem. 1999;274:584–94.
71. Letamendia A, Lastres P, Botella LM, Raab U, Langa C, Velasco B, et al. Role of endoglin in cellular responses to transforming growth factor-beta. A comparative study with betaglycan. J Biol Chem. 1998;273:33011–9.
72. Chaiworapongsa T, Romero R, Kim YM, Kim GJ, Kim MR, Espinoza J, et al. Plasma soluble vascular endothelial growth factor receptor-1 concentration is elevated prior to the clinical diagnosis of pre-eclampsia. J Matern Fetal Neonatal Med. 2005;17:3–18.
73. Romero R, Nien JK, Espinoza J, Todem D, Fu W, Chung H, et al. A longitudinal study of angiogenic (placental growth factor) and anti-angiogenic (soluble endoglin and soluble vascular endothelial growth factor receptor-1) factors in normal pregnancy and patients destined to develop preeclampsia and deliver a small for gestational age neonate. J Matern Fetal Neonatal Med. 2008;21:9–23.

74. Rizos D, Eleftheriades M, Karampas G, Rizou M, Haliassos A, Hassiakos D, et al. Placental growth factor and soluble fms-like tyrosine kinase-1 are useful markers for the prediction of preeclampsia but not for small for gestational age neonates: a longitudinal study. Eur J Obstet Gynecol Reprod Biol. 2013;171:225–30.
75. Bakalis S, Peeva G, Gonzalez R, Poon LC, Nicolaides KH. Prediction of small-for-gestational-age neonates: screening by biophysical and biochemical markers at 30–34 weeks. Ultrasound Obstet Gynecol. 2015;46:446–51.
76. Geva E, Ginzinger DG, Zaloudek CJ, Moore DH, Byrne A, Jaffe RB. Human placental vascular development: vasculogenic and angiogenic (branching and nonbranching) transformation is regulated by vascular endothelial growth factor-A, angiopoietin-1, and angiopoietin-2. J Clin Endocrinol Metab. 2002;87:4213–24.
77. Zhang EG, Smith SK, Baker PN, Charnock-Jones DS. The regulation and localization of angiopoietin-1, -2, and their receptor Tie2 in normal and pathologic human placentae. Mol Med. 2001;7:624–35.
78. Dunk C, Shams M, Nijjar S, Rhaman M, Qiu Y, Bussolati B, et al. Angiopoietin-1 and angiopoietin-2 activate trophoblast Tie-2 to promote growth and migration during placental development. Am J Pathol. 2000;156:2185–99.
79. Oike Y, Yasunaga K, Suda T. Angiopoietin-related/angiopoietin-like proteins regulate angiogenesis. Int J Hematol. 2004;80:21–8.
80. Wang Q, Lash GE. Angiopoietin 2 in placentation and tumor biology: the yin and yang of vascular biology. Placenta. 2017;56:73–8.
81. Morisada T, Kubota Y, Urano T, Suda T, Oike Y. Angiopoietins and angiopoietin-like proteins in angiogenesis. Endothelium. 2006;13:71–9.
82. Aggarwal PK, Jain V, Srinivasan R, Jha V. Maternal EDN1 G5665T polymorphism influences circulating endothelin-1 levels and plays a role in determination of preeclampsia phenotype. J Hypertens. 2009;27:2044–50.
83. Dieber-Rotheneder M, Beganovic S, Desoye G, Lang U, Cervar-Zivkovic M. Complex expression changes of the placental endothelin system in early and late onset preeclampsia, fetal growth restriction and gestational diabetes. Life Sci. 2012;91:710–5.
84. Margarit L, Griffiths AN, Tsapanos V, Tsakas S, Gumenos D, Decavalas G. Second trimester amniotic fluid endothelin-1 concentrations and subsequent development of intrauterine growth restriction. Eur J Obstet Gynecol Reprod Biol. 2007;134:192–5.
85. Thaete LG, Kushner DM, Dewey ER, Neerhof MG. Endothelin and the regulation of uteroplacental perfusion in nitric oxide synthase inhibition-induced fetal growth restriction. Placenta. 2005;26:242–50.
86. Thaete LG, Dewey ER, Neerhof MG. Endothelin and the regulation of uterine and placental perfusion in hypoxia-induced fetal growth restriction. J Soc Gynecol Investig. 2004;11:16–21.
87. Arslan M, Yazici G, Erdem A, Erdem M, Arslan EO, Himmetoglu O. Endothelin 1 and leptin in the pathophysiology of intrauterine growth restriction. Int J Gynaecol Obstet. 2004;84:120–6.
88. Erdem M, Erdem A, Erdem O, Yildirim G, Memis L, Himmetoğlu O. Immunohistochemical localization of endothelin-1 in human placenta from normal and growth-restricted pregnancies. Pediatr Dev Pathol. 2003;6:307–13.
89. Molvarec A, Jermendy A, Nagy B, Kovács M, Várkonyi T, Hupuczi P. Association between tumor necrosis factor (TNF)-alpha G-308A gene polymorphism and preeclampsia complicated by severe fetal growth restriction. Clin Chim Acta. 2008;392:52–7.
90. Ghulmiyyah L, Sibai B. Maternal mortality from preeclampsia/eclampsia. Semin Perinatol. 2012;38:56–9.
91. Zarate A, Saucedo R, Valencia J, Manuel L, Hernández M. Early disturbed placental ischemia and hypoxia creates immune alteration and vascular disorder causing preeclampsia. Arch Med Res. 2014;45:519–24.
92. Redline RW, Patterson P. Pre-eclampsia is associated with an excess of proliferative immature intermediate trophoblast. Hum Pathol. 1995;26:594–600.
93. Myatt L. Role of placenta in preeclampsia. Endocrine. 2002;19:103–11.

94. de Groot CJ, O'Brien TJ, Taylor RN. Biochemical evidence of impaired trophoblastic invasion of decidual stroma in women destined to have preeclampsia. Am J Obstet Gynecol. 1996;175:24–9.
95. Derrien T, Johnson R, Bussotti G, Tanzer A, Djebali S, Tilgner H, et al. The GENCODE v7 catalog of human long noncoding RNAs: analysis of their gene structure, evolution, and expression. Genome Res. 2012;22:1775–89.
96. Shi X, Sun M, Liu H, Yao Y, Song Y. Long non-coding RNAs: a new frontier in the study of human diseases. Cancer Lett. 2013;339:159–66.
97. Zou Y, Jiang Z, Yu X, Zhang Y, Zuo Q, Zhou J, et al. Upregulation of long noncoding RNA SPRY4-IT1 modulates proliferation, migration, apoptosis, and network formation in trophoblast cells HTR-8SV/neo. PLoS One. 2013;8:e79598–11.
98. Zhang Y, Zou Y, Wang W, Zuo Q, Jiang Z, Sun M, et al. Downregulated long non-coding RNA MEG3 and its effect on promoting apoptosis and suppressing migration of trophoblast cells. J Cell Biochem. 2015;116:542–50.
99. Yuan SX, Yang F, Yang Y, Tao QF, Zhang J, Huang G, et al. Long noncoding RNA associated with microvascular invasion in hepatocellular carcinoma promotes angiogenesis and serves as a predictor for hepatocellular carcinoma patients' poor recurrence-free survival after hepatectomy. Hepatology. 2012;56:2231–41.
100. Zou Y, Li Q, Xu Y, Yu X, Zuo Q, Huang S, et al. Promotion of trophoblast invasion by lncRNA MVIH through inducing Jun-B. J Cell Mol Med. 2018;22:1214–23.
101. Nausch N, Florin L, Hartenstein B, Angel P, Schorpp-Kistner M, Cerwenka A. Cutting edge: the AP-1 subunit JunB determines NK cell-mediated target cell killing by regulation of the NKG2D-ligand RAE-1epsilon. J Immunol. 2006;176:7–11.
102. Jochum W, Passegue E, Wagner EF. AP-1 in mouse development and tumorigenesis. Oncogene. 2001;20:2401–12.
103. Maitre JL. Mechanics of blastocyst morphogenesis. Biol Cell. 2017;109:323–38.
104. Genbacev O, Joslin R, Damsky CH, Polliotti BM, Fisher SJ. Hypoxia alters early gestation human cytotrophoblast differentiation/invasion in vitro and models the placental defects that occur in preeclampsia. J Clin Invest. 1996;97:540–50.
105. Genbacev O. Regulation of human placental development by oxygen tension. Science. 1997;277:1669–72.
106. Huppertz B, Gauster M, Orendi K, König J, Moser G. Oxygen as modulator of trophoblast invasion. J Anat. 2009;215:14–20.
107. McNally R, Alqudah A, Obradovic D, McClements L. Elucidating the pathogenesis of preeclampsia using in vitro models of spiral uterine artery remodelling. Curr Hypertens Rep. 2017;19:93.
108. Holtan SG, Creedon DJ, Haluska P, Markovic SN. Cancer and pregnancy: parallels in growth, invasion, and immune modulation and implications for cancer therapeutic agents. Mayo Clin Proc. 2009;84:985–1000.
109. Desforges M, Harris LK, Aplin JD. Elastin-derived peptides stimulate trophoblast migration and invasion: a positive feedback loop to enhance spiral artery remodelling. Mol Hum Reprod. 2015;21:95–104.
110. Liu X, Li Z, Song Y, Wang R, Han L, Wang Q, et al. AURKA induces EMT by regulating histone modification through Wnt/beta-catenin and PI3K/Akt signaling pathway in gastric cancer. Oncotarget. 2016;7:33152–64.
111. Bernaudo S, Salem M, Qi X, Zhou W, Zhang C, Yang W, et al. Cyclin G2 inhibits epithelial-to-mesenchymal transition by disrupting Wnt/beta-catenin signaling. Oncogene. 2016;35:4816–27.
112. Zuo Q, Huang S, Zou Y, Xu Y, Jiang Z, Zou S, et al. The Lnc RNA SPRY4-IT1 modulates trophoblast cell invasion and migration by affecting the epithelial-mesenchymal transition. Sci Rep. 2016;6:37183.
113. Klein R. Bidirectional modulation of synaptic functions by Eph/ephrin signaling. Nat Neurosci. 2009;12:15–20.

114. Liu X, Luo Q, Zheng Y, Liu X, Hu Y, Wang F, et al. The role of delta-like 4 ligand/notch-ephrin-B2 cascade in the pathogenesis of preeclampsia by regulating functions of endothelial progenitor cell. Placenta. 2015;36:1002–10.
115. Wang Y, Nakayama M, Pitulescu ME, Schmidt TS, Bochenek ML, Sakakibara A, et al. Ephrin-B2 controls VEGF-induced angiogenesis and lymphangiogenesis. Nature. 2010;465: 483–6.
116. You LR, Lin FJ, Lee CT, DeMayo FJ, Tsai MJ, Tsai SY. Suppression of Notch signalling by the COUP-TFII transcription factor regulates vein identity. Nature. 2005;435:98–104.
117. Williams CK, Li JL, Murga M, Harris AL, Tosato G. Upregulation of the Notch ligand Delta-like 4 inhibits VEGF induced endothelial cell function. Blood. 2006;107:931–9.
118. Hunkapiller NM, Gasperowicz M, Kapidzic M, Plaks V, Maltepe E, Kitajewski J, et al. A role for Notch signaling in trophoblast endovascular invasion and in the pathogenesis of pre-eclampsia. Development. 2011;138:2987–98.
119. Haider S, Meinhardt G, Velicky P, Otti GR, Whitley G, Fiala C, et al. Notch signaling plays a critical role in motility and differentiation of human first-trimester cytotrophoblasts. Endocrinology. 2014;55:263–74.
120. Velicky P, Haider S, Otti GR, Fiala C, Pollheimer J, Knöfler M. Notch-dependent RBPJκ inhibits proliferation of human cytotrophoblasts and their differentiation into extravillous trophoblasts. Mol Hum Reprod. 2014;20:756–66.
121. Kopan R, Ilagan MX. The canonical Notch signaling pathway: unfolding the activation mechanism. Cell. 2009;137:216–33.
122. Haider S, Meinhardt G, Saleh L, Fiala C, Pollheimer J, Knöfler M. Notch1 controls development of the extravillous trophoblast lineage in the human placenta. Proc Natl Acad Sci U S A. 2016;113:E7710–9.
123. Page-McCaw A, Ewald AJ, Werb Z. Matrix metalloproteinases and the regulation of tissue remodelling. Nat Rev Mol Cell Biol. 2007;8:221–33.
124. Majali-Martinez A, Velicky P, Pollheimer J, Knöfler M, Yung HW, Burton GJ, et al. Endothelin-1 down-regulates matrix metalloproteinase 14 and 15 expression in human first trimester trophoblasts via endothelin receptor type B. Hum Reprod. 2017;32:46–54.
125. Kusuma GD, Manuelpillai U, Abumaree MH, Pertile MD, Brennecke SP, Kalionis B. Mesenchymal stem cells reside in a vascular niche in the decidua basalis and are absent in remodelled spiral arterioles. Placenta. 2015;36:312–21.
126. Muñoz-Hernandez R, Miranda ML, Stiefel P, Lin RZ, Praena-Fernández JM, Dominguez-Simeon MJ, et al. Decreased level of cord blood circulating endothelial colony-forming cells in preeclampsia. Hypertension. 2014;64:165–71.
127. Cartwright JE, James-Allan L, Buckley RJ, Wallace AE. The role of decidual NK cells in pregnancies with impaired vascular remodelling. J Reprod Immunol. 2017;119:81–4.
128. Williams PJ, Bulmer JN, Searle RF, Innes BA, Robson SC. Altered decidual leucocyte populations in the placental bed in pre-eclampsia and foetal growth restriction: a comparison with late normal pregnancy. Reproduction. 2009;138:177–84.
129. Fraser R, Whitley GS, Thilaganathan B, Cartwright JE. Decidual natural killer cells regulate vessel stability: implications for impaired spiral artery remodelling. J Reprod Immunol. 2015;110:54–60.
130. DeFranco EA. Influence of paternal age on perinatal outcomes. Am J Obstet Gynecol. 2017;217:566.e1–6.
131. Johnston LB, Clark AJ, Savage MO. Genetic factors contributing to birth weight. Arch Dis Child Fetal Neonatal Ed. 2002;86:F2–3.
132. Maccani MM. Epigenetics in the Placenta. Am J Reprod Immunol. 2009;62:78.
133. McMinn J, Wei M, Schupf N, Cusmai J, Johnson EB, Smith AC, et al. Unbalanced placental expression of imprinted genes in human intrauterine growth restriction. Placenta. 2006;27:540–9.
134. Hillman SL, Finer S, Smart MC, Mathews C, Lowe R, Rakyan VK, et al. Novel DNA methylation profiles associated with key gene regulation and transcription pathways in blood and placenta of growth-restricted neonates. Epigenetics. 2015;10:50–61.

135. Han VK, Bassett N, Walton J, Challis JR. The expression of insulin-like growth factor (IGF) and IGF-binding protein (IGFBP) genes in the human placenta and membranes: evidence for IGF-IGFBP interactions at the feto-maternal interface. J Clin Endocrinol Metab. 1996;812:680–93.
136. Oh Y, Müller HL, Lee DY, Fielder PJ, Rosenfeld RG. Characterization of the affinities of insulin-like growth factor (IGF)-binding proteins 1-4 for IGF-I, IGF-II, IGF-I/insulin hybrid, and IGF-I analogs. Endocrinology. 1993;132:1337–44.
137. Nawathe AR, Christian M, Kim SH, Johnson M, Savvidou MD, Terzidou V. Insulin-like growth factor axis in pregnancies affected by fetal growth disorders. Clin Epigenetics. 2016;8:11.
138. Stewart PM, Murry BA, Mason JI. Type 2 11 betahydroxysteroid dehydrogenase in human fetal tissues. J Clin Endocrinol Metab. 1994;78:1529–32.
139. Marsit CJ, Maccani MA, Padbury JF, Lester BM. Placental 11-beta hydroxysteroid dehydrogenase methylation is associated with newborn growth and a measure of neurobehavioral outcome. PLoS One. 2012;7:e33794.
140. Zhao Y, Gong X, Chen L, Li L, Liang Y, Chen S, et al. Site-specific methylation of placental HSD11B2 gene promoter is related to intrauterine growth restriction. Eur J Hum Genet. 2014;22:734–40.
141. Tycko B. Imprinted genes in placental growth and obstetric disorders. Cytogenet Genome Res. 2006;113:271–8.
142. Hemberger M. Epigenetic landscape required for placental development. Cell Mol Life Sci. 2007;64:2422–36.
143. Giabicani É, Brioude F, Le Bouc Y, Netchine I. Imprinted disorders and growth. Ann Endocrinol (Paris). 2017;78:112–3.
144. Du M, Zhou W, Beatty LG, Weksberg R, Sadowski PD. The KCNQ1OT1 promoter, a key regulator of genomic imprinting in human chromosome 11p15.5. Genomics. 2004;84:288–300.
145. Netchine I, Rossignol S, Azzi S, Brioude F, Le Bouc Y. Imprinted anomalies in fetal and childhood growth disorders: the model of Russell-Silver and Beckwith-Wiedemann syndromes. Endocr Dev. 2012;23:60–70.
146. Bell AC, West AG, Felsenfeld G. The protein CTCF is required for the enhancer blocking activity of vertebrate insulators. Cell. 1999;98:387–96.
147. Demars J, Shmela ME, Rossignol S, Okabe J, Netchine I, Azzi S, et al. Analysis of the IGF2/H19 imprinting control region uncovers new genetic defects, including mutations of OCT-binding sequences, in patients with 11p15 fetal growth disorders. Hum Mol Genet. 2010;19:803–14.
148. Abi Habib W, Brioude F, Edouard T, Bennett JT, Lienhardt-Roussie A, Tixier F, et al. Genetic disruption of the oncogenic HMGA2-PLAG1-IGF2 pathway causes fetal growth restriction. Genet Med. 2017;20:250.
149. Ferreira JC, Choufani S, Grafodatskaya D, Butcher DT, Zhao C, Chitayat D, et al. WNT2 promoter methylation in human placenta is associated with low birthweight percentile in the neonate. Epigenetics. 2011;6:440–9.
150. Leeuwerke M, Eilander MS, Pruis MG, Lendvai Á, Erwich JJ, Scherjon SA, et al. DNA methylation and expression patterns of selected genes in first-trimester placental tissue from pregnancies with small-for-gestational-age infants at birth. Biol Reprod. 2016;94:37.
151. Tabano S, Colapietro P, Cetin I, Grati FR, Zanutto S, Mandò C, et al. Epigenetic modulation of the IGF2/H19 imprinted domain in human embryonic and extra-embryonic compartments and its possible role in fetal growth restriction. Epigenetics. 2010;5:313–24.
152. Bourque DK, Avila L, Peñaherrera M, von Dadelszen P, Robinson WP. Decreased placental methylation at the H19/IGF2 imprinting control region is associated with normotensive intrauterine growth restriction but not preeclampsia. Placenta. 2010;31:197–202.
153. Reshetnikov E, Zarudskaya O, Polonikov A, Bushueva O, Orlova V, Krikun E, et al. Genetic markers for inherited thrombophilia are associated with fetal growth retardation in the population of Central Russia. J Obstet Gynaecol Res. 2017;43:1139–44.

154. Kumar N, Leverence J, Bick D, Sampath V. Ontogeny of growth-regulating genes in the placenta. Placenta. 2012;33:94–9.
155. Jensen AB, Tunster SJ, John RM. The significance of elevated placental PHLDA2 in human growth restricted pregnancies. Placenta. 2014;35:528–32.
156. Ishida M, Monk D, Duncan AJ, Abu-Amero S, Chong J, Ring SM, et al. Maternal inheritance of a promoter variant in the imprinted PHLDA2 gene significantly increases birth weight. Am J Hum Genet. 2012;90:715–9.

Classification

5

Talita Micheletti Helfer, Elisenda Eixarch,
Francesc Figueras, and Eduard Gratacós

Introduction

Fetal growth restriction (FGR) is a common complication of pregnancy that has been associated with several adverse outcomes [1, 2]. Despite advances in fetal medicine, there is still lack of consensus regarding definition and diagnostic criteria for fetal growth restriction [3] with uncertainty surrounding the optimal management and timing of delivery for the growth-restricted fetus [1].

In light of these facts, standardized classification of FGR represents an important tool not only for clinical and management reasons but also for research and epidemiological purposes. Throughout time, FGR classification has evolved from one rooted in the phases of fetal growth (hyperplasia/hypertrophy) – in which the antepartum or postpartum morphometric measurements of the fetal head and abdomen distinguish symmetric (type I) from asymmetric (type II) growth-restricted fetuses and neonates [4] – to those based on the onset during pregnancy and the clinical stages of the condition [5]. Therefore, the objective of this chapter is to present current classification of FGR.

It is important to highlight that, since failure to achieve growth potential is a concept difficult to gauge, fetal size is used in the definition of FGR, with all its limitations. Therefore, traditionally, a small for gestational age (SGA) fetus has

T. M. Helfer (✉)
Fetal i+D Fetal Medicine Research Center, BCNatal | Barcelona Center for Maternal Fetal and Neonatal Medicine - Hospital Clínic and Hospital Sant Joan de Déu, IDIBAPS, University of Barcelona, Barcelona, Spain

E. Eixarch · F. Figueras · E. Gratacós
Fetal i+D Fetal Medicine Research Center, BCNatal | Barcelona Center for Maternal Fetal and Neonatal Medicine - Hospital Clínic and Hospital Sant Joan de Déu, IDIBAPS, University of Barcelona and Centre for Biomedical Research on Rare Diseases (CIBER-ER), Barcelona, Spain

L. M. M. Nardozza et al. (eds.), *Fetal Growth Restriction*,
https://doi.org/10.1007/978-3-030-00051-6_5

been regarded as equivalent of FGR. However, a distinction between FGR (with an increased risk of perinatal complications) and low-risk SGA is desirable [6].

Classification According to the Onset of Fetal Growth Restriction

FGR can be classified according to the onset, if early or late in pregnancy. Specialist consensus agrees that the demarcation should be gestational age at diagnosis before or after 32 weeks [3]. This classification differentiates two phenotypes determined

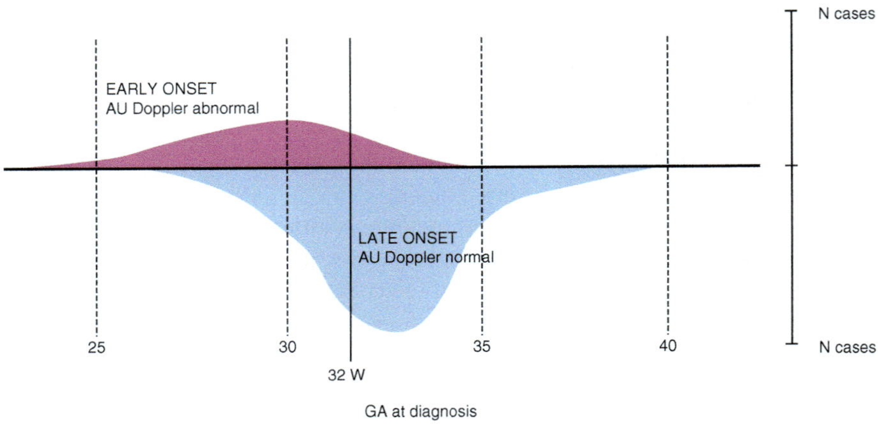

Fig. 5.1 Distribution of early- and late-onset fetal growth restriction. (Adapted from Savchev et al. [8])

Table 5.1 Main differences between early- and late-onset forms of fetal growth restriction

	Early-onset FGR	Late-onset FGR
Prevalence	0.5–1%	5–10%
Challenge	Management (GA at delivery, balancing risk of fetal compromise and risks of prematurity)	Detection and diagnosis
Evidence of placental disease	High (abnormal UA Doppler, higher association with PE, severe angiogenic disbalance)	Low (normal UA Doppler, lower association with PE, mild angiogenic disbalance)
Pathophysiology	Severe hypoxia (systemic CV adaptation)	Mild hypoxia (central CV adaptation)
Clinical course	Higher tolerance to hypoxia (sequence of Doppler alterations)	Lower tolerance to hypoxia (shorter natural history)
Clinical impact	Higher mortality and morbidity	Lower mortality and morbidity but higher prevalence

Adapted from Figueras et al. [6]

FGR fetal growth restriction, *GA* gestational age, *UA* umbilical artery, *PE* preeclampsia, *CV* cardiovascular

by the severity of placental disease and the adaptive response and deterioration [7, 8]. Consequently, late FGR does not present the same Doppler sequence of alterations as early FGR [9]. Figure 5.1 represents the distribution, and Table 5.1 depicts the main differences between these two phenotypes of FGR.

Early-Onset Fetal Growth Restriction

Early-onset FGR is less prevalent and represents 20–30% of all FGR cases. The association with early preeclampsia is common [5, 10], and the association with severe placental insufficiency and chronic fetal hypoxia is high [5]. Placental histology of preterm FGR neonates reveals numerous pathologies that reflect uteroplacental insufficiency and abnormal blood supply [11].

Because the fetus is still immature, there is a higher tolerance to hypoxia, and deterioration normally takes weeks [5, 12]. This explains the natural history of the disease, when the umbilical artery (UA) Doppler is abnormal in a high proportion of cases [5, 13]. Fetal condition deteriorates with progression to decompensated hypoxia and acidosis, which is reflected by escalating abnormalities in the UA (from elevated pulsatility index [PI] to absent and reversed end-diastolic velocity [AEDV/REDV]) and increased PI in the ductus venosus (DV) [5]. This cascade of

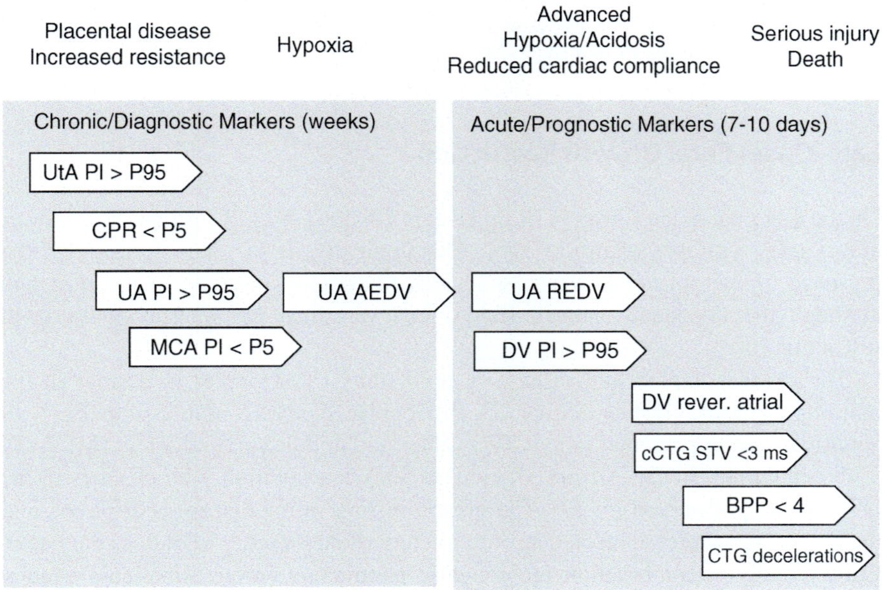

Fig. 5.2 Cascade of events in early fetal growth restriction. *UtA* uterine artery, *PI* pulsatility index, *CPR* cerebroplacental ratio, *UA* umbilical artery, *MCA* middle cerebral artery, *AEDV* absent end-diastolic velocity, *REDV* reverse end-diastolic velocity, *DV* ductus venosus, *cCTG* computerized cardiotocography, *STV* short-term variation, *BPP* biophysical profile. (Adapted from Figueras and Gratacos [5])

changes reflected in the pattern of Doppler changes allows for monitoring the progression of fetal deterioration and tailoring elective delivery. Figure 5.2 represents the sequence of events that is commonly observed in early FGR. Individual parameters are explained in other sections of this book.

The screening of early FGR in first or second trimester is more feasible than for the late-onset one. A model that combines uterine Doppler velocimetry, biochemical markers (angiogenic factors), and maternal characteristics may detect early-onset growth restriction in up to 90%. Such result could be explained, at least in part, by the strong association between early SGA and preeclampsia [10].

Even though the diagnosis and detection of early-onset FGR based on ultrasound and Doppler parameters are relatively easy, the management is challenging, because it frequently requires striking a balance between the risk of intrauterine fetal compromise and the risks of extreme prematurity [5].

In the early-onset form of the disease, there is a high rate of perinatal morbidity and mortality [5]. The best results in terms of short-term and 2-year outcomes were reported by the TRUFFLE study. Perinatal death occurred in 8%, and 31% of babies met criteria for a composite outcome of death or severe morbidity. Major contributors to severe morbidity were sepsis (18%) and bronchopulmonary dysplasia (10%). Less frequent complications were germinal matrix hemorrhage (2%) and cystic periventricular leukomalacia (1%). Maternal hypertension, in particular if severe, shortens the interval to delivery and influences neonatal outcome negatively [14]. In addition, extremes of blood flow resistance and cardiovascular deterioration, prematurity, and intracranial hemorrhage increase the risks for psychomotor delay and cerebral palsy in early FGR [15].

Late-Onset Fetal Growth Restriction

On the other hand, late-onset FGR represents 70–80% of FGR [16] and has a lower association with preeclampsia [16]. Histologically, it is characterized by the presence of uteroplacental vascular lesions (especially infarcts) in the placenta, although the incidence of such lesions is lower than in preterm fetal growth restriction [6].

The degree of placental disease is mild; thus UA Doppler is normal in the majority of cases. Despite normal UA PI Doppler, there is a high association with abnormal cerebroplacental ratio (CPR) values and middle cerebral artery (MCA) PI <5th percentile [5, 17]. Advanced signs of fetal deterioration with changes in the DV are rarely observed [5, 17]. The natural history of the disease is different, and the cascade of sequential fetal deterioration described for early FGR does not occur. Consequently, a combination of biometric parameters (severe smallness usually defined as estimated fetal weight or abdominal circumference <3rd centile) with Doppler criteria of placental insufficiency (either in the maternal [uterine Doppler] or fetal [cerebroplacental ratio] compartments) is needed as a classification tool that correlates with the risk for adverse perinatal outcome [6]. Because the fetus is more mature, there is a lower tolerance to hypoxia and a higher risk of acute fetal deterioration and intrapartum fetal distress. Therefore, late FGR may undergo rapid deterioration leading to severe injury or death without predictable deterioration pattern, as in early FGR [5, 18].

Late-onset growth restriction is still largely unpredicted by first- or second-trimester screening; for this reason, early screening for late FGR is of limited value. However, at third trimester, compared to clinically indicated ultrasonography, universal screening triples the detection rate of late SGA/FGR [6, 19]. In addition, as opposed to early third-trimester ultrasound, scanning late in pregnancy (around 37 weeks) increases the detection rate for birth weight <3rd centile [6, 20].

Compared with early-onset FGR, diagnosis of late-onset one is more challenging, while the management should not present difficulties [5]. There is association between late-onset FGR and cesarean delivery for fetal distress, neonatal acidosis, and admission to the neonatal unit [21]. Moreover, not only is late smallness associated with hypoxic neonatal complications and cerebral palsy but also with altered brain metabolites and poorer neurodevelopmental scores. At long term, late-onset compromise of fetal growth seems to be associated with poorer school performance, and as a consequence of fetal programing, such late small fetuses may have higher incidence of metabolic syndrome [6].

Classification According to Clinical Stages of Fetal Growth Restriction

Even though the classification according to the gestational age of diagnosis (onset) is important for the understanding of different clinical presentations of FGR as well as for standardizing study of the disease, from a clinical perspective, it is helpful to classify small fetuses in stages according to indices or signs that are associated with similar fetal risks and prognosis. Such approach indicates similar follow-up intervals, timing of delivery, and other management strategies, depending on the stratification of risk. A stage-based classification was proposed by Figueras and Gratacos [5, 7]:

SGA: Includes those fetuses with EFW <10th and >=3rd percentile with normal Doppler parameters including mean uterine artery (UtA) PI, UA PI, MCA PI, and CPR. Perinatal results of this group are good. Follow-up every 2 weeks is safe and induction of labor at 40 weeks is recommended [7].

Stage I FGR: Includes fetuses with EFW <3rd percentile or <10th percentile with abnormalities in at least one of the following Doppler parameters: mean UtA PI, UA PI, MCA PI, or CPR. Evidence suggests a low risk of fetal deterioration before term [22]. Weekly monitoring seems reasonable. Delivery beyond 37 weeks is acceptable, and induction of labor is not contraindicated, even though the risk of intrapartum fetal distress is increased [7].

Stage II FGR: This stage is defined by the presence of AEDV in UA. Twice-weekly monitoring is recommended and delivery should be after 34 weeks. The risk of emergency cesarean section in labor induction exceeds 50%. Therefore, elective cesarean section is a reasonable option [7].

Stage III FGR: The stage is defined by REDV in AU or DV PI >95th centile. There is an association with higher risk of stillbirth and poorer neurological outcome. However, since signs suggesting a very high risk of stillbirth within days are not present yet, it seems reasonable to delay elective delivery to reduce the possible effects of severe prematurity. Monitoring every 24–48 hour is recommended. Delivery should be recommended by cesarean section after 30 weeks [7].

Stage IV FGR: It is defined by the presence of abnormal cardiotocography (CTG) (spontaneous FHR decelerations or reduced short-term variation [<3 ms] in the computerized CTG) or reverse atrial flow in the DV. FHR deceleration is an ominous sign, normally preceded by the other two signs, and thus it is rarely observed, but if persistent it may justify emergency cesarean section. Abnormal cCTG and DV are associated with very high risks of stillbirth within the next 3–7 days or disability; therefore, monitoring every 12–24 hour should be performed until delivery. Cesarean section at a tertiary center after 26 weeks' gestation is recommended. Intact survival exceeds 50% only after 26–28 weeks' gestation, and, before this threshold, parents should be counseled by multidisciplinary teams [7].

Particularly at early gestational ages, and at whatever stage, coexistence of severe PE may distort the natural history, and strict fetal monitoring is warranted since fetal deterioration may occur unexpectedly at any time [7].

Further management aspects of FGR according to clinical classification are discussed in other sections. However, it is important to mention that FGR cases seem to benefit from close monitoring by expert obstetric and neonatal care teams. When a protocol of classification and follow-up is established, there is an improvement in care [14].

Conclusion

Classification of FGR is an important aspect of the management and study of the disease. Globally, there is still lack of standard classification. Nevertheless, even if evidence-based protocols are somehow adapted to local context, when a protocol is established, there are benefits and the clinical care is optimized.

References

1. Manning FA. Practice bulletin – fetal growth restriction. Curr Opin Obstet Gynecol. 1995;7:146–9.
2. Demicheva E, Crispi F. Long-term follow-up of intrauterine growth restriction: Cardiovascular disorders. Fetal Diagn Ther. 2014;36:143–53.
3. Gordijn SJ, Beune IM, Thilaganathan B, Papageorghiou A, Baschat AA, Baker PN, et al. Consensus definition of fetal growth restriction: a Delphi procedure. Ultrasound Obstet Gynecol. 2016;48:333–9.

4. Lin CC, Santolaya-Forgas J. Current concepts of fetal growth restriction: part II. Diagnosis and management. Obstet Gynecol. 1999;93:140–6.
5. Figueras F, Gratacós E. Update on the diagnosis and classification of fetal growth restriction and proposal of a stage-based management protocol. Fetal Diagn Ther. 2014;36:86–98.
6. Figueras F, Caradeux J, Crispi F, Eixarch E, Peguero A, Gratacos E. Diagnosis and surveillance of late-onset fetal growth restriction. Am J Obstet Gynecol. 2018;218:S790–S802.e1.
7. Figueras F, Gratacos E. Stage-based approach to the management of fetal growth restriction. Prenat Diagn. 2014;34:655–9.
8. Savchev S, Figueras F, Sanz-Cortes M, Cruz-Lemini M, Triunfo S, Botet F, et al. Evaluation of an optimal gestational age cut-off for the definition of early- and late-onset fetal growth restriction. Fetal Diagn Ther. 2014;36:99–105.
9. Unterscheider J, Daly S, Geary MP, Kennelly MM, McAuliffe FM, O'Donoghue K, et al. Optimizing the definition of intrauterine growth restriction: the multicenter prospective PORTO Study. Am J Obstet Gynecol. 2013;208:290.e1–6.
10. Crovetto F, Triunfo S, Crispi F, Rodriguez-Sureda V, Roma E, Dominguez C, et al. First-trimester screening with specific algorithms for early- and late-onset fetal growth restriction. Ultrasound Obstet Gynecol. 2016;48:340–8.
11. Apel-Sarid L, Levy A, Holcberg G, Sheiner E. Term and preterm (<34 and <37 weeks gestation) placental pathologies associated with fetal growth restriction. Arch Gynecol Obstet. 2010;282:487–92.
12. Hecher K, Bilardo CM, Stigter RH, Ville Y, Hackelöer BJ, Kok HJ, et al. Monitoring of fetuses with intrauterine growth restriction: a longitudinal study. Ultrasound Obstet Gynecol. 2001;18:564–70.
13. Turan OM, Turan S, Gungor S, Berg C, Moyano D, Gembruch U, et al. Progression of Doppler abnormalities in intrauterine growth restriction. Ultrasound Obstet Gynecol. 2008;32:160–7.
14. Lees C, Marlow N, Arabin B, Bilardo CM, Brezinka C, Derks JB, et al. Perinatal morbidity and mortality in early-onset fetal growth restriction: cohort outcomes of the trial of randomized umbilical and fetal flow in Europe (TRUFFLE). Ultrasound Obstet Gynecol. 2013;42:400–8.
15. Baschat AA. Neurodevelopment after Fetal Growth Restriction. Fetal Diagn Ther. 2014;36:136–42.
16. Crovetto F, Crispi F, Scazzocchio E, Mercade I, Meler E, Figueras F, et al. First-trimester screening for early and late small-for-gestational-age neonates using maternal serum biochemistry, blood pressure and uterine artery Doppler. Ultrasound Obstet Gynecol. 2014;43:34–40.
17. Oros D, Figueras F, Cruz-Martinez R, Meler E, Munmany M, Gratacos E. Longitudinal changes in uterine, umbilical and fetal cerebral Doppler indices in late-onset small-for-gestational age fetuses. Ultrasound Obstet Gynecol. 2011;37:191–5.
18. Hershkovitz R, Kingdom JCP, Geary M, Rodeck CH. Fetal cerebral blood flow redistribution in late gestation: identification of compromise in small fetuses with normal umbilical artery Doppler. Ultrasound Obstet Gynecol. 2000;15:209–12.
19. Sovio U, Smith GCS. The effect of customization and use of a fetal growth standard on the association between birthweight percentile and adverse perinatal outcome. Am J Obstet Gynecol. 2018;218(2S):S738–44.
20. Roma E, Arnau A, Berdala R, Bergos C, Montesinos J, Figueras F. Ultrasound screening for fetal growth restriction at 36 vs 32 weeks' gestation: a randomized trial (ROUTE). Ultrasound Obstet Gynecol. 2015;46:391–7.
21. Figueras F, Gardosi J. Intrauterine growth restriction: new concepts in antenatal surveillance, diagnosis, and management. Am J Obstet Gynecol. 2011;204:288–300.
22. Cruz-Martínez R, Figueras F, Hernandez-Andrade E, Oros D, Gratacos E. Fetal brain Doppler to predict cesarean delivery for nonreassuring fetal status in term small-for-gestational-age fetuses. Obstet Gynecol. 2011;117:618–26.

Prediction

6

Ana Cristina Perez Zamarian, Jader de Jesus Cruz,
and Luciano Marcondes Machado Nardozza

Introduction

Fetal growth restriction (FGR) is considered as the most common and complex problem of modern obstetrics by the American College of Obstetricians and Gynecologists [1]. It is associated with increased fetal and neonatal morbidity and mortality, accounting for up to 50% of fetal deaths. It is also linked to diseases in childhood (such as delayed psychomotor development, learning disabilities, and language disorders) and in adulthood (obesity, hypertension, and type 2 diabetes) [1].

It is known that the majority of deaths with fetal growth problems are potentially avoidable through better assessment of risk factors and surveillance of growth during pregnancy. Antenatal detection of the fetuses with growth restriction can lead to appropriate investigations during pregnancy and improve outcome by reducing the stillbirth risk through appropriate timely delivery (Fig. 6.1) [2, 3].

Recent studies have demonstrated that aspirin started before 16 week's gestation can significantly reduce the incidence of small for gestational age (SGA) and FGR (Table 6.1). The clinical impact of such finding is important because screening in the first trimester can identify women at higher risk of developing FGR, thus selecting the pregnancies who would potentially benefit from the use of aspirin [4, 5].

Screening for FGR and SGA in the first trimester can be achieved by a combination of maternal characteristics, biophysical parameters, and biochemical factors. Reported detection rates for such screening range between 20% and 67%, being the performance lower for SGA than for FGR [5, 6].

A. C. P. Zamarian (✉) · L. M. M. Nardozza
Discipline of Fetal Medicine, Department of Obstetrics, Paulista School of Medicine, Federal University of São Paulo (EPM-UNIFESP), São Paulo, SP, Brazil
e-mail: acrispz@uol.com.br

J. de Jesus Cruz
Fetal Medicine Unit, Maternidade Alfredo da Costa, Centro Hospitalar Lisboa Central, Lisbon, Portugal

L. M. M. Nardozza et al. (eds.), *Fetal Growth Restriction*,
https://doi.org/10.1007/978-3-030-00051-6_6

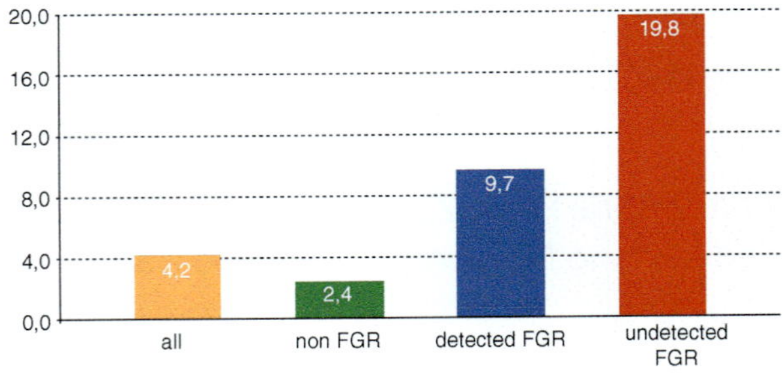

Fig. 6.1 Rate of stillbirth per 1000 birth in England (FGR defined as BW <10th centile corrected by GA at delivery)

Table 6.1 Aspirin in prevention of FGR (FGR defined as BW <10th centile)

Started aspirin	Dose	Relative risk
Before/at 16 weeks	100 mg	0.45
	150 mg	0.29
After 16 weeks	100 mg	0.96
	150 mg	0.90

Table 6.2 Odds ratio for maternal characteristic in screening for small for gestational age (SGA)

Maternal characteristics	Odds ratio
Age (years)	1.03
Weight (kg)	0.99
Height (cm)	0.97
Previous SGA	2.1
Smoking	3.5
Chronic hypertension	4.2
Type 2 diabetes mellitus	3.8
Systemic lupus erythematosus	4.8

Clinical Findings

Clinical findings include maternal factors, personal and family history, and fetal factors.

The association between maternal characteristics and fetal birth weight has been extensively studied and reported. Some studies have shown that the likelihood of SGA or FGR fetuses increases with maternal age and decreased with maternal weight and height. The risk appears to be higher in women of Afro-Caribbean and South Asian ethnic background compared to Caucasian women. The likelihood of being affected by SGA or FGR also increases in parous women with prior SGA or FGR, in cigarette smokers and illicit drugs users, and in women with a history of chronic hypertension, type 2 diabetes mellitus, and systemic lupus erythematosus. The use of ovulation drugs also has an influence on this risk (Table 6.2). In relation to fetal factors, multiple pregnancies, congenital infections, and aneuploidies are the most common and important variables related to fetal growth restriction [1]. Maternal factors alone can provide a detection rate of about 37%, for a 10% false positive for SGA and FGR fetuses [7, 8].

Studies show that the accuracy in predicting FGR at birth through ultrasound measurements, such as estimated fetal weight below the 10th percentile (p), is associated with a sensitivity ranging from 49% to 59%. Other measures, such as abdominal circumference (AC) and AC development, can also be evaluated. However, the study concludes that further research should focus on the use of biomarkers associated with fetal biometry [9].

Biophysical Markers

Uterine Artery Doppler

It is thought that one of the mechanisms for fetal growth restriction is the impaired placentation. Uterine artery (UtA) Doppler examination provides important information on the conversion process of spiral arteries into uteroplacental arteries. Reflecting the underlying process of placentation therefore provides a noninvasive method for evaluating uteroplacental blood flow (Figs. 6.2 and 6.3) [10]. Several studies conducted since the 1980s have shown the importance of this marker in both the first and second trimesters.

The pulsatility index (PI) and resistance index (RI) have been the most commonly used measurable indices. PI is better as it is the one who describes the shape of the waveform better, as it includes the area below the curve in the formula [11]. In the first trimester, uterine artery pulsatility index (UtAPI) is increased in FGR and SGA pregnancies. A screening for preterm SGA and FGR at 11–13 weeks by a

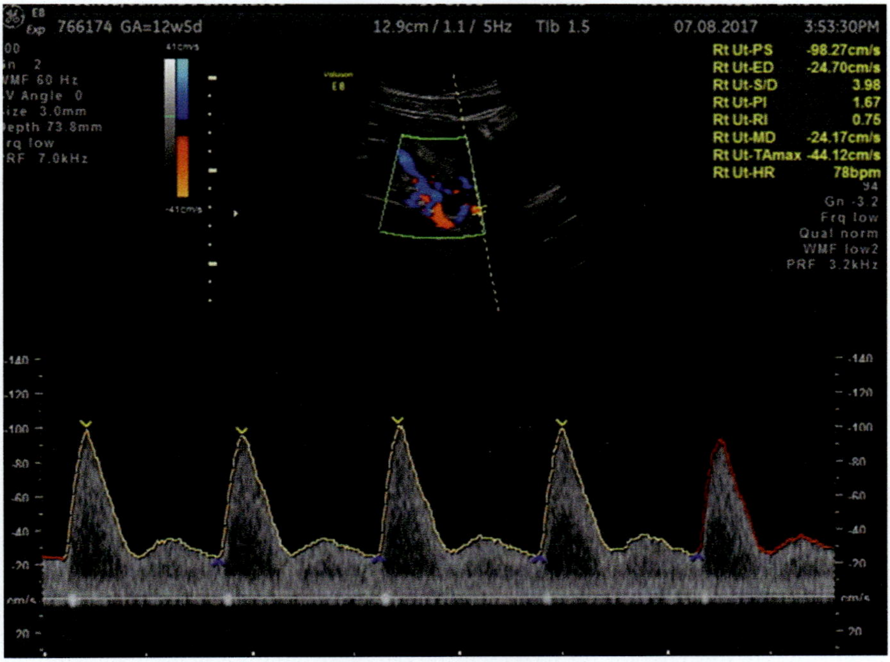

Fig. 6.2 Doppler velocimetry of the right uterine artery in the first trimester

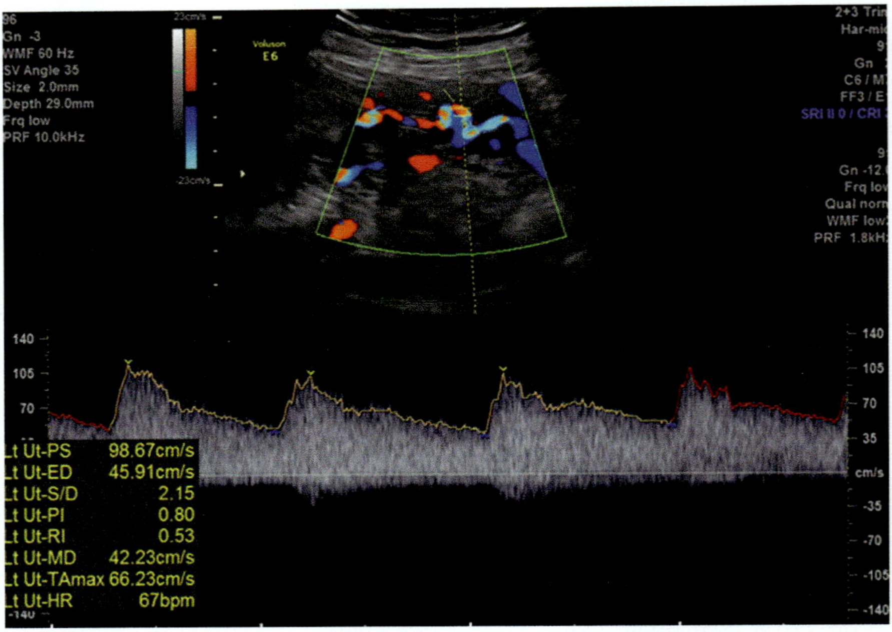

Fig. 6.3 Doppler velocimetry of the right uterine artery in the second trimester

combination of maternal characteristics and UtAPI has a detection rate of about 43% for a 10% false-positive rate (FPR) [12].

It is possible to include the assessment of UtAPI in the second and third trimester of pregnancy routine ultrasound. Such evaluation, in the second trimester, when combined with maternal characteristics and other biophysical and biochemical markers, can detect about 88% of the preterm SGA fetuses for a 10% FPR. In the routine third-trimester ultrasound examination (30–34 weeks), about 32% of the pregnancies resulting in preterm SGA fetuses will have an UtAPI above the 95 centile [13, 14].

Biochemical Markers

In an attempt to improve the prediction of FGR, biochemical markers were introduced in the early 2000s. Placental function is critical for fetal growth; therefore, placental insufficiency is an important component of intrauterine fetal growth restriction. A vast array of biochemical markers are present in maternal blood and are determinants of placental function and angiogenic factors. These metabolites have been described and studied as potential markers for SGA and FGR, like A disintegrin and metalloprotease-12 (ADAM-12), placental protein 13 (PP13), soluble endoglin (sEng), placental growth factor (PlGF), soluble fms-like tyrosine kinase-1 (sFlt-1), and pregnancy-associated plasma protein-A (PAPP-A). In this chapter we will focus on the more commonly used and studied markers: placental growth factor (PlGF), soluble fms-like tyrosine kinase-1 (sFlt-1), and pregnancy-associated plasma protein-A (PAPP-A) as they are, to

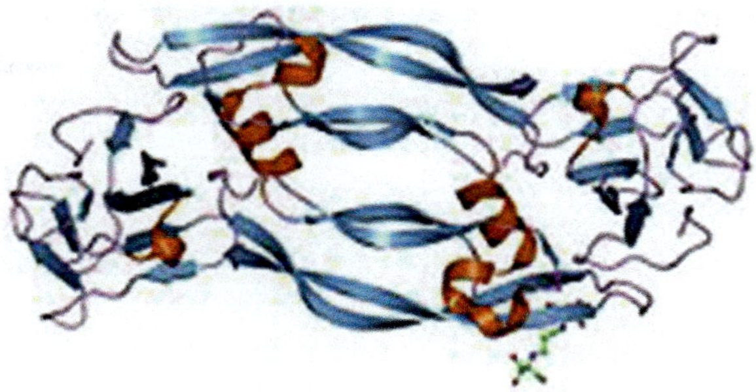

Fig. 6.4 Three-dimensional (3D) representation of PlGF structure

the date, the most relevant in respect of prediction of FGR and SGA. Another advantage of PlGF, sFlt-1, and PAPP-A is that they are known to be useful in screening for aneuploidies and preeclampsia. This makes easier to incorporate a screening for SGA and FGR in a daily clinic as the biochemical markers used are, in many countries, already in use.

The levels of pregnancy-associated plasma protein-A (PAPP-A) depend on placental function and volume; therefore, decreased levels of this protein are described in the literature as possible predictors of FGR, with sensitivity ranging from 8% to 33% [1]. Poon et al. [7] described that in the first trimester, the association of maternal characteristics and PAPP-A can predict 44% of preterm SGA fetuses for a 10% FPR. There is currently no evidence that PAPP-A can be useful in prediction of SGA or FGR if measured in the second or third trimester.

PlGF (Fig. 6.4) is reduced in pregnancies resulting in fetal growth restriction, particularly preterm FGR and SGA (requiring delivery before 37 weeks). This biochemical marker has high levels of specificity (98%), medium sensitivity (75%), high negative predictive values (99.2%), and low positive predictive values (58%) for preterm FGR [15]. The association of PlGF with maternal factors and biophysical markers in the first trimester can predict about 62% of the pregnancies resulting in FGR and about 48% of SGA for a 10% FPR [6, 7, 16]. It is also possible to use PlGF in the second and third trimester of pregnancy to predict SGA. In the second trimester, the association of PlGF with maternal factors and biophysical markers can predict 64% of the preterm SGA fetuses for a 10% FPR. In the third trimester, a similar association can predict 88% of the preterm SGA and 51% of the term SGA (birth after 37 weeks) [8, 12–14].

Soluble fms-like tyrosine kinase-1 (sFlt-1) is useful in the prediction of FGR. In the first trimester, the ratio between sFlt-1 and PlGF (sFlt-1/PlGF ratio) is a better predictor than sFlt-1 alone. The sFlt-1/PlGF ratio at 11–13 weeks can detect 61% of the pregnancies resulting in fetal growth restriction for a 10% false-positive rate [8].

Combined Screening

There is a significant variation in relation to detection rates in different studies. This can be partially explained by the different classifications in terms of FGR and the combination of markers used.

First-Trimester Screening for SGA, Early FGR, and Late FGR

Poon et al. [7] demonstrated that a combination of maternal characteristics and biophysical (uterine artery PI, mean arterial pressure) and biochemical markers (PAPP-A and PlGF) in the first trimester can be used as a screening method for SGA. The detection rates of such screening are 52% and 32% for preterm and term SGA, respectively, for a 10% FPR. Crovetto et al. [8] show a similar result for total SGA (term and preterm) with a detection rate of 42% for 10% FPR, although this study used different biochemical markers (sFlt-1/PlGF ratio) compared with Poon et al. [7].

For FGR, a similar screening test can be used; the detection rate is higher when compared to the detection rates of SGA. In the first trimester, the detection rate for FGR based on a combination of maternal characteristics and biophysical (uterine artery PI, mean arterial pressure) and biochemical markers (sFlt-1/PlGF ratio) is about 62% for a 10% false-positive rate. If the FGR is divided into early and late onset, the detection rate increases for early (71%) without changing significantly for late FGR (61%) for the same 10% FPR. This shows that it is better to use specific algorithms for early and late FGR rather than using an overall algorithm.

Second-Trimester Screening for SGA

Screening can also be conducted in the second trimester. Familiari et al. retrospectively evaluated 23,894 women between 19 and 24 weeks of pregnancy. The study included maternal characteristics (age, body mass index, and ethnicity), fetal biometry, birth weight, and uterine artery PI. The results showed that the combination of all markers led to detection rates of 40%, 66%, and 89% for small for gestational age (births below the 5th percentile) at term, preterm, and early preterm, respectively, with 10% false-positive rates [17]. In 2015, Poon et al. have shown a statistical model to predict pregnancies with small-for-gestational-age fetuses based on maternal characteristics, biophysical markers (fetal biometry and uterine artery Doppler), PlGF and alpha-fetoprotein (AFP) levels in the second trimester. This screening method has a detection rate of 100% for severe SGA requiring delivery before 32 weeks, 78% for the ones requiring delivery between 32 and 36 weeks, and 42% for the ones requiring delivery after 37 weeks for a 10% FPR [18].

Third-Trimester Screening for SGA

The prediction of late FGR in the third trimester is also important. Late restriction is often difficult to diagnose, being unnoticed by the obstetrician, and it is responsible for a considerable percentage of near-term fetal deaths.

Longitudinal monitoring of only the measurement of AC and estimated fetal weight showed a very low sensitivity of 28%, with 10% false positives [19]. Miranda et al. developed a screening model for the prognosis of adverse perinatal events in fetuses of adequate weight and small-for-gestational-age fetuses in the third trimester (between 32 and 36 weeks). The model considered maternal characteristics, estimated fetal weight, maternal-fetal Doppler velocimetry, and levels of estriol, PlGF, lipocalin-2, and inhibin-A. The prevalence of adverse perinatal events was 9.3% in the adequate weight group and 27.4% in the SGA fetus group. The adverse effects prediction model had a detection rate of only 26% in the general population and 62% in the SGA group [20]. Bakalis et al. conducted a study with 9472 women between 30 and 34 weeks of pregnancy in order to evaluate a model intended to predict small-for-gestational-age fetuses in the absence of PE. The model included maternal characteristics, estimated fetal weight, uterine artery Doppler, mean arterial pressure, PlGF, and sFlt-1. With 10% false positives, the prediction rate for neonates born between 32 and 36 weeks was 89% for those whose weight was below the 10th percentile and 96% for those whose weight was below the 3rd percentile. For neonates born after 37 weeks, the prediction rate was 57% for those whose weight was below the 10th percentile and 72% for those whose weight was below the 3rd percentile [21].

Main results of the studies are summarized in Table 6.3.

Table 6.3 Main results of the studies presented in the chapter

Author	Markers	Results
Papageorghiou et al. [10]	Uterine artery Doppler	Prediction rate: 20%
Benton et al. [15]	PlGF	Sensitivity: 75% Specificity: 98%
Albu et al. [1]	PAPP-A	Sensitivity: 8–33%
Albu et al. [1]	ADAM-12	Sensitivity: 7.16–20%
Karagiannis et al. [16]	1° trimester: Maternal characteristics, biophysical and biochemical markers	Detection rate: 73%
Crovetto et al. [8]	1° trimester: Maternal characteristic, mean blood pressure, uterine artery Doppler, PlGF, and sFlt-1	Detection rate for SGA: 42% Detection rate for FGR: 67%
Familiari et al. [17]	2° trimester: Maternal characteristic, fetal biometry, birth weight, uterine artery PI	Detection rates for SGA births are 40% for terms, 66% for preterm, and 89% for early preterm
Poon et al. [18]	2° trimester: Maternal factors, fetal biometry, uterine artery Doppler, PlGF, and PAPP-A	Detection rates for SGA births are 100% for <32 w, 78% for 32–36 w, and 42% for >37 w
Miranda et al. [20]	3° trimester: Maternal characteristic, estimated fetal weight, maternal-fetal Doppler, estriol, PlGF, lipocalin-2, and inhibin-A	Detection rate for adverse effects: 62% in SGA group
Bakalis et al. [21]	3° trimester: Maternal factors, estimated fetal weight, uterine artery Doppler, mean blood pressure, PlGF, and sFlt-1	Prediction rates for SGA births are: Between 32 and 36 w: 89% for <p10th and 96% for <p3rd After 37 w: 57% for <p10th and 72% for <p3rd

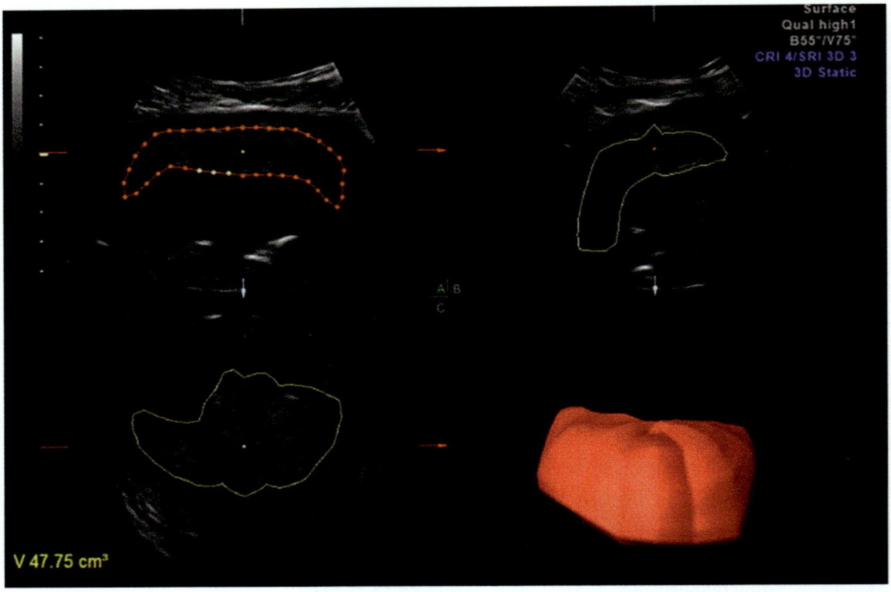

Fig. 6.5 Calculation of first-trimester placental volume using virtual organ computer-aided analysis (VOCAL)

Other Markers

In addition to maternal, biometric, and Doppler velocimetry findings and angiogenic factors, other markers were studied in order to assist in predicting the FGR. Placental volume determined by three-dimensional (3D) ultrasound in the first trimester was studied for predicting pregnancies with small-for-gestational-age fetuses. A systematic review conducted by Farina et al. analyzed 12 studies on placental volume between 11 and 14 weeks. They concluded that placental volume as an isolated marker shows very low prediction rates and can be better used in combination with other markers [22]. Virtual organ computer-aided analysis (VOCAL) software can be used to measure blood volume and flow in a region of interest (Fig. 6.5). A 2008 study by Guiot et al. showed that blood flow changes can be identified by 3D power Doppler before abnormalities are diagnosed using conventional umbilical artery Doppler [23].

Conclusion

FGR is a complex obstetric condition responsible for a considerable percentage of perinatal morbidity and mortality. Screening for FGR remains a challenge, and numerous studies are being conducted with an aim of improving its sensitivity. Effective screening helps to identify patients at risk, who would then be monitored more frequently in an attempt to minimize adverse perinatal effects. After a well-established prediction model of good accuracy is achieved, the challenge will be to identify interventions that can modify the history of the condition that justify population screening. To this date, studies show that aspirin started before 16 weeks may reduce the prevalence of this condition.

References

1. Albu A, Anca A, Horhoianu V, Horhoianu I. Predictive factors for intrauterine growth restriction. J Med Life. 2014;7:165–71.
2. Gardosi J, Madurasinghe V, Williams M, Malik A, Francis A. Maternal and fetal risk factors for stillbirth. Obstet Gynecol Surv. 2013;68:329–31.
3. Gardosi J, Giddings S, Clifford S, Wood L, Francis A. Association between reduced stillbirth rates in England and regional uptake of accreditation training in customised fetal growth assessment. BMJ Open. 2013;3:e003942.
4. Roberge S, Nicolaides K, Demers S, Hyett J, Chaillet N, Bujold E. The role of aspirin dose on the prevention of preeclampsia and fetal growth restriction: systematic review and meta-analysis. Am J Obstet Gynecol. 2017;216:110–120.e6.
5. Tan MY, Poon LC, Rolnik DL, Syngelaki A, de Paco Matallana C, Akolekar R, et al. Prediction and prevention of small-for-gestational-age neonates: evidence from SPREE and ASPRE. Ultrasound Obstet Gynecol. 2018;52:52–9.
6. Crovetto F, Triunfo S, Crispi F, Rodriguez-Sureda V, Dominguez C, Figueras F, et al. Differential performance of first-trimester screening in predicting small-for-gestational-age neonate or fetal growth restriction. Ultrasound Obstet Gynecol. 2017;49:349–56.
7. Poon LC, Syngelaki A, Akolekar R, Lai J, Nicolaides KH. Combined screening for preeclampsia and small for gestational age at 11–13 weeks. Fetal Diagn Ther. 2013;33:16–27.
8. Crovetto F, Triunfo S, Crispi F, Rodriguez-Sureda V, Roma E, Dominguez C, et al. First-trimester screening with specific algorithms for early- and late-onset fetal growth restriction. Ultrasound Obstet Gynecol. 2016;48:340–8.
9. Poljak B, Agarwal U, Jackson R, Alfirevic Z, Sharp A. Diagnostic accuracy of individual antenatal tools for prediction of small-for-gestational age at birth. Ultrasound Obstet Gynecol. 2017;49:493–9.
10. Papageorghiou AT, Yu CK, Cicero S, Bower S, Nicolaides KH. Second-trimester uterine artery Doppler screening in unselected populations: a review. J Mater Fetal Neonatal Med. 2002;12:78–88.
11. Gómez O, Figueras F, Fernández S, Bennasar M, Martínez JM, Puerto B, et al. Reference ranges for uterine artery mean pulsatility index at 11–41 weeks of gestation. Ultrasound Obstet Gynecol. 2008;32:128–32.
12. Crovetto F, Figueras F, Triunfo S, Crispi F, Rodriguez-Sureda V, Dominguez C, et al. First trimester screening for early and late preeclampsia based on maternal characteristics, biophysical parameters, and angiogenic factors. Prenat Diagn. 2015;35:183–91.
13. Valiño N, Giunta G, Gallo DM, Akolekar R, Nicolaides KH. Biophysical and biochemical markers at 30–34 weeks' gestation in the prediction of adverse perinatal outcome. Ultrasound Obstet Gynecol. 2016;47:194–202.
14. Valiño N, Giunta G, Gallo DM, Akolekar R, Nicolaides KH. Biophysical and biochemical markers at 35–37 weeks' gestation in the prediction of adverse perinatal outcome. Ultrasound Obstet Gynecol. 2016;47:203–9.
15. Benton SJ, McCowan LM, Heazell AE, Grysnpan D, Hutcheon JA, Senger C, et al. Placental growth factor as a marker of fetal growth restriction caused by placental dysfunction. Placenta. 2016;42:1–8.

16. Karagiannis G, Akolekar R, Sarquis R, Wright D, Nicolaides KH. Prediction of small-for-gestation neonates from biophysical and biochemical markers at 11–13 weeks. Fetal Diagn Ther. 2011;29:148–54.
17. Familiari A, Bhide A, Morlando M, Scala C, Khalil A, Thilaganathan B. Mid-pregnancy fetal biometry, uterine artery Doppler indices and maternal demographic characteristics: role in prediction of small-for-gestational-age birth. Acta Obstet Gynecol Scand. 2016;95:238–44.
18. Poon LC, Lesmes C, Gallo DM, Akolekar R, Nicolaides KH. Prediction of small-for-gestational-age neonates: screening by biophysical and biochemical markers at 19–24 weeks. Ultrasound Obstet Gynecol. 2015;46:437–45.
19. Basuki TR, Caradeux J, Eixarch E, Gratacós E, Figueras F. Longitudinal assessment of abdominal circumference versus estimated fetal weight in the detection of late fetal growth restriction. Fetal Diagn Ther. 2018; https://doi.org/10.1159/000485889.
20. Miranda J, Triunfo S, Rodriguez-Lopez M, Sairanen M, Kouru H, Parra-Saavedra M, et al. Performance of third-trimester combined screening model for prediction of adverse perinatal outcome. Ultrasound Obstet Gynecol. 2017;50:353–60.
21. Bakalis S, Peeva G, Gonzalez R, Poon LC, Nicolaides KH. Prediction of small-for-gestational-age neonates: screening by biophysical and biochemical markers at 30–34 weeks. Ultrasound Obstet Gynecol. 2015;46:446–51.
22. Farina A. Systematic review on first trimester three-dimensional placental volumetry predicting small for gestational age infants. Prenat Diagn. 2016;36:135–41.
23. Guiot C, Gaglioti P, Oberto M, Piccoli E, Rosato R, Todros T. Is three-dimensional power Doppler ultrasound useful in the assessment of placental perfusion in normal and growth-restricted pregnancies? Ultrasound Obstet Gynecol. 2008;31:171–6.

Biochemical Assessment of Placental Function

7

Irene Martín-Estal, Miguel Angel Rodriguez-Zambrano, and Inma Castilla-Cortázar

Abbreviations

ADAM12	A disintegrin and metalloprotease 12
AFP	A-fetoprotein
AGEs	Advanced glycation end products
eNOS	Endothelial nitric oxide synthase
FGR	Fetal growth restriction
GDM	Gestational diabetes mellitus
GLUTs	Glucose transporters
GRP78	Glucose-regulated protein 78
HbA	Maternal hemoglobin
HbF	Fetal hemoglobin
hCG	Human chorionic gonadotropin
HIF-1	Hypoxia-inducible factor-1
Hsp70	Heat shock protein 70
IGF-1	Insulin-like growth factor-1
IGF-2	Insulin-like growth factor-2
IGFBPs	Insulin-like binding proteins
IGFs	Insulin-like growth factors

I. Martín-Estal
Tecnologico de Monterrey, Escuela de Medicina y Ciencias de la Salud, Monterrey, NL, Mexico
e-mail: i.mdelestal@itesm.mx

M. A. Rodriguez-Zambrano
Fundacion de Investigacion HM Hospitales, Madrid, Spain

I. Castilla-Cortázar (✉)
Tecnologico de Monterrey, Escuela de Medicina y Ciencias de la Salud, Monterrey, NL, Mexico

Fundacion de Investigacion HM Hospitales, Madrid, Spain

L. M. M. Nardozza et al. (eds.), *Fetal Growth Restriction*,
https://doi.org/10.1007/978-3-030-00051-6_7

LDLs	Low-density lipoproteins
LGA	Large for gestational age
mtDNA	Mitochondrial DNA
NO	Nitric oxide
NPY	Neuropeptide Y
NTDs	Neural tube defects
PAPP-A	Pregnancy-associated plasma protein A
pGF	Placental growth factor
pGH	Placental growth hormone
pL	Placental lactogen
pO_2	Partial pressure of oxygen
PP13	Placental protein 13
PSG1	Glycosylated pregnancy-specific glycoprotein 1
PTH-rP	Parathyroid hormone-related protein
RAAS	Renin-angiotensin-aldosterone system
RFM	Reduced fetal movements
ROS	Reactive oxygen species
sENG	Soluble endoglin
sFLT1/sVEGFR-1	Soluble fms-like tyrosine kinase-1 or soluble VEGF receptor-1
SGA	Small for gestational age
VEGF	Vascular endothelial growth factor
β-hCG	β-Human chorionic gonadotropin

The Placenta: A Key Organ in Fetal Programming

As is well-known, the placenta is an intrauterine organ with central functions in pregnancy, supporting normal growth and development of the fetus [1]. The main placental functions will be discussed in the subsequent sections, including nutrient and oxygen supply to the fetus, as well as hormone and growth factor production and secretion that may affect mother, fetus, or both [2–4]. Changes in placental development, physiology, and function have notable effects on the intrauterine environment, the fetus, and its ability to deal with such environments [1, 4].

The placenta participates in fetal nutrition by providing oxygen, water, carbohydrates, amino acids, lipids, vitamins, minerals, and other nutrients to the fetus, as well as removing carbon dioxide and other waste products. Moreover, this organ metabolizes several molecules to generate metabolic products that will be released into maternal and/or fetal circulations. In addition to metabolic and transport functions, the placenta can operate as a barrier: it can prevent infections, the dispersion of maternal diseases, and fetal transport of certain xenobiotics that could be harmful for fetal development [1]. Additionally, the placenta can produce and secrete several hormones into both maternal and fetal circulations, thus affecting pregnancy outcomes, fetal growth and development, and parturition [1, 4].

Functions of the Human Placenta During Pregnancy

Nutrient Transport and Metabolism

Several decades ago, it was believed that the placenta only functioned as a passive barrier, preventing transfer of maternal metabolites, hormones, proteins, bacteria, viruses, xenobiotics, and drugs to the fetus and the simultaneous transport of essential nutrients [1, 5]. This concept has evolved to provide greater emphasis on other placental functions: proper implantation and placental development is needed to ensure the suitable enlargement of the fetoplacental unit necessary for fetal growth and development. Obviously, placental expansion is a regulated process where several mechanisms take part. It becomes more noticeable in the second and third trimesters of human pregnancy where nutrient uptake and metabolism generate the cellular energy essential for protein synthesis [5].

The primary determinant for fetal growth is the nutrient concentration in the maternal circulation and the blood supply to the placenta. This organ responds to environmental prompts such as maternal stress, energy intake, and dietary composition by adapting its morphological and functional phenotype to optimize fetal development in relation to the availability of existing resources [6–9]. Therefore, the placenta is metabolically active; it can sense nutrient availability and adapt placental metabolism to sustain fetal growth in the different stages of pregnancy, maintaining the maternofetal nutrient transport [10]. This flux is essential to preserve nutrient intraplacental levels, being crucial for cell growth and survival in deprivation conditions [5]. It is important to notice that nutrient transport in early pregnancy is different from that observed at term [1, 11]. This alteration could be due to changes in the expression of transporter proteins as a result of oxygen tension and blood flow to the intervillous space [1, 12]. During the first trimester of pregnancy, nutrition is histotrophic with trophoblast phagocytosis of glycogen and several glycoproteins [1, 12]. After the onset of maternal blood flow to the intervillous space (10–12 weeks), maternal blood is in contact with the terminal villi of the placenta and consequently leads to the transport of respiratory gases, nutrients, and waste products between mother and fetus across the placental membrane. The following is a detailed description of the transport and metabolism of several compounds crucial for the development of pregnancy.

Transport and Metabolism of Respiratory Gases

Nutrient and oxygen supply are the primary determinants for fetal growth and development [13, 14]. Like other cellular membranes, the placental membrane is extremely permeable to respiratory gases, allowing the rapid exchange of oxygen and carbon dioxide from maternal to fetal blood and vice versa (Fig. 7.1) [1, 5, 15, 16]. There are two factors that facilitate the movement of oxygen in the maternofetal direction: (1) a marked difference in pO_2 between maternal and fetal blood, as a result of a high

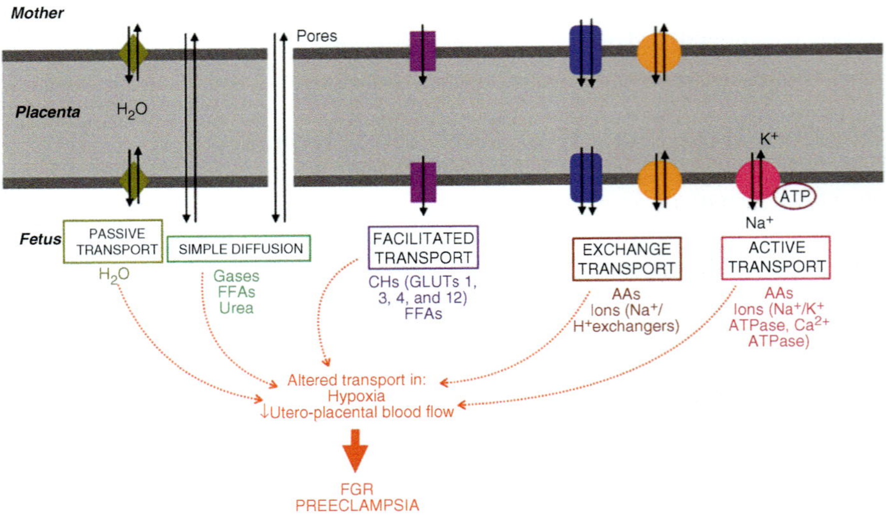

Fig. 7.1 Placental transport of nutrients, ions, and respiratory gases during pregnancy. *AAs*, amino acids; *CHs*, carbohydrates; *FFAs*, fatty acids; *FGR*, fetal growth restriction; *GLUTs*, glucose transporters

oxygen consumption by the placenta itself and/or the mixture of arterial and venous bloods in the intervillous space, causing a significantly lower pO_2 in the umbilical vein (34–41 mmHg) than that observed in maternal arterial blood (100 mmHg); and (2) a higher hemoglobin concentration in fetal blood [1, 13]. Also, fetal hemoglobin (HbF) has a higher affinity for oxygen as compared to maternal hemoglobin (HbA), favoring oxygen transport to the fetus.

Alterations in respiratory gases supply, specially oxygen, could lead to pregnancy complications, such as fetal growth restriction (FGR) and preeclampsia. Both pathologies have direct adverse consequences in the neonate, disturbing its growth and development and also increasing adult morbidity and mortality [17–20]. One of these stated neonatal alterations is hypoxia, a common complication of pregnancy as a result of several exogenous insults, such as smoking, anemia, cord occlusion, and/or poor placental vascularity [9, 21–23]. Hypoxia responses are mediated by HIF-1 (hypoxia-inducible factor-1), and it would be activated in the placenta as a result of the diminution in oxygen supply and the reduced intervillous pO_2 that takes place in FGR and preeclampsia pregnancies [5]. Several adaptations are observed in in vivo experimental models, such as adjustments in placental nutrient transport capacity, helping to maintain fetal growth and development in the abovementioned situations. Studies in human and ovine placentas have revealed that, at high altitude, both types of placentas can increase fetal vascularity and a thinning of the diffusion barrier between maternal and fetal circulations, hence improving oxygen diffusion capacity [23–28]. Likewise, studies in rodents disclosed that in hypoxic conditions, there are several modifications in placental vascularity, barrier thickness, passive diffusion, nutrient transport, and nutrient transporter expression which compromise placental growth and development depending on the severity of the hypoxic insult

[25, 29–42]. All these studies demonstrate that the placenta can sense oxygen signals, possibly through the insulin-IGFs (insulin-like growth factors) pathway. This adaption of phenotype optimizes maternal resource allocation to fetal growth during these abnormal circumstances [9].

Transport and Metabolism of Carbohydrates
Glucose is the primary source of energy for the fetus and the placenta; the majority of fetal glucose comes from maternal carbohydrate metabolism. This demand is highly increased during the third trimester of pregnancy [43]. The maternal circulation is the only supply for fetoplacental glucose, as there is no gluconeogenesis in the fetus and placental gluconeogenesis contributes slightly [1, 5, 10]. Glucose transport across the placenta occurred generally via facilitated diffusion by several glucose transporters (GLUTs), due to the low permeability of syncytiotrophoblast plasma membranes (Fig. 7.1) [43–45]. Five isoforms of these transporters (GLUT1, 3, 4, 8, and 12) have been identified in human and rodent placentas, where they are found embedded asymmetrically in both microvillous (maternal-facing) and basal (fetal-facing) membranes of the syncytiotrophoblast, the main placental barrier

Table 7.1 Characteristics and localization of glucose transporters (GLUTs) in the placenta

Glucose transporter	Localization	Characteristics	References
GLUT1	Syncytiotrophoblast, cytotrophoblast, endothelium, vascular smooth muscle, stromal cells *At term*: microvillous and basal membranes with an asymmetric distribution	Involved in glucose transport across the term placenta	Gude et al. [1]; Baumann et al. [43]; Illsley (2007)
GLUT3	*First trimester*: extravillous trophoblast, cytotrophoblast *At term*: endothelial cells lining the fetal capillaries	Regulation of glucose levels	Baumann et al. [43]; Illsley (2007)
GLUT4	Placental stromal cells	Insulin-responsive glucose transporter Involved in glucose transport and its conversion to glycogen in response to insulin in fetal circulation	Baumann et al. [43]; Xing et al. [47]
GLUT8	Blastocyst	Involved in glucose uptake within the placenta and transport to the fetus	Baumann et al. [43]
GLUT12	*First trimester*: extravillous trophoblast, cytotrophoblast, syncytiotrophoblast *At term*: vascular smooth muscle, stromal cells	Involved in facilitation of glucose transport	Baumann et al. [43]

layer (Table 7.1) [1, 43, 46, 47]. As expected, there are several differences in cellular distribution of these GLUTs between the first trimester of pregnancy and term placentas, suggesting divergences in function in early and late pregnancy [1, 43].

Maternal-fetal glucose transfer is regulated by several factors: (1) glucose supply, determined by both blood glucose concentration and blood flow; (2) placental glucose metabolism; and (3) placental glucose transporter density. Glucose transfer across the placental barrier is a prompt process limited by the movement to and from the transfer site [43]. Alterations in maternal or fetal plasma glucose concentrations will change the maternal-fetal glucose concentration gradient, hence varying glucose transfer. In this way, changes in blood glucose will modify glucose delivery to the fetus, as seen in diabetic hyperglycemia and hypoglycemia, where glucose deprivation can disturb fetal growth [10]. The reduction in uteroplacental blood flow observed in FGR will also alter glucose supply, changing glucose transfer to the fetus [48]. Likewise, the reduction in oxygen delivery under hypoxic conditions will change placental metabolic demand for glucose, producing alterations in maternal transport [49]. For example, *GLUT1* gene transcription is increased in hypoxic conditions [50] in order to try to compensate the high glucose consumption [43]. Also, GLUT1 is positively regulated by IGF-1 (insulin-like growth factor-1), placental growth hormone (pGH), and hypoxia [43].

The placenta has a very high rate of glucose consumption. In the syncytiotrophoblast, glucose can have different destinies: (1) it can be metabolized via glycolysis to obtain energy; (2) it can be converted in placental glycogen (non-triose phosphate pathways); (3) it can be metabolized into pentose phosphate; and (4) it can be transported to fetal circulation [1, 5]. As expected, the aforementioned glucose destinies vary throughout pregnancy. In early pregnancy, almost 75% of glucose is metabolized through the glycolytic pathway, 15% via non-triose phosphate pathways and 10% via the pentose phosphate pathway. At term, the glycolytic pathway reaches 90% and 10% for non-triose phosphate and pentose phosphate pathways [5]. Alterations in these metabolic pathways, such as glycogen depositions, have been observed in diabetic and preeclamptic pregnancies at term, possibly as a response to hyperglycemia, suggesting how important is the metabolic and transport capacity of the placenta itself for suitable fetal growth and development [5]. Placental glucose consumption is reduced during periods of maternal undernutrition, where maternal hypoglycemia induces uteroplacental tissues to use less glucose due to its low availability, hence saving glucose for the fetus [10, 51].

The high rate of placental glucose consumption has led to an increased placental production of lactate; at least 70% of syncytial glucose consumption ends up as lactate in normal pregnancy. This metabolite is also transported to the fetus by the placenta as the lactate transport capacity of the syncytial microvillous membrane is greater than the fetal-facing basal membrane. Under hypoxic conditions, such transport arrangement changes because the fetus becomes a net lactate producer and the placenta removes lactate from the fetus [1, 5, 51, 52]. As stated with glucose metabolism, placental lactate production in sheep decreases under maternal nutrient deprivation making glucose less promptly available for fetal consumption and producing fetal malnutrition [10, 51].

Transport and Metabolism of Amino Acids

Amino acids are required by the fetus for protein synthesis and energy purposes. Fetal amino acids come from maternal amino acid pools, where essential amino acids (obtained from the diet) and others can be synthetized by the placenta from metabolic intermediates, such as glycine and serine [1, 5, 10]. Fetal concentrations of virtually all amino acids are greater than maternal concentrations, suggesting that the placenta dynamically transports amino acids from the maternal compartment to the developing fetus [53–55]. Some of these amino acids taken up by the placenta may return to the maternal circulation rather than being transported to the fetus [56–58]. Consequently, amino acid transport from maternal to fetal circulation occurs by a concentration gradient along with transporters located in the microvillous and basal membranes of the syncytiotrophoblast (Fig. 7.1) [59]. These transporters interact not only with their principal substrates but also with ions (co-substrates) and other amino acids present in the intrauterine environment. Such interactions stimulate or inhibit plasma membrane and trans-syncytial transport [60].

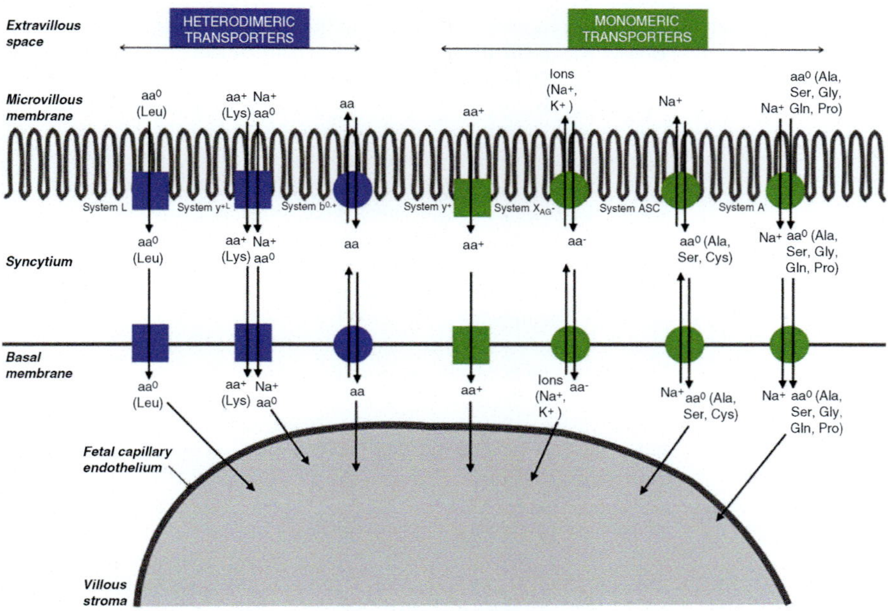

Fig. 7.2 Amino acid transport between mother and fetus during pregnancy. There are two types of amino acid transporters: (1) heterodimeric transporters, such as system L that transports neutral amino acids, system y^+L that uses the inwardly directed Na^+ gradient and neutral amino acids to drive cationic amino acids into the syncytial cells, and system $b^{0,+}$ that uses the outwardly directed gradients of specific amino acids to drive the inward transport of other amino acids with related structures, and (2) monomeric transporters, such as system y^+ that transports cationic amino acids, system X_{AG}^- that uses the ionic gradient for active transport of anionic amino acids (Glu, Asp), system ASC that transports short-chain neutral amino acids (Ala, Ser, Cys), and system A that transports neutral amino acids. Na^+-dependent transporters are represented with squares, and Na^+-independent transporters are represented with circles

These transporters involved in amino acid transport can be classified in heterodimeric and monomeric transporters (Fig. 7.2) [1, 5, 58, 60–67]. Many of them have overlapping specificities; that is why the net flux of specific amino acids will depend on the amino acid concentration at both sides of the membrane through which the transport of these molecules is taking place [5].

In addition to the amino acid transport across the placenta, there are several placental metabolic processes concerning these molecules: amino acid metabolism for energy production (besides there is significant amino acid oxidation in the fetus), amino acid utilization for the synthesis of other constituents (tetrahydrofolate,

Table 7.2 Amino acid metabolic processes in the human placenta

Energy generation		
Amino acid	*Metabolic processes*	*Destination*
Branched-chain amino acids (Leu, Val, Ile)	Transamination in the placenta to branched-chain keto acids and decarboxylation to produce acyl-CoA derivatives	Tricarboxylic acid cycle
Biosynthesis		
Amino acid	*Metabolic processes*	*What is it for?*
Ser	Conversion to Gly in the carbon cycle where THF is converted to methylene-THF	Supplies methyl groups for folate cofactors necessary for nucleotide synthesis and homocysteine remethylation to Met
Ser	Synthesis of phosphatidylserine (major membrane component)	
Gly	Produced in the placenta as the primary source for transfer to the fetus via the action of the enzyme serine hydroxymethyltransferase	
Pro	Synthesis of polyamines (spermidine, spermine)	
Arg	Essential for placental generation of NO	
Ala	Production from Glu and pyruvate to provide a source of Ala to be transferred to the fetus	
Ser	Cofactor in transsulfuration pathways responsible for the interconversion of Met, homocysteine, and Cys	
Amino acid shuttling		
Amino acid	*Metabolic processes*	*Destination*
Glu	Taken up from the placenta from both maternal and fetal circulations and conversion to Gln	Released into the fetal circulation
Gln	Conversion to Glu by the fetal liver	Released into the fetal circulation and shuttle back to the placenta
Ser	Taken up from the placenta from both maternal and fetal circulations and conversion to Gly	Released into the fetal circulation
Gly	Conversion to Ser by the fetal liver	
Protein synthesis and degradation (catabolism)		
Protein synthesis	Under hypoxic conditions, it is supported by glycolytic generation of energy. It is higher in term placentas	
Protein catabolism	It may not be a significant process	
FGR	Diminution in protein synthesis due to substrate restriction	
	Increase in protein catabolism in order to provide substrates for oxidative metabolism	

FGR fetal growth restriction, *NO* nitric oxide, *THF* tetrahydrofolate

phosphatidylserine, nitric oxide), conversion as a part of the placental-fetal shuttle system, and protein synthesis in the syncytiotrophoblast supported by both oxidative and anaerobic metabolism [5] (Table 7.2).

Alterations in maternal and/or fetal amino acid circulating levels would change their transport characteristics, leading to modifications in the efflux of amino acids into the fetal circulation and the alteration of placental amino acid metabolism, thus manipulating the availability of substrates for metabolism. All of these variations lead to insufficient amino acid fetal supply. Consequently, fetal growth and development would be compromised, resulting in several pregnancy pathologies such as FGR.

Transport and Metabolism of Lipids

Numerous lipids (including free fatty acids, essential fatty acids obtained from diet – linoleic and linolenic acids – triacylglycerols, phospholipids, glycolipids, sphingolipids, cholesterol, cholesterol esters, fat-soluble vitamins, etc.) are bound to transport proteins in plasma; e.g., free fatty acids bind to serum albumin, while phospholipids, cholesterol, and triacylglycerols bind different proteins to form several types of lipoprotein complexes. Hence, the maternal surface of the placenta expresses lipoprotein lipase, an enzyme that can release free fatty acids and glycerol from the maternal circulating lipoprotein complexes. Both lipophilic molecules can cross the placental syncytiotrophoblast membranes via simple diffusion and membrane-bound, cytosolic fatty acid-binding proteins [1, 10, 68]. Long-chain polyunsaturated fatty acids are preferably transported by the placenta, enriching fetal blood in such molecules, compared to maternal blood [69]. In addition to the placental role in fatty acid transport, the placenta can synthetize substantial concentrations of fatty acids, this process being less active in term human placentas than their oxidation [10].

As soon as fatty acids reach the cytoplasm of the placental trophoblast, they can undergo three pathways: (1) they can bind to cytosolic binding proteins, (2) they can be transported out of the trophoblast, and/or (3) they can be oxidized or esterified [1, 70]. Placental microsomes contain enzymes necessary for the synthesis of glycolipids from glycerol-3-phosphate, free fatty acids, and other precursors. Also, the placenta can synthetize cholesterol. However, under normal circumstances cholesterol is derived from maternal circulating LDLs (low-density lipoproteins). Essential fatty acid consumption is an essential process, as is seen in low birth weight neonates where low intake of essential fatty acids corresponds with the observed low birth weight at term [10]. FGR placentas usually show a deficiency in oxidative enzymes, bringing about an excess in lipid peroxidation and reactive oxygen species (ROS) formation, both processes injurious to maternal endothelial cells [10].

Transport of Water, Inorganic Ions, Minerals, and Vitamins

In addition to the aforementioned transported molecules, water transport across the placenta is also important and depends on hydrostatic and osmotic pressures. Water moves passively throughout the placenta across a water channel-forming integral protein expressed in the trophoblast (Fig. 7.1) [71]. Ions, such as potassium, magnesium, calcium, and phosphate, are transported through the placenta actively, whereas sodium and chloride are transported passively [71]. In consequence, there are several active ion-transporting systems in the placenta, e.g., Na^+/K^+ ATPase, Ca^{2+} ATPase, and Na^+/H^+ exchangers, among others [72]. As a result of this placental transport, sodium and chloride levels in fetal and maternal blood are similar, unlike potassium, calcium, and phosphate levels, which are higher in fetal blood [73]. Conversely, vitamins and minerals are transferred from the maternal to the fetal circulation. For example, iron dissociates from transferrin at the placental interface and is transported through the placenta [1].

All of these transport systems are crucial for appropriate placental and fetal development. The malfunction of one of these transport systems or a combination of several of them would be detrimental to placental and fetal growth and development, leading to the occurrence of several pregnancy disorders, such as FGR.

Endocrine Functions of the Placenta

The placenta is a neuroendocrine organ that produces several hormones to manage the communication between mother and fetus. Such hormones have endocrine, paracrine, and/or autocrine purposes. The placenta releases these hormones into both maternal and fetal circulations, and their synthesis and secretion are responsive to environmental changes. A dysregulated placental hormone secretion is associated with FGR, among other abnormalities [1, 74].

Most placental hormones are synthetized and secreted from cytotrophoblast, syncytiotrophoblast, or both throughout pregnancy. Hofbauer cells (villous stromal cells and macrophages) are also a source of hormones and growth factors [74]. These placental hormones include protein hormones, e.g., chorionic gonadotropin, IGFs, placental lactogen, placental growth hormone, and glucocorticoids, and steroid hormones, e.g., estrogen and progesterone (Table 7.3) [2, 4, 75–101]. For example, placental lactogen and progesterone affect maternal metabolism to support glucose delivery to the fetus [102]; IGF-1 modulates growth, cell division, and differentiation [103]; IGF-2 (insulin-like growth factor-2) modulates trophoblast development at the feto-maternal interface [103]; and glucocorticoids regulate organ development and maturation [104].

Analysis of altered maternal serum levels of placental hormones is helpful for risk assessment in prenatal diagnosis; their measurement is less harmful than amniocentesis for predicting pregnancy abnormalities such as aneuploidy, FGR, preterm birth, and placental abnormalities. In the first trimester of pregnancy, several maternal serum parameters have been analyzed to determine the risk for aneuploidy, preeclampsia, FGR, trisomies 21 and 18, and fetal demise. These parameters include hCG (human chorionic gonadotropin), PAPP-A (pregnancy-associated plasma protein A), a disintegrin and metalloprotease 12 (ADAM12), and placental protein 13 (PP-13) [74, 105]. During the second trimester of pregnancy, altered maternal serum levels in parameters such as hCG (human chorionic gonadotropin), inhibin A, and unconjugated estriol are suitable for risk assessment of trisomies 21 and 18, anencephaly, steroid sulfatase deficiency, and Smith-Lemli-Opitz syndrome [74, 105].

Table 7.3 Placental hormones

Hormone	Site of production in placenta	Production during normal pregnancy	Functions
Activin	Syncytiotrophoblast and cytotrophoblast	At term, labor	Stimulates FSH, prostaglandins, and oxytocin secretion Modulates cytotrophoblast proliferation and differentiation
CRH (corticotropin-releasing hormone)	Syncytiotrophoblast, amnion, musculature of umbilical vessels, maternal decidua	Late pregnancy	Stimulates ACTH and DHEA-S secretion Promotes labor and initiation of parturition Vasodilation of placental vessels Accelerates pulmonary maturation Promotes myometrium contractility
Eicosanoids	Chorionic membranes and the decidua	Late pregnancy	Controls blood flow in the placenta
Estrogens (estrone, estradiol, and estriol)	Placenta?	From 6 to 8 weeks	Influences uterine blood flow Progesterone production and steroid metabolism Prepares breasts for lactation Initiation of labor
GHRH (growth hormone releasing hormone)	?	?	Stimulates fetal pituitary Regulates fetal and placental growth
hCG (human chorionic gonadotropin)	Trophectoderm and syncytiotrophoblast	Preimplantation embryo and from 1 to 12 weeks with a rise late in pregnancy	Stimulates corpus luteum to produce progesterone Increases fetal testosterone production, affecting male sexual development Prolongs the corpus luteum life in early pregnancy Vasodilation and smooth muscle relaxation
hPGH (human placental growth hormone)	Syncytiotrophoblast	From 13 to 28 weeks	Somatogenic, lactogenic, and lipolytic functions Regulates IGF-1 levels Increases the availability of glucose and amino acids for the fetus
hPL (human placental lactogen)	Syncytiotrophoblast	Early in pregnancy (from 13 to 28 weeks)	Stimulates maternal food intake and maternal weight gain *Fetus*: increases insulin, IGFs, adrenocortical hormones, and pulmonary surfactant levels Modulates embryonic development Involved in angiogenesis Participates in calcium absorption and breast development Increases the availability of glucose and amino acids for the fetus

(continued)

Table 7.3 (continued)

Hormone	Site of production in placenta	Production during normal pregnancy	Functions
IGF-1	Syncytiotrophoblast	During pregnancy	Stimulates placental growth Involved in steroidogenesis Glucose and amino acid uptake Fetal and placental growth, differentiation, and development Its concentrations correlate with fetal body weight
IGF-2	Trophoblast	From 1 to 10 weeks	Stimulates placental growth Participates in embryonic development Modulates trophoblast development at the feto-maternal interface Key role in placental growth
Inhibin A	Syncytiotrophoblast and cytotrophoblast	Increases during pregnancy	Inhibits FSH release Controls steroidogenesis, peptide hormone, and prostaglandin secretion
Leptin	Syncytiotrophoblast and cytotrophoblast	From 1 to 40 weeks	Regulates maternal food intake Inhibits insulin secretion In the fetus, mediates insulin's anabolic actions
NPY (neuropeptide Y)	Cytotrophoblast	Early pregnancy until term, decreases after delivery	Regulates placental and uterine blood flow Stimulates CRH from placental cells Contributes to uterine contractility
Oxytocin	Uterus	Increases throughout pregnancy	Myometrium contractions
PAPP-A (pregnancy-associated plasma protein A)	Syncytiotrophoblast and maternal decidua	Increases throughout pregnancy	It is an IGFBP-4 proteinase: increases IGF bioavailability
Progesterone	Syncytiotrophoblast	From 6 to 8 weeks, increases during pregnancy and labor	Maintenance of uterine quiescence Prime breasts for lactation Stimulates weight gain and fat deposition Inhibits uterine contraction Increases the availability of glucose for the fetus
Prolactin	Trophoblast	At term	Influences successful implantation Stimulates maternal hyperphagia Regulates fetal growth and development
PTH-rP (parathyroid hormone-related protein)	Syncytiotrophoblast, trophoblast, and cytotrophoblast	Decrease during pregnancy	Promotes maternal gastrointestinal absorption of calcium Increases insulin production in pregnancy Primes the breast for lactation

Table 7.3 (continued)

Hormone	Site of production in placenta	Production during normal pregnancy	Functions
Relaxin	Endometrium and decidua	?	Softens the symphysis pubis during pregnancy Reduces collagen synthesis in the cervix Increases water, protein, collagen, and glycogen levels in the uterus Promotes angiogenesis
Renin	Trophoblasts and decidua	Increases during pregnancy (after the 6th week)	Regulates maternal blood pressure and uteroplacental blood flow
VEGF (vascular endothelial growth factor)	Decidua and trophoblast villi	Increases during pregnancy; important during first trimester	Initiates vasculogenesis Stimulates angiogenesis Modulates trophoblast survival and function

All these analyses support the idea that a suitable and worldwide placental profile measurement of several placental hormones will be useful in the early diagnoses of common pregnancy disorders.

Protective Functions of the Placenta

In addition to the aforementioned functions, the placenta has a role in protecting the fetus from small xenobiotics that could circulate in maternal blood, due to their simple diffusion across the placenta via transcellular or paracellular routes and/or their transport by one or more placental transport systems [1]. To exert such protective function, the placenta exhibits several features that could reduce placental transport of toxic substances: export pumps in the maternal-facing membrane of the syncytiotrophoblast and cytochrome P450 enzymes that can metabolize drugs and other xenobiotics (alcohol, thalidomide, anticonvulsants, lithium, warfarin, and isotretinoin) which, if not degraded, can cross the placenta and have damaging effects on the fetus [1, 106, 107].

To strengthen the protective functions of the placenta, several proteins, including maternal antibodies, are transported throughout the placenta by pinocytosis. Such transport is responsible for providing passive immunity to the neonate [1, 108]. Also, the placenta forms an obstacle against bacterial, protozoal, and viral infection from mother to fetus, infections that could be detrimental and related to poor pregnancy outcomes [109].

Regulation of Maternal and Fetal Blood Supplies to the Placenta

One of the crucial roles of the placenta is to provide a physiological communication mechanism between mother and fetus, which serves as an exchange system for numerous substances (nutrients, oxygen, hormones, water, and waste products) between both units. All of these substances are necessary for proper fetal and placental growth and development [110]. For this reason, an appropriate placental circulation is necessary for a successful pregnancy [111–113].

Uterine and umbilical blood flows, which are responsible for the circulation to the maternal and fetal portions of the placenta, respectively, increase exponentially during pregnancy, facilitated by the decrease in umbilical blood resistance throughout the third trimester of pregnancy in humans [110, 113, 114]. In addition to changes in the placental circulation, an increase in the rate of substance extraction from uterine or umbilical blood permits an augmented oxygen, glucose, and water transport necessary for increased fetal growth [110, 113, 115]. All these observations suggest that increased placental blood flow is the key mechanism of transplacental exchange during gestation.

A suitable blood flow to the placenta could be decisive for normal fetal growth, as observed in normal pregnancies where there is an increase of specific transporters and a rise in the maternofetal concentration gradient of several metabolites. In pregnancies compromised nutritionally or by environmental heat stress, a reduced placental mass and blood flow leads to FGR [113, 116–118]. In conclusion, angiogenesis is responsible for the increase in placental blood flow throughout pregnancy [113, 119–121].

It has been observed in several animal models that diminished uterine and/or umbilical blood flows lead to reduced fetal growth due to the decrease in nutrient transport between mother and fetus. These results suggest that alterations in fetal growth are associated with altered placental development and may be due to an altered expression of angiogenic factors, which results in fetal hypoxia [113, 121, 122]. Several of these altered angiogenic factors, such as vascular endothelial growth factor (VEGF) and endothelial nitric oxide synthase (eNOS), can be modified due to a distorted placental blood flow. It should be noted that eNOS produces nitric oxide (NO), a key regulator of angiogenesis and vasodilatation [111, 123, 124]. This molecule regulates normal blood flow to the uterus and contributes to low fetoplacental vascular resistance during pregnancy. In several models of compromised pregnancy in humans and sheep (e.g., FGR conditions and multiple fetuses), eNOS placental expression is reduced, whereas circulating NO and its metabolites are elevated, suggesting that impaired NO synthesis could provide the explanation of the development of FGR during pregnancy [125–133]. This suggests that restoration of placental blood flow and proper placental vascularity could provide an optimal therapeutic target in compromised pregnancies. Placental expression and production of angiogenic and vasoactive factors could be powerful indicators of pathologies associated with FGR.

Placental Biomarkers: Their Usefulness in the Diagnosis of Pregnancy Disorders

During pregnancy, there is an increase in the labor of almost every maternal organ along with the concurrence of several physiological changes in order to develop an appropriate environment for fetal and placental growth and development [134–136]. However, these physiological changes and the inability of an organ system to meet the increased physiological requirements, which increase throughout pregnancy, could enhance the risk of developing several disorders, impairing fetal development and resulting in acute and/or chronic diseases during adult life [134]. Truthfully, pregnancy is the supreme physiological "stress assessment" that a woman can experience in her life.

Most pregnancy syndromes develop in the third trimester of pregnancy, and most could be due to the dysfunctional regulation of trophoblast invasion and placental development in early pregnancy [134, 137]. Until now, expected traditional risk factors and maternal history are not enough to predict complications during pregnancy, such as preeclampsia, FGR, gestational diabetes, hypertension, preterm birth, and thyroid, liver, and kidney diseases [134, 138–140]. There are numerous factors that raise the risk for development of pregnancy complications (e.g., advanced maternal age, undernutrition, maternal obesity, poor cardiovascular or metabolic health, maternal parity, and pregnancy history) [141, 142]. It is important to state that, unexpectedly, numerous women may develop pregnancy difficulties without any known risk factors. For this reason, the detection and analysis of placental biomarkers, which are released by the placenta into the maternal circulation, could be useful in the diagnosis and prediction of the incidence and severity of the aforementioned diseases and might contribute to the development of numerous therapies to prevent maternal and fetal consequences related to pregnancy disorders [134, 143, 144].

To date, even though several placental biomarkers have been associated with pregnancy complications, no biomarker has been effectively used in clinical practice to diagnose and predict such diseases. Table 7.4 shows the existing placental biomarkers that are measured during gestation and related to several pregnancy disorders [145–161].

Abnormal Placental Biomarker Expression in the Development of Pregnancy Diseases

There are several placental biomarkers whose altered levels are related to a particular pregnancy disorder (Tables 7.4 and 7.5). One of the most common syndromes during pregnancy that has several complications in fetal and adult life is FGR. This is an important obstetric condition defined as the inability to achieve the expected weight or size for gestational age [162, 163]. FGR has a multifactorial etiology, and its incidence embraces approximately 5–10% of newborns worldwide, the frequency being greater in underdeveloped and South American countries [4]. This pregnancy disorder is the second greatest cause of perinatal mortality and morbidity

Table 7.4 Placental biomarkers and their implication in pregnancy disorders

Placental biomarker	Pregnancy disorder	Levels in pregnancy disorder	Characteristics of the placental biomarker
Placental hormones and proteins			
Activin A	Preeclampsia, FGR, and gestational hypertension	Increased	Produced by the decidua, placenta, and fetal membranes; regulates menstrual cycle and enhances FSH biosynthesis. It is a biomarker for the diagnose of trophoblast dysfunction
A disintegrin and metalloprotease 12 (ADAM12)	Preeclampsia, SGA, and FGR	Reduced	Synthetized by trophoblasts, involved in growth and differentiation; screened for Down syndrome
	LGA	Increased	
A-fetoprotein (AFP)	Open spina bifida, preeclampsia, and FGR	Increased	Produced by the fetal liver and gastrointestinal tract; important in the maintenance of uteroplacental blood flow
Angiotensin I	Preeclampsia	Reduced	Components of the renin-angiotensin-aldosterone system (RAAS) that acts as a mediator of fluid homeostasis
Angiotensin II	Preeclampsia	Reduced	
	GDM	Increased	
Angiotensin I–VII (the smaller angiotensin fragment)	GDM and preterm birth	Reduced	
	Preeclampsia	Increased	
Autoantibodies against angiotensin II type 1 receptor	Preeclampsia and FGR	Increased	
C-type natriuretic peptide	Hypertension, preeclampsia, placental disorders, SGA, LGA, and GDM	Unchanged	Role in maintaining fetal-maternal homeostasis
Corticotropin-releasing hormone (CRH)	Preterm birth, preeclampsia, and FGR	Increased	Regulates parturition
Folic acid	Preeclampsia, spontaneous abortion, placental abruption, and FGR	Reduced	Important in the proper development of spinal cord and placenta; prevents defects at birth
Glycosylated pregnancy-specific glycoprotein 1 (PSG1)	GDM	Increased	Produced by the syncytiotrophoblast, role in the establishment of the vasculature at the maternal-fetal interface
Homocysteine	Preeclampsia, spontaneous abortion, placental abruption, and FGR	Increased	Correlated with the occurrence of blood clots; related to placental vascular diseases
β-Human chorionic gonadotropin (β-hCG)	Preeclampsia and preterm birth	Increased	Secreted by the trophoblast; important in the implantation and maintenance of the blastocyst and corpus luteum at the beginning of pregnancy. Marker for Down syndrome in pregnancies
	FGR	Reduced	

Table 7.4 (continued)

Placental biomarker	Pregnancy disorder	Levels in pregnancy disorder	Characteristics of the placental biomarker
IGF-1	Acromegaly	Increased	Regulator of placental and fetal development. In FGR increases arterial resistance
	Preeclampsia and FGR	Reduced	
IGF-2	Preeclampsia	Unchanged	Important in the stimulation of placental growth
	FGR	Reduced	
IGFBP-1	Preeclampsia	Increased	Important in differentiation, proliferation, and decidualization of the endometrium, as well as in trophoblast invasion, implantation, and fetal growth
IGFBP-3	Preeclampsia, gestational hypertension, and FGR	Reduced	Major carrier protein for IGF-1 and IGF-2
Inhibin A	Miscarriage	Reduced	Modulates the secretion of other placental hormones and maintains the ovarian quiescence throughout pregnancy; biomarker for placental function produced by the decidua, placenta, and fetal membranes. It is a hormonal marker of placental oxidative stress
	Preeclampsia, FGR, and gestational hypertension	Increased	
Leptin	FGR	Reduced	Produced by the trophoblast during late pregnancy; role in implantation, placental endocrine function, and conceptus and fetal development
	Type 1 diabetes, preeclampsia, and GDM	Increased	
Placental growth factor (pGF)	Preeclampsia, SGA, and FGR	Reduced	Biomarker of syncytial stress and placental dysfunction
Placental lactogen	GDM and FGR	Reduced	Role in β-cell expansion that occurs during pregnancy, biomarker of placental dysfunction. Its levels correlate with RFM
Placental protein 13 (PP13)	Preeclampsia and FGR	Reduced	Modulator of immune function, expressed by the syncytiotrophoblast
Placental vascular endothelial growth factor (VEGF)	Preeclampsia and FGR	Increased	Involved in angiogenesis and vasculogenesis; important in proliferation, migration, and metabolic activity of the trophoblasts. It is expressed in the syncytiotrophoblast and invasive chorionic trophoblast
Pregnancy-associated plasma protein A (PPAP-A)	Preeclampsia, FGR, infant death, preterm birth, and SGA	Reduced	Important during villous differentiation and trophoblastic invasion of the decidua, produced by trophoblasts; biomarker for placental dysfunction, commonly screened for Down syndrome

(continued)

Table 7.4 (continued)

Placental biomarker	Pregnancy disorder	Levels in pregnancy disorder	Characteristics of the placental biomarker
Progesterone	FGR	Reduced	Important role in implantation, pregnancy, menstrual cycle, and embryogenesis. Its levels correlate with RFM
Prorenin	Preeclampsia	Increased	Components of the renin-angiotensin-aldosterone system (RAAS) that acts as a mediator of fluid homeostasis
Prorenin receptor	Preeclampsia	Increased	
Soluble endoglin (sENG)	Preeclampsia, SGA, and preterm delivery	Increased	Biomarker of syncytial stress
Soluble fms-like tyrosine kinase-1 (sFLT1) or soluble VEGF receptor-1 (sVEGFR-1)	Preeclampsia, SGA, FGR, and late miscarriage	Increased	Biomarker of syncytial stress; it is an indicator of placental disease
Placental stress markers			
Advanced glycation end products (AGEs)	GDM	Increased	Oxidative stress products
Glucose-regulated protein 78 (GRP78)	GDM and preeclampsia	Low GRP78 C-terminal/ full length	Tissue marker of endoplasmic reticulum stress, expressed by cytotrophoblasts in the placenta
Heat shock protein 70 (Hsp70)	Preeclampsia and preterm birth	Increased	Marker of cellular stress, systemic inflammation, and hepatocellular injury
Oxidized DNA (8-hydroxydeoxy-guanosine)	GDM and FGR	Increased	Oxidized nucleoside of DNA, detected in urine, biomarker for DNA lesion, oxidative stress, and a risk factor for cancer, atherosclerosis, and diabetes
Protein carbonyls	Preeclampsia, GDM, FGR, and preterm birth	Increased	Biomarker of oxidative stress
Placental debris and extracellular vesicles			
Mitochondrial DNA (mtDNA)	Preeclampsia and FGR	Increased	Indicates mitochondrial dysfunction, leading to placental anomalies
Placenta-derived exosomes	Preeclampsia and GDM	Increased	Indicate placental metabolic state and function; these bodies include proteins, RNAs, and DNA. Preeclampsia is associated with increased DNA-positive and altered lipid composition microvesicles

RFM reduced fetal movements, *FGR* fetal growth restriction, *GDM* gestational diabetes mellitus, *SGA* small for gestational age, *LGA* large for gestational age

Table 7.5 Altered levels of placental biomarkers in fetal growth restriction, preeclampsia, and other important pregnancy disorders

		FGR		Preeclampsia		Other pregnancy disorders
Placental biomarker levels	Reduced levels	Placental lactogen Progesterone PP13 Leptin pGF PAPP-A Estriol	ADAM12 Folic acid IGF-1 IGF-2 IGFBP-3 β-hCG hCG GH	PP13 pGF Angiotensin I and II Angiotensin I–VII PPAP-A	ADAM12 Folic acid IGF-1 IGFBP-3 GRP78	*GDM:* Placental lactogen, angiotensin I-VII, GRP78 *Preterm birth:* Angiotensin 1-7, PPAP-A *Down Syndrome:* PPAP-A, AFP, pGF *Late miscarriage:* Inhibin A *Placental abruption and spontaneous abortion:* Folic acid *Infant death:* PPAP-A *SGA:* pGF, PPAP-A, ADAM12 *Gestational hypertension:* IGFBP-3
	Increased levels	CRH sFLT1/sVEGFR-1 VEGF Autoantibodies against angiotensin II type I receptor Inhibin A Activin A Homocysteine	AFP IGFBP-1 Protein carbonyls Oxidized DNA mtDNA	Leptin CRH IGFBP-1 sFLT1/sVEGFR-1 VEGF sENG Autoantibodies against angiotensin II type I receptor Prorenin Prorenin receptor Inhibin A Homocysteine	AFP Activin A β-hCG hCG Protein carbonyls Hsp70 Placenta-derived exosomes mtDNA	*GDM:* Leptin, angiotensin II, oxidized DNA, AGEs, placenta-derived exosomes *Placental abruption and spontaneous abortion:* Homocysteine *Preterm birth:* sENG, protein carbonyls, Hsp70, CRH, β-hCG, activin A, estriol *Down syndrome:* hCG, β-hCG, inhibin A *Late miscarriage:* sFLT1/sVEGFR-1 *SGA:* sENG, sFLT1/sVEGFR-1 *LGA:* ADAM12 *Gestational hypertension:* Inhibin A, activin A *Type 1 diabetes:* Leptin *Acromegaly:* IGF-1 *Open spina bifida:* AFP
	Unchanged levels			IGF-2 C-type natriuretic peptide		C-type natriuretic peptide Hypertension, preeclampsia, placental disorders, SGA, LGA, GDM

FGR fetal growth restriction, *GDM* gestational diabetes mellitus, *SGA* small for gestational age, *LGA* large for gestational age

[164]. FGR newborns could experience several clinical complications (hypoglycemia, neonatal asphyxia, hypothermia, ventricular hemorrhage, polycythemia, etc.) that can result in pathological conditions during early life, thus affecting height, weight, and neurological development [165, 166]. Consequently, FGR newborns might have medical problems during adult life, such as cardiovascular disease, insulin resistance, diabetes, hypertension, and obesity [166, 167].

In FGR pregnancies, several anatomical abnormalities in the placenta have been observed, such as inadequate trophoblastic invasion, abnormal insertion of the umbilical cord, and placental thrombosis, among others. These abnormalities produce an atypical distribution of amino acid transporters and an aberrant endocrine function, leading to an abnormal expression of placental biomarkers [4]. In accordance with the literature, reduced or increased levels of several hormones important in implantation and placental and fetal growth and development have been found. For example, it has been observed in FGR a decrease in placental lactogen, leptin, placental growth factor (pGF), IGF-1, IGF-2, and IGFBP-3 (insulin-like growth factor-binding protein-3), suggesting an abnormal placental development and implantation of the embryo. These aberrations result in anatomical placental alterations that could restrict nutrient and oxygen exchange between mother and fetus, hence producing a hypoxic intrauterine environment that compromises blood supply, growth, and development of the fetus. Augmented concentrations of placental VEGF, inhibin A, and activin A have been observed in FGR pregnancies, suggesting that the hyper-expression of hormones involved in placental growth and development is also harmful and leads to placental defects that affect fetal development.

Another common pregnancy disorder is preeclampsia. As with FGR, preeclampsia is a heterogeneous syndrome that impinges on multiple organs, hence progressing to maternal multiorgan failure, coagulopathy, and maternal and fetal death in its acute form [168, 169]. For this reason, preeclampsia is a complicated pathology to be diagnosed or treated. Even though its incidence is unknown, it has been estimated that this disorder affects approximately 2–8% of all pregnancies worldwide [170]. The physiopathology of preeclampsia is not completely understood, but it includes an atypical placentation (trophoblast invasion and impairment of the maternal-fetal interface) and an intensified vascular reactivity that result in endothelial damage, as observed several weeks or months prior to the clinical recognition of the disease [169, 171, 172].

It has been shown that numerous placental biomarkers affecting the progression of pregnancy and fetal growth and development are altered throughout gestation in preeclampsia. Decreased levels of placental protein 13 (PP13), pGF, angiotensin I and II, angiotensin I–VII, pregnancy-associated plasma protein 12 (PAPP-A), and a disintegrin and metalloprotease 12 (ADAM12) are observed. All of these hormones are related to placental growth and development, and decreased levels indicate placental dysfunction that could compromise fetal blood flow and further development. Analogous to FGR, increased levels of soluble fms-like tyrosine kinase-1 or soluble VEGF receptor-1 (sFLT1/sVEGFR-1), VEGF, soluble endoglin (sENG), inhibin A, activin A, A-fetoprotein (AFP), and β-human chorionic gonadotropin (β-hCG) are found in pregnant women with preeclampsia. All of them are implicated in placental growth and development, the progression of implantation, and blastocyst maintenance during pregnancy. As a result, altered levels of these placental biomarkers may produce a distorted fetal blood flow with the consequences that are found in this disease state. Several studies previously disclosed that IGFs and their binding proteins (IGFBPs) may play a key role in paracrine functions at the maternal-fetal interface throughout pregnancy [173, 174]. Reduced levels of IGF-1 and IGFBP-3 and increased levels of IGFBP-1 are crucial for proper fetal development and placental progression (appropriate differentiation, proliferation, decidualization of the endometrium, trophoblast invasion, and implantation), respectively, all indispensable for the suitable advance of pregnancy [159, 161, 175].

In conclusion, these placental biomarkers could be effective in the detection and analysis of pregnancy disorders and, also, may be used as markers for worsening severity. Nevertheless, the observed biomarker levels in pregnancy disorders such as FGR and preeclampsia could be confused with chronic medical diseases (e.g., chronic hypertension, collagen vascular diseases, renal diseases, etc.) where altered concentrations determine exacerbations of such chronic disorders. Therefore, it is important to avoid the confusion between pregnancy disorders and chronic diseases that might be present in the mother even long before the onset of gestation, preventing inadequate treatments and their future consequences.

Biochemical Placental Function Profile as a Proposal for the Diagnosis of Pregnancy Disorders

Prenatal screening is a reputable part of antenatal care in developed countries. It allows the detection of abnormalities in the fetus before birth. This routine arose due to the amount of information acquired over the last few years about hormone and cytokine production by intrauterine tissues (placenta, amnion, chorion, and decidua), thus playing an important role in maternal-fetal physiological interactions, the reprogramming of maternal endocrine system, and the signaling mechanisms that determine parturition [176]. It is known that in several pregnancy disorders, there is a disproportionate release of various placental hormones, being a placental and fetal adaptive response to hostile intrauterine environmental conditions, e.g., hypertension, hypoxia, infections, and/or placental and fetal malformations. For this reason, placental hormones have been investigated as biochemical markers of pregnancy disorders, because there are quite a lot of experimental assays that can detect high levels of these hormones in maternal serum, umbilical cord blood, and amniotic fluid. The frequent disorders being screened include fetal neural tube defects (NTDs), chromosomal and structural abnormalities, and maternal conditions such as preeclampsia [177]. A screening test can be based on a single marker or a combination of several markers, the latter being most recommended for use due to the validity of the results obtained (<7% of false-positive results observed in pregnant women) [178].

Standard Biochemical Components Measured in Maternal Serum
Ordinarily, between 15 and 21 weeks of gestation, a maternal serum sample is screened for four different hormones: AFP, estriol, hCG, and inhibin A. AFP was the primary protein marker to be screened and is associated with fetal aberrations: increased AFP levels in maternal serum are associated with open NTDs, spina bifida, and anencephaly, whereas reduced AFP levels are associated with Down syndrome. Conversely, estriol, hCG, and inhibin A are markers used in the diagnosis of chromosome and pregnancy abnormalities, such as Down syndrome, preeclampsia, FGR, and preterm birth. Table 7.5 shows the principal placental biomarkers evaluated in the diagnosis of the aforementioned pregnancy disorders. As it can be noticed, several placental biomarkers have the same altered levels in the studied pregnancy disorders (Down syndrome, preeclampsia, FGR, and preterm birth), suggesting that the evaluation of more than one biomarker could be more useful to diagnose and prevent such diseases. Otherwise, there are some placental biomarkers, such as hCG, β-hCG, pGF, and estriol, among others, that have different altered levels in the abovementioned diseases, suggesting that these biomarkers are not specific enough for the diagnosis of these pregnancy disorders. Conclusively, the diagnosis and prevention of conventional screened disorders throughout pregnancy would be more functional and advantageous if an analysis of a set of placental biomarkers is used [176].

For example, in Down syndrome, the screening of AFP levels along with maternal age, at a fixed 5% false-positive rate, has an average detection rate of 28% of pregnancies. If in this screening the measurement of more placental biomarkers is combined, the results are better: the determination of hCG plus unconjugated estriol and inhibin A levels shows an average detection rate of 60% and 70% of pregnancies with Down syndrome, respectively [177, 179]. These data suggest that the association of maternal age with different serum protein levels would be suitable for the screening of this disorder throughout pregnancy (Table 7.6). Furthermore, an expanded Down syndrome screening protocol may lead to the early identification of preeclampsia, another pregnancy disorder [180].

In preeclampsia the screening of several placental biomarker levels (PAPP-A and pGF) along with maternal characteristics, uterine artery Doppler pulsatility index, and mean arterial pressure can detect approximately 90% of early-onset preeclampsia pregnancies in the first trimester (Table 7.6) [176, 180].

However, not all placental biomarkers are powerful indexes of placental function, e.g., maternal serum progesterone and 5α-dihydroprogesterone levels are useless index markers of the abnormal placental function developed in preeclampsia [176, 180]. Similarly, maternal leptin levels do not predict fetal birth weight as this placental biomarker is ineffective for the antenatal detection of FGR [176, 180]).

Table 7.6 Placental biochemical biomarkers related to pregnancy disorders

Pregnancy disorder	Placental biomarker and other measurements	Altered levels	Trimester of pregnancy where the biomarker is altered	Observations
Down syndrome	hCG	Increased	Second trimester	
	Free subunit β-hCG	Increased	First trimester	
	PAPP-A	Reduced	–	Provides the highest detection rate for Down syndrome at early screening
	Inhibin A	Increased	Second trimester	
	Ultrasound nuchal translucency (NT)	–	–	
	AFP	Reduced	Second trimester	In the mid-1980s, AFP was shown to be a Down syndrome marker, only used in young women. Both markers have high risk to justify amniocentesis, an invasive test to observe the presence of Down syndrome
	Maternal age (>35 years)	–	–	
	pGF	Reduced	First trimester	
	Dehydroepiandrosterone sulfate (DHEA-S)	Reduced	–	DHEA-S levels are reduced in maternal serum, placental tissue, and fetal liver. This suggest that the reduction of estriol levels is linked to the reduced fetal DHEA-S synthesis
Fetal growth restriction (FGR)	PAPP-A	Reduced	First trimester	
	AFP	Increased	Third trimester	
	hCG	Reduced	Second trimester	It is important to notice that during the third trimester, there is an increase in hCG levels together with pathological umbilical artery flow cytometry
	Unconjugated estriol	Reduced	Second trimester	
	Inhibin A	Increased	Third trimester	
	Free subunit β-hCG	Reduced	First trimester	It is associated with poor pregnancy outcome and IUGR
	Estriol	Reduced	Third trimester	Reduced maternal serum and urinary estriol and placental lactogen levels are tools for the monitoring of fetal welfare and fetal growth
	Placental lactogen	Reduced	Third trimester	
	GH	Reduced	Second trimester	GH levels are reduced in maternal serum and placental tissues
	IGF-1	Reduced	Third trimester	IGF-1 levels are reduced in maternal serum
	IGFBP-1	Increased	Second trimester	
Neural tube defects (NTDs)	AFP	Increased	Second trimester	Marker screened for anencephaly and spina bifida

(continued)

Table 7.6 (continued)

Pregnancy disorder	Placental biomarker and other measurements	Altered levels	Trimester of pregnancy where the biomarker is altered	Observations
Preeclampsia	PAPP-A	Reduced	First trimester	It is more associated with preeclampsia
	pGF	Reduced	First trimester	
	Mean arterial pressure (MAP)	–	First trimester	
	Uterine artery Doppler	–	First trimester	
	Free subunit β-hCG	Increased	First trimester	
	hCG	Increased	Second and third trimesters	
	Activin A	Increased	First trimester	Marker screened in hypertensive disorders and preeclampsia
	Inhibin A	Increased	First trimester	Marker screened in hypertensive disorders and preeclampsia. It is a more accurate marker than hCG and other routine markers in predicting preeclampsia
	Angiotensin I and II	Reduced	Third trimester	In hypertensive disorders, there is a diminution of vasoactive system and an augmented response to the pressor effect of angiotensin II
	Active renin	Reduced	Third trimester	
	Aldosterone	Reduced	Third trimester	
	Activity of angiotensin-converting enzyme	Reduced	Third trimester	
	N-terminal peptide of pro-ANP (atrial natriuretic peptide)	Increased	Third trimester	
	Endothelin-1 mRNA and immunoreactive proteins	Increased	–	
	Allopregnanolone	Increased	–	Promising marker for preeclampsia
	CRH	Increased	Second trimester	CRH levels are increased in maternal serum, umbilical cord plasma, and venous cord blood. During pregnancy, it is observed the secretion of CRH from the placenta into fetal circulation
	Leptin	Increased	Third trimester	
Preterm birth	Short cervix	–	–	Detects approximately 1/3 of the preterm births
	PAPP-A	Reduced	First trimester	
	Plasma granulocyte colony-stimulating factor levels	Increased	Third trimester	
	CRH	Increased	Third trimester	
	Angiogenin	Increased	Second trimester	Angiogenin levels are increased in amniotic fluid. It is a potential prognostic marker of preterm labor
	Activin A	Increased	–	Activin A levels are increased in maternal serum
	Estriol	Increased	Second and third trimesters	
	Free subunit β-hCG	Increased	Second trimester	

The Next Step: Proposal of a Profile of Placental Specific Components to Be Used for the Diagnosis of Pregnancy Disorders

In order to maximize the performance of routine serum tests during pregnancy, it would be beneficial to include in this analysis the study of various placental biomarker levels that can be related to the most common diseases found during pregnancy (FGR, preeclampsia, gestational diabetes mellitus, and Down syndrome), avoiding in this way invasive techniques. For example, the inclusion of leptin and β-hCG serum levels could discern the possible occurrence of FGR or preeclampsia during the first and second trimesters of pregnancy, and their levels change in opposite directions in these diseases. Moreover, IGF-1, IGF-2, IGFBP-3, pGF, placental lactogen (pL), and leptin serum levels can detect abnormal placental development and implantation of the embryo that could lead to nutrient and oxygen restriction between mother and fetus, resulting in a hypoxic intrauterine environment which would compromise fetal perfusion. Likewise, circulating levels of sFLT1/sVEGFR-1, VEGF, inhibin A, activin A, AFP, and β-hCG can identify placental defects that alter fetal development. It should be noticed that almost all placental biomarkers are important during the first trimester of pregnancy, where most fetal development takes place and where the fetus is more susceptible to external and/or internal risk factor exposure. For this reason, the first trimester of pregnancy is the period of maximum care for pregnant women. In this fashion, the measurement of the abovementioned placental biomarker serum levels plus hematological and endocrine parameters, maternal history, and ultrasound tests during gestation could provide significant information about the presence or absence of numerous pregnancy disorders, such as FGR, preeclampsia, gestational diabetes mellitus, and Down syndrome, thus avoiding invasive techniques (Table 7.7).

A novel biomarker that is becoming important during pregnancy in recent years is IGF-1 circulating levels. This hormone is an unusual placental biomarker to be evaluated in gestational serum tests, mainly due to its cost. So, why is IGF-1 getting this relevance? This anabolic hormone is secreted throughout pregnancy and is produced mainly by the placenta, but also there is a limited production by the mother and the fetus. For instance, an alteration in its production and/or secretion by any of the three gestation entities (placenta, mother, or fetus) could lead to the development of FGR, a disease characterized by placental IGF-1 deficiency that compromises fetal perfusion, resulting in a hypoxic intrauterine environment that enhances oxidative stress and produces an abnormal fetal growth and development (Table 7.7).

In conclusion, although anatomical and physiological consequences of pregnancy disorders do not manifest themselves until the third trimester, it is important to discern their existence from the first trimester, in order to initiate the treatment to prevent their fetal consequences. For this reason, the analysis of placental biomarker serum levels is an important tool that could allow the clinicians to rule out or suggest the presence of a particular pregnancy disease. Almost all biomarkers are secreted by the placenta; hence placental anomalies during gestation (e.g., unusual trophoblast invasion, spiral artery disorganization, etc.) could produce an excess or decrease in the expression of certain biomarkers, indicating in this way the importance of such analysis.

Table 7.7 Proposal of a profile of several placental biomarker levels screened during first trimester of pregnancy for common pregnancy disorders

Screened placental biomarker	Abnormality detected	Pregnancy disorder	In combination with…
Activin A	Placental defects	Preeclampsia, FGR, gestational hypertension	Measurement of hematological and endocrine parameters Maternal history Ultrasound tests (nuchal translucency, chromosomal abnormalities)
A-fetoprotein (AFP)		Open spina bifida, preeclampsia, FGR	
Inhibin A		Preeclampsia, FGR, gestational hypertension, miscarriage	
Soluble fms-like tyrosine kinase-1/soluble VEGF receptor-1 (sFLT1/sVEGFR-1)		Preeclampsia, SGA, FGR, late miscarriage	
Placental vascular endothelial growth factor (VEGF)		Preeclampsia, FGR	
β-Human chorionic gonadotropin (β-hCG)		Preeclampsia, preterm birth, infant death	
IGF-1	Abnormal placental development and implantation of the embryo, leading to hypoxic conditions	Acromegaly, preeclampsia, FGR	
IGF-2		Preeclampsia, FGR	
IGFBP-3		Preeclampsia, gestational hypertension, FGR	
Leptin		FGR, Type 1 diabetes, preeclampsia, GDM	
Pregnancy-associated plasma protein A (PAPP-A)		Preeclampsia, FGR, preterm birth, SGA, infant death	
Placental growth factor (pGF)		Preeclampsia, SGA, FGR	
Placental lactogen (pL)		GDM, FGR	

FGR fetal growth restriction, *GDM* gestational diabetes mellitus, *SGA* small for gestational age

In future years, it will be necessary to establish a worldwide clinical profile of these biomarker levels in order to analyze and detect pregnancy disorders. Until now, different clinicians only study some placental biomarkers, based on the suspicion of a particular disease, avoiding the analysis of other placental biomarkers of potentially greater importance. Consequently, it is crucial to unify the placental biomarker levels of scrutiny, because a complete analysis of such biomarkers in early pregnancy could allow the clinicians to identify and start the appropriate treatment or, at least, minimize and/or prevent pregnancy complications related to risk factors.

References

1. Gude NM, Roberts CT, Kalionis B, King RG. Growth and function of the normal human placenta. Thromb Res. 2004;114:397–407.
2. Hiden U, Glitzner E, Hartmann M, Desoye G. Insulin and the IGF system in the human placenta of normal and diabetic pregnancies. J Anat. 2009;215:60–8.
3. Murphy VE, Smith R, Giles WB, Clifton VL. Endocrine regulation of human fetal growth: the role of the mother, placenta, and fetus. Endocr Rev. 2006;27:141–69.
4. Martín-Estal I, de la Garza RG, Castilla-Cortázar I. Intrauterine growth retardation (IUGR) as a novel condition of insulin-like growth factor-1 (IGF-1) deficiency. Rev Physiol Biochem Pharmacol. 2016;170:1–35.
5. Illsley NP. Placental metabolism. In: Kay HH, Nelson DM, Wang Y, editors. Placenta. 1st ed. Oxford: Wiley-Blackwell; 2011. p. 50–6.
6. Fowden AL, Sferruzzi-Perri AN, Coan PM, Constancia M, Burton GJ. Placental efficiency and adaptation: endocrine regulation. J Physiol. 2009;587:3459–72.
7. Vaughan OR, Sferruzzi-Perri AN, Coan PM, Fowden AL. Environmental regulation of placental phenotype: implications for fetal growth. Reprod Fertil Dev. 2011;24:80–96.
8. Sferruzzi-Perri AN, Vaughan OR, Forhead AJ, Fowden AL. Hormonal and nutritional drivers of intrauterine growth. Curr Opin Clin Nutr Metab Care. 2013;16:298–309.
9. Higgins JS, Vaughan OR, Fernandez de Liger E, Fowden AL, Sferruzzi-Perri AN. Placental phenotype and resource allocation to fetal growth are modified by the timing and degree of hypoxia during mouse pregnancy. J Physiol. 2016;594:1341–56.
10. Belkacemi L, Nelson DM, Desai M, Ross MG. Maternal undernutrition and fetal programming: role of the placenta. In: Placenta. Oxford: Wiley-Blackwell; 2011. p. 1–9.
11. Glazier JD, Jansson T. Placental transport in early pregnancy – a workshop report. Placenta. 2004;25(Suppl A):S57–9.
12. Burton GJ, Watson AL, Hempstock J, Skepper JN, Jauniaux E. Uterine glands provide histiotrophic nutrition for the human fetus during the first trimester of pregnancy. J Clin Endocrinol Metab. 2002;87:2954–9.
13. Glazier JD, Harrington B, Sibley CP, Turner M. Placental function in maternofetal exchange. In: Rodeck CH, Whittle M, editors. Fetal medicine: basic science and clinical practice. London: Churchill Livingstone; 1999. p. 111–26.
14. Burton GJ, Fowden AL. The placenta: a multifaceted, transient organ. Philos Trans R Soc Lond Ser B Biol Sci. 2015;370:20140066.
15. Carter AM. Placental oxygen consumption. Part I: in vivo studies – a review. Placenta. 2000;21(Suppl A):S31–7.
16. Schneider H. Placental oxygen consumption. Part II: in vitro studies – a review. Placenta. 2000;21(Suppl A):S38–44.
17. McMillen IC, Robinson JS. Developmental origins of the metabolic syndrome: prediction, plasticity, and programming. Physiol Rev. 2005;85:571–633.
18. Myatt L. Placental adaptive responses and fetal programming. J Physiol. 2006;572:25–30.
19. Giussani DA, Davidge ST. Developmental programming of cardiovascular disease by prenatal hypoxia. J Dev Orig Health Dis. 2013;4:328–37.
20. Zhang S, Regnault TR, Barker PL, Botting KJ, McMillen IC, McMillan CM, et al. Placental adaptations in growth restriction. Nutrients. 2015;7:360–89.
21. Hutter D, Kingdom J, Jaeggi E. Causes and mechanisms of intrauterine hypoxia and its impact on the fetal cardiovascular system: a review. Int J Pediatr. 2010;2010:401323.
22. Zamudio S. The placenta at high altitude. High Alt Med Biol. 2003;4:171–91.
23. Tissot van Patot M, Grilli A, Chapman P, Broad E, Tyson W, Heller DS, et al. Remodelling of uteroplacental arteries is decreased in high altitude placentae. Placenta. 2003;24:326–35.
24. Ali KZ, Burton GJ, Morad N, Ali ME. Does hypercapillarization influence the branching pattern of terminal villi in the human placenta at high altitude? Placenta. 1996;17:677–82.
25. Krebs C, Macara LM, Leiser R, Bowman AW, Greer IA, Kingdom JC. Intrauterine growth restriction with absent end-diastolic flow velocity in the umbilical artery is associated with maldevelopment of the placental terminal villous tree. Am J Obstet Gynecol. 1996;175:1534–42.

26. Mayhew TM. Thinning of the intervascular tissue layers of the human placenta is an adaptive response to passive diffusion in vivo and may help to predict the origins of fetal hypoxia. Eur J Obstet Gynecol Reprod Biol. 1998;81:101–9.
27. Tissot van Patot MC, Murray AJ, Beckey V, Cindrova-Davies T, Johns J, Zwerdlinger L, et al. Human placental metabolic adaptation to chronic hypoxia, high altitude: hypoxic preconditioning. Am J Physiol Regul Integr Comp Physiol. 2010;298:R166–R72.
28. Parraguez VH, Atlagich M, Díaz R, Cepeda R, González C, De los Reyes M, et al. Ovine placenta at high altitudes: comparison of animals with different times of adaptation to hypoxic environment. Anim Reprod Sci. 2006;95:151–7.
29. Jansson N, Pettersson J, Haafiz A, Ericsson A, Palmberg I, Tranberg M, et al. Down-regulation of placental transport of amino acids precedes the development of intrauterine growth restriction in rats fed a low protein diet. J Physiol. 2006;576:935–46.
30. Jones HN, Woollett LA, Barbour N, Prasad PD, Powell TL, Jansson T. High-fat diet before and during pregnancy causes marked up-regulation of placental nutrient transport and fetal overgrowth in C57/BL6 mice. FASEB J. 2009;23:271–8.
31. Coan PM, Vaughan OR, Sekita Y, Finn SL, Burton GJ, Constancia M, et al. Adaptations in placental phenotype support fetal growth during undernutrition of pregnant mice. J Physiol. 2010;588:527–38.
32. Rosario FJ, Jansson N, Kanai Y, Prasad PD, Powell TL, Jansson T. Maternal protein restriction in the rat inhibits placental insulin, mTOR, and STAT3 signaling and down-regulates placental amino acid transporters. Endocrinology. 2011;152:1119–29.
33. Sferruzzi-Perri AN, Vaughan OR, Coan PM, Suciu MC, Darbyshire R, Constancia M, et al. Placental-specific Igf2 deficiency alters developmental adaptations to undernutrition in mice. Endocrinology. 2011;152:3202–12.
34. Sferruzzi-Perri AN, Vaughan OR, Haro M, Cooper WN, Musial B, Charalambous M, et al. An obesogenic diet during mouse pregnancy modifies maternal nutrient partitioning and the fetal growth trajectory. FASEB J. 2013;27:3928–37.
35. Bacon BJ, Gilbert RD, Kaufmann P, Smith AD, Trevino FT, Longo LD. Placental anatomy and diffusing capacity in guinea pigs following long-term maternal hypoxia. Placenta. 1984;5:475–87.
36. Gheorghe CP, Mohan S, Oberg KC, Longo LD. Gene expression patterns in the hypoxic murine placenta: a role in epigenesis? Reprod Sci. 2007;14:223–33.
37. Hvizdošová-Klesčová A, Uhlík J, Malina M, Vulterinová H, Novotný T, Vajner L. Remodeling of fetoplacental arteries in rats due to chronic hypoxia. Exp Toxicol Pathol. 2013;65:97–103.
38. Zhou J, Xiao D, Hu Y, Wang Z, Paradis A, Mata-Greenwood E, et al. Gestational hypoxia induces preeclampsia-like symptoms via heightened endothelin-1 signaling in pregnant rats. Hypertension. 2013;62:599–607.
39. Cuffe JS, Walton SL, Singh RR, Spiers JG, Bielefeldt-Ohmann H, Wilkinson L, et al. Mid- to late term hypoxia in the mouse alters placental morphology, glucocorticoid regulatory pathways and nutrient transporters in a sex-specific manner. J Physiol. 2014;592:3127–41.
40. Jacobs R, Robinson JS, Owens JA, Falconer J, Webster ME. The effect of prolonged hypobaric hypoxia on growth of fetal sheep. J Dev Physiol. 1988;10:97–112.
41. Penninga L, Longo LD. Ovine placentome morphology: effect of high altitude, long-term hypoxia. Placenta. 1998;19:187–93.
42. Parraguez VC, Atlagich M, Díaz R, Bruzzone ME, Behn C, Raggi LA. Effect of hypobaric hypoxia on lamb intrauterine growth: comparison between high- and low-altitude native ewes. Reprod Fertil Dev. 2005;17:497–505.
43. Baumann MU, Deborde S, Illsley NP. Placental glucose transfer and fetal growth. Endocrine. 2002;19:13–22.
44. Illsley NP, Hall S, Penfold P, Stacey TE. Diffusional permeability of the human placenta. Contrib Gynecol Obstet. 1985;13:92–7.
45. Jansson T, Powell TL, Illsley NP. Non-electrolyte solute permeabilities of human placental microvillous and basal membranes. J Physiol. 1993;468:261–74.
46. Illsley NP. Glucose transporters in the human placenta. Placenta. 2000;21:14–22.

47. Xing AY, Challier JC, Lepercq J, Caüzac M, Charron MJ, Girard J, et al. Unexpected expression of glucose transporter 4 in villous stromal cells of human placenta. J Clin Endocrinol Metab. 1998;83:4097–101.
48. Illsley N, Hall S, Stacey T. The modulation of glucose transfer across the human placenta by intervillous flow rates: an in vitro perfusion study. Troph Res. 1987;2:535–44.
49. Johnson LW, Smith CH. Monosaccharide transport across microvillous membrane of human placenta. Am J Phys. 1980;238:C160–8.
50. Semenza GL. Expression of hypoxia-inducible factor 1: mechanisms and consequences. Biochem Pharmacol. 2000;59:47–53.
51. Hay WW. Regulation of placental metabolism by glucose supply. Reprod Fertil Dev. 1995;7:365–75.
52. Piquard F, Schaefer A, Dellenbach P, Haberey P. Lactate movements in the term human placenta in situ. Biol Neonate. 1990;58:61–8.
53. Yudilevich DL, Sweiry JH. Transport of amino acids in the placenta. Biochim Biophys Acta. 1985;822:169–201.
54. Cetin I, de Santis MS, Taricco E, Radaelli T, Teng C, Ronzoni S, et al. Maternal and fetal amino acid concentrations in normal pregnancies and in pregnancies with gestational diabetes mellitus. Am J Obstet Gynecol. 2005;192:610–7.
55. Philipps AF, Holzman IR, Teng C, Battaglia FC. Tissue concentrations of free amino acids in term human placentas. Am J Obstet Gynecol. 1978;131:881–7.
56. Cetin I, Fennessey PV, Sparks JW, Meschia G, Battaglia FC. Fetal serine fluxes across fetal liver, hindlimb, and placenta in late gestation. Am J Phys. 1992;263:E786–93.
57. Lewis RM, Glazier J, Greenwood SL, Bennett EJ, Godfrey KM, Jackson AA, et al. L-serine uptake by human placental microvillous membrane vesicles. Placenta. 2007;28:445–52.
58. Cleal JK, Lewis RM. The mechanisms and regulation of placental amino acid transport to the human foetus. J Neuroendocrinol. 2008;20:419–26.
59. Cetin I. Amino acid interconversions in the fetal-placental unit: the animal model and human studies in vivo. Pediatr Res. 2001;49:148–54.
60. Cariappa R, Heath-Monnig E, Smith CH. Isoforms of amino acid transporters in placental syncytiotrophoblast: plasma membrane localization and potential role in maternal/fetal transport. Placenta. 2003;24:713–26.
61. Battaglia FC, Regnault TR. Placental transport and metabolism of amino acids. Placenta. 2001;22:145–61.
62. Jansson T. Amino acid transporters in the human placenta. Pediatr Res. 2001;49:141–7.
63. Kudo Y, Boyd CA. Human placental amino acid transporter genes: expression and function. Reproduction. 2002;124:593–600.
64. Regnault TRH, de Vrijer B, Battaglia FC. Transport and metabolism of amino acids in placenta. Endocrine. 2002;19:23–41.
65. Chillarón J, Roca R, Valencia A, Zorzano A, Palacín M. Heteromeric amino acid transporters: biochemistry, genetics, and physiology. Am J Physiol Renal Physiol. 2001;281:F995–F1018.
66. Wagner CA, Lang F, Bröer S. Function and structure of heterodimeric amino acid transporters. Am J Physiol Cell Physiol. 2001;281:C1077–93.
67. Palacín M, Estévez R, Bertran J, Zorzano A. Molecular biology of mammalian plasma membrane amino acid transporters. Physiol Rev. 1998;78:969–1054.
68. Haggarty P. Placental regulation of fatty acid delivery and its effect on fetal growth – a review. Placenta. 2002;23(Suppl A):S28–38.
69. Dutta-Roy AK. Transport mechanisms for long-chain polyunsaturated fatty acids in the human placenta. Am J Clin Nutr. 2000;71:315S–22S.
70. Coleman RA, Haynes EB. Synthesis and release of fatty acids by human trophoblast cells in culture. J Lipid Res. 1987;28:1335–41.
71. Stulc J. Placental transfer of inorganic ions and water. Physiol Rev. 1997;77:805–36.
72. Sibley CP, Glazier JD, Greenwood SL, Lacey H, Mynett K, Speake P, et al. Regulation of placental transfer: the Na(+)/H(+) exchanger – a review. Placenta. 2002;23(Suppl A):S39–46.
73. Shennan DB, Boyd CA. Ion transport by the placenta: a review of membrane transport systems. Biochim Biophys Acta. 1987;906:437–57.

74. McNamara JM, Kay HH. Placental hormones: physiology, disease, and prenatal diagnosis. Placenta. Wiley-Blackwell: Oxford; 2011. p. 57–65.
75. Rabinovici J, Goldsmith PC, Librach CL, Jaffe RB. Localization and regulation of the activin-A dimer in human placental cells. J Clin Endocrinol Metab. 1992;75:571–6.
76. Petraglia F. Inhibin, activin and follistatin in the human placenta – a new family of regulatory proteins. Placenta. 1997;18:3–8.
77. Florio P, Luisi S, Ciarmela P, Severi FM, Bocchi C, Petraglia F. Inhibins and activins in pregnancy. Mol Cell Endocrinol. 2004;180:93–100.
78. Grammatopoulos DK. Placental corticotrophin-releasing hormone and its receptors in human pregnancy and labour: still a scientific enigma. J Neuroendocrinol. 2008;20:433–8.
79. Karteris E, Grammatopoulos DK, Randeva HS, Hillhouse EW. The role of corticotropin-releasing hormone receptors in placenta and fetal membranes during human pregnancy. Mol Genet Metab. 2001;72:287–96.
80. Florio P, Severi FM, Ciarmela P, Fiore G, Calonaci G, Merola A, et al. Placental stress factors and maternal-fetal adaptive response: the corticotropin-releasing factor family. Endocrine. 2002;19:91–102.
81. Muyan M, Boime I. Secretion of chorionic gonadotropin from human trophoblasts. Placenta. 1997;18:237–41.
82. Kurtzman JT, Wilson H, Rao CV. A proposed role for hCG in clinical obstetrics. Semin Reprod Med. 2001;19:63–8.
83. Lacroix MC, Guibourdenche J, Frendo JL, Muller F, Evain-Brion D. Human placental growth hormone – a review. Placenta. 2002;23(Suppl A):S87–94.
84. Freemark M. Regulation of maternal metabolism by pituitary and placental hormones: roles in fetal development and metabolic programming. Horm Res. 2006;65(Supp 6):41–9.
85. Handwerger S, Freemark M. The roles of placental growth hormone and placental lactogen in the regulation of human fetal growth and development. J Pediatr Endocrinol Metab. 2000;13:343–56.
86. Riley SC, Leask R, Balfour C, Brennand JE, Groome NP. Production of inhibin forms by the fetal membranes, decidua, placenta and fetus at parturition. Hum Reprod. 2000;15:578–83.
87. Reis FM, Florio P, Cobellis L, Luisi S, Severi FM, Bocchi C, et al. Human placenta as a source of neuroendocrine factors. Biol Neonate. 2001;79:150–6.
88. Ashworth CJ, Hoggard N, Thomas L, Mercer JG, Wallace JM, Lea RG. Placental leptin. Rev Reprod. 2000;5:18–24.
89. Petraglia F, Calza L, Giardino L, Sutton S, Marrama P, Rivier J, et al. Identification of immunoreactive neuropeptide-γ in human placenta: localization, secretion, and binding sites. Endocrinology. 1989;124:2016–22.
90. Kaludjerovic J, Ward WE. The interplay between estrogen and fetal adrenal cortex. J Nutr Metab. 2012;2012:837901.
91. Albrecht ED, Pepe GJ. Estrogen regulation of placental angiogenesis and fetal ovarian development during primate pregnancy. Int J Dev Biol. 2010;54:397–407.
92. Kallen CB. Steroid hormone synthesis in pregnancy. Obstet Gynecol Clin N Am. 2004;31:795–816.
93. Shanker YG, Rao AJ. Progesterone receptor expression in the human placenta. Mol Hum Reprod. 1999;5:481–6.
94. Iliodromiti Z, Antonakopoulos N, Sifakis S, Tsikouras P, Daniilidis A, Dafopoulos K, et al. Endocrine, paracrine, and autocrine placental mediators in labor. Hormones. 2012;11:397–409.
95. Grill S, Rusterholz C, Zanetti-Dällenbach R, Tercanli S, Holzgreve W, Hahn S, et al. Potential markers of preeclampsia – a review. Reprod Biol Endocrinol. 2009;7:70.
96. Malassiné A, Cronier L. Hormones and human trophoblast differentiation: a review. Endocrine. 2002;19:3–11.
97. Corbacho AM, Martínez De La Escalera G, Clapp C. Roles of prolactin and related members of the prolactin/growth hormone/placental lactogen family in angiogenesis. J Endocrinol. 2002;173:219–38.

98. Gude NM, King RG, Brennecke SP. Autacoid interactions in the regulation of blood flow in the human placenta. Clin Exp Pharmacol Physiol. 1998;25:706–11.
99. Fialova L, Malbohan IM. Pregnancy-associated plasma protein A (PAPP-A): theoretical and clinical aspects. Bratisl Lek Listy. 2002;103:194–205.
100. Lawrence JB, Oxvig C, Overgaard MT, Sottrup-Jensen L, Gleich GJ, Hays LG, et al. The insulin-like growth factor (IGF)-dependent IGF binding protein-4 protease secreted by human fibroblasts is pregnancy-associated plasma protein-A. Proc Natl Acad Sci U S A. 1999;96:3149–53.
101. Sun IYC, Overgaard MT, Oxvig C, Giudice LC. Pregnancy-associated plasma protein A proteolytic activity is associated with the human placental trophoblast cell membrane. J Clin Endocrinol Metab. 2002;87:5235–40.
102. Fowden AL, Forhead AJ. Endocrine mechanisms of intrauterine programming. Reproduction. 2004;127:515–26.
103. Fowden AL. The insulin-like growth factors and feto-placental growth. Placenta. 2003;24:803–12.
104. Fowden AL, Li J, Forhead AJ. Glucocorticoids and the preparation for life after birth: are there long-term consequences of the life insurance? Proc Nutr Soc. 1998;57:113–22.
105. Gagnon A, Wilson RD, Audibert F, Allen VM, Blight C, Brock JA, et al. Obstetrical complications associated with abnormal maternal serum markers analytes. J Obstet Gynaecol Can. 2008;30:918–49.
106. Marin JJ, Macias RI, Serrano MA. The hepatobiliary-like excretory function of the placenta. A review. Placenta. 2003;24:431–8.
107. Pasanen M. The expression and regulation of drug metabolism in human placenta. Adv Drug Deliv Rev. 1999;38:81–97.
108. Moffett A, Loke YW. The immunological paradox of pregnancy: a reappraisal. Placenta. 2004;25:1–8.
109. Arechavaleta-Velasco F, Koi H, Strauss JF 3rd, Parry S. Viral infection of the trophoblast: time to take a serious look at its role in abnormal implantation and placentation? J Reprod Immunol. 2002;55:113–21.
110. Reynolds LP, Redmer DA. Utero-placental vascular development and placental function. J Anim Sci. 1995;73:1839–51.
111. Reynolds LP, Borowicz PP, Vonnahme KA, Johnson ML, Grazul-Bilska AT, Redmer DA, et al. Placental angiogenesis in sheep models of compromised pregnancy. J Physiol. 2005;565:43–58.
112. Reynolds LP, Borowicz PP, Vonnahme KA, Johnson ML, Grazul-Bilska AT, Wallace JM, et al. Animal models of placental angiogenesis. Placenta. 2005;26:689–708.
113. Reynolds LP, Caton JS, Redmer DA, Grazul-Bilska AT, Vonnahme KA, Borowicz PP, et al. Evidence for altered placental blood flow and vascularity in compromised pregnancies. J Physiol. 2006;572:51–8.
114. Konje JC, Howarth ES, Kaufmann P, Taylor DJ. Longitudinal quantification of uterine artery blood volume flow changes during gestation in pregnancies complicated by intrauterine growth restriction. BJOG. 2003;110:301–5.
115. Molina RD, Meschia G, Battaglia FC, Hay WW. Gestational maturation of placental glucose transfer capacity in sheep. Am J Phys. 1991;261:R697–704.
116. Thureen PJ, Trembler KA, Meschia G, Makowski EL, Wilkening RB. Placental glucose transport in heat-induced fetal growth retardation. Am J Phys. 1992;263:R578–85.
117. Wallace JM, Bourke DA, Aitken RP, Leitch N, Hay WW. Blood flows and nutrient uptakes in growth-restricted pregnancies induced by overnourishing adolescent sheep. Am J Physiol Regul Integr Comp Physiol. 2002;282:R1027–36.
118. Wallace JM, Regnault TR, Limesand SW, Hay WW, Anthony RV. Investigating the causes of low birth weight in contrasting ovine paradigms. J Physiol. 2005;565:19–26.
119. Charnock-Jones DS, Kaufmann P, Mayhew TM. Aspects of human fetoplacental vasculogenesis and angiogenesis. I. Molecular regulation. Placenta. 2004;25:103–13.

120. Kaufmann P, Mayhew TM, Charnock-Jones DS. Aspects of human fetoplacental vasculogenesis and angiogenesis. II. Changes during normal pregnancy. Placenta. 2004;25:114–26.
121. Mayhew TM, Charnock-Jones DS, Kaufmann P. Aspects of human fetoplacental vasculogenesis and angiogenesis. III. Changes in complicated pregnancies. Placenta. 2004;25:127–39.
122. Huppertz B, Peeters LL. Vascular biology in implantation and placentation. Angiogenesis. 2005;8:157–67.
123. Reynolds LP, Redmer DA. Angiogenesis in the placenta. Biol Reprod. 2001;64:1033–40.
124. Redmer DA, Aitken RP, Milne JS, Reynolds LP, Wallace JM. Influence of maternal nutrition on messenger RNA expression of placental angiogenic factors and their receptors at midgestation in adolescent sheep. Biol Reprod. 2005;72:1004–9.
125. Magness RR, Sullivan JA, Li Y, Phernetton TM, Bird IM. Endothelial vasodilator production by uterine and systemic arteries. VI. Ovarian and pregnancy effects on eNOS and NO(x). Am J Physiol Heart Circ Physiol. 2001;280:H1692–8.
126. Itoh H, Bird IM, Nakao K, Magness RR. Pregnancy increases soluble and particulate guanylate cyclases and decreases the clearance receptor of natriuretic peptides in ovine uterine, but not systemic, arteries. Endocrinology. 1998;139:3329–41.
127. Vagnoni KE, Shaw CE, Phernetton TM, Meglin BM, Bird IM, Magness RR. Endothelial vasodilator production by uterine and systemic arteries. III. Ovarian and estrogen effects on NO synthase. Am J Phys. 1998;275:H1845–56.
128. Zheng J, Li Y, Weiss AR, Bird IM, Magness RR. Expression of endothelial and inducible nitric oxide synthases and nitric oxide production in ovine placental and uterine tissues during late pregnancy. Placenta. 2000;21:516–24.
129. Joyce JM, Phernetton TM, Shaw CE, Modrick ML, Magness RR. Endothelial vasodilator production by uterine and systemic arteries. IX. eNOS gradients in cycling and pregnant ewes. Am J Physiol Heart Circ Physiol. 2002;282:H342–8.
130. Vonnahme KA, Wilson ME, Li Y, Rupnow HL, Phernetton TM, Ford SP, et al. Circulating levels of nitric oxide and vascular endothelial growth factor throughout ovine pregnancy. J Physiol. 2005;565:101–9.
131. Bird IM, Zhang L, Magness RR. Possible mechanisms underlying pregnancy-induced changes in uterine artery endothelial function. Am J Physiol Regul Integr Comp Physiol. 2003;284:R245–58.
132. Maul H, Longo M, Saade GR, Garfield RE. Nitric oxide and its role during pregnancy: from ovulation to delivery. Curr Pharm Des. 2003;9:359–80.
133. Wu G, Bazer FW, Cudd TA, Meininger CJ, Spencer TE. Maternal nutrition and fetal development. J Nutr. 2004;134:2169–72.
134. Williams D. Pregnancy: a stress test for life. Curr Opin Obstet Gynecol. 2003;15:465–71.
135. Torgersen KL, Curran CA. A systematic approach to the physiologic adaptations of pregnancy. Crit Care Nurs Q. 2006;29:2–19.
136. Weissgerber TL, Wolfe LA. Physiological adaptation in early human pregnancy: adaptation to balance maternal-fetal demands. Appl Physiol Nutr Metab. 2006;31:1–11.
137. Norwitz ER. Defective implantation and placentation: laying the blueprint for pregnancy complications. Reprod Biomed Online. 2006;13:591–9.
138. Joshi D, James A, Quaglia A, Westbrook RH, Heneghan MA. Liver disease in pregnancy. Lancet. 2010;375:594–605.
139. Steegers EAP, von Dadelszen P, Duvekot JJ, Pijnenborg R. Pre-eclampsia. Lancet. 2010;376:631–44.
140. Acharya A, Santos J, Linde B, Anis K. Acute kidney injury in pregnancy-current status. Adv Chronic Kidney Dis. 2013;20:215–22.
141. Villar J, Carroli G, Wojdyla D, Abalos E, Giordano D, Ba'aqeel H, et al. Preeclampsia, gestational hypertension and intrauterine growth restriction, related or independent conditions? Am J Obstet Gynecol. 2006;194:921–31.

142. Ben-Haroush A, Yogev Y, Hod M. Epidemiology of gestational diabetes mellitus and its association with Type 2 diabetes. Diabet Med. 2004;21:103–13.
143. Cuffe JS, Holland O, Salomon C, Rice GE, Perkins AV. Placental derived biomarkers of pregnancy disorders. Placenta. 2017;54:104–10.
144. Sattar N, Greer IA. Pregnancy complications and maternal cardiovascular risk: opportunities for intervention and screening? BMJ. 2002;325:157–60.
145. Irani RA, Xia Y. Renin angiotensin signaling in normal pregnancy and preeclampsia. Semin Nephrol. 2011;31:47–58.
146. Ha CT, Wu JA, Irmak S, Lisboa FA, Dizon AM, Warren JW, et al. Human pregnancy specific beta-1-glycoprotein 1 (PSG1) has a potential role in placental vascular morphogenesis. Biol Reprod. 2010;83:27–35.
147. Henson MC, Castracane VD. Leptin in pregnancy: an update. Biol Reprod. 2006;74:218–29.
148. Patil M, Panchanadikar TM, Wagh G. Variation of PAPP-A level in the first trimester of pregnancy and its clinical outcome. J Obstet Gynaecol India. 2014;64:116–9.
149. Cowans NJ, Spencer K. First-trimester ADAM12 and PAPP-A as markers for intrauterine fetal growth restriction through their roles in the insulin-like growth factor system. Prenat Diagn. 2007;27:264–71.
150. Kasimis C, Evangelinakis N, Rotas M, Georgitsi M, Pelekanos N, Kassanos D. Predictive value of biochemical marker ADAM-12 at first trimester of pregnancy for hypertension and intrauterine growth restriction. Clin Exp Obstet Gynecol. 2016;43:43–7.
151. Muttukrishna S. Role of inhibin in normal and high-risk pregnancy. Semin Reprod Med. 2004;22:227–34.
152. Barut F, Barut A, Gun BD, Kandemir NO, Harma MI, Harma M, et al. Intrauterine growth restriction and placental angiogenesis. Diagn Pathol. 2010;5:24.
153. Tandon V, Hiwale S, Amle D, Nagaria T, Patra PK. Assessment of serum vascular endothelial growth factor levels in pregnancy-induced hypertension patients. J Pregnancy. 2017;2017:3179670.
154. Bredaki FE, Mataliotakis M, Wright A, Wright D, Nicolaides KH. Maternal serum alpha-fetoprotein at 12, 22 and 32 weeks' gestation in screening for pre-eclampsia. Ultrasound Obstet Gynecol. 2016;47:466–71.
155. Audibert F, Benchimol Y, Benattar C, Champagne C, Frydman R. Prediction of preeclampsia or intrauterine growth restriction by second trimester serum screening and uterine Doppler velocimetry. Fetal Diagn Ther. 2005;20:48–53.
156. Rondo PH, Tomkins AM. Folate and intrauterine growth retardation. Ann Trop Paediatr. 2000;20:253–8.
157. Pandey K, Dubay P, Bhagoliwal A, Gupta N, Tyagi G. Hyperhomocysteinemia as a risk factor for IUGR. J Obstet Gynaecol India. 2012;62:406–8.
158. Florio P, Luisi S, Ciarmela P, Severi FM, Bocchi C, Petraglia F. Inhibins and activins in pregnancy. Mol Cell Endocrinol. 2004;225:93–100.
159. Ingec M, Gursoy HG, Yildiz L, Kumtepe Y, Kadanali S. Serum levels of insulin, IGF-1, and IGFBP-1 in pre-eclampsia and eclampsia. Int J Gynaecol Obstet. 2004;84:214–9.
160. Laway BA. Pregnancy in acromegaly. Ther Adv Endocrinol Metab. 2015;6:267–72.
161. Cooley SM, Donnelly JC, Geary MP, Rodeck CH, Hindmarsh PC. Maternal insulin-like growth factors 1 and 2 (IGF-1, IGF-2) and IGF BP-3 and the hypertensive disorders of pregnancy. J Matern Fetal Neonatal Med. 2010;23:658–61.
162. Collins S, Arulkumaran S, Hayes K, Jackson S, Impey L. Oxford handbook of obstetrics and gynaecology. Oxford: Oxford University Press; 2013.
163. Goldenberg RL, Cliver SP. Small for gestational age and intrauterine growth restriction: definitions and standards. Clin Obstet Gynecol. 1997;40:704–14.
164. Kramer MS, Olivier M, McLean FH, Willis DM, Usher RH. Impact of intrauterine growth retardation and body proportionality on fetal and neonatal outcome. Pediatrics. 1990;86:707–13.

165. Maulik D. Management of fetal growth restriction: an evidence-based approach. Clin Obstet Gynecol. 2006;49:320–34.
166. Bamfo JE, Odibo AO. Diagnosis and management of fetal growth restriction. J Pregnancy. 2011;2011:640715.
167. Hattersley AT, Tooke JE. The fetal insulin hypothesis: an alternative explanation of the association of low birthweight with diabetes and vascular disease. Lancet. 1999;353:1789–92.
168. Friedman SA, Taylor RN, Roberts JM. Pathophysiology of preeclampsia. Clin Perinatol. 1991;18:661–82.
169. Barron WM. The syndrome of preeclampsia. Gastroenterol Clin N Am. 1992;21:851–72.
170. Jeyabalan A. Epidemiology of preeclampsia: impact of obesity. Nutr Rev. 2013;71(Suppl 1):S18–25.
171. Roberts JM, Taylor RN, Musci TJ, Rodgers GM, Hubel CA, McLaughlin MK. Preeclampsia: an endothelial cell disorder. Am J Obstet Gynecol. 1989;161:1200–4.
172. Zhou Y, Damsky CH, Fisher SJ. Preeclampsia is associated with failure of human cytotrophoblasts to mimic a vascular adhesion phenotype. One cause of defective endovascular invasion in this syndrome? J Clin Invest. 1997;99:2152–64.
173. Irwin JC, Suen LF, Martina NA, Mark SP, Giudice LC. Role of the IGF system in trophoblast invasion and pre-eclampsia. Hum Reprod. 1999;14(Suppl 2):90–6.
174. Chard T. Insulin-like growth factors and their binding proteins in normal and abnormal human fetal growth. Growth Regul. 1994;4:91–100.
175. Halhali A, Tovar AR, Torres N, Bourges H, Garabedian M, Larrea F. Preeclampsia is associated with low circulating levels of insulin-like growth factor I and 1,25-dihydroxyvitamin D in maternal and umbilical cord compartments. J Clin Endocrinol Metab. 2000;85:1828–33.
176. Reis FM, D'Antona D, Petraglia F. Predictive value of hormone measurements in maternal and fetal complications of pregnancy. Endocr Rev. 2002;23:230–57.
177. Cuckle H. Prenatal screening using maternal markers. J Clin Med. 2014;3:504–20.
178. Appendix F. Maternal serum marker screening. Understanding genetics: a district of Columbia guide for patients and health professionals. Washington, DC: Genetic Alliance; 2010.
179. Johnson J, Pastuck M, Metcalfe A, Connors G, Krause R, Wilson D, et al. First-trimester Down syndrome screening using additional serum markers with and without nuchal translucency and cell-free DNA. Prenat Diagn. 2013;33:1044–9.
180. Krantz D, Hallahan T, Janik D, Carmichael J. Maternal serum screening markers and adverse outcome: a new perspective. J Clin Med. 2014;3:693–712.

Clinical Diagnosis

8

Alberto Borges Peixoto, Laudelino Marques Lopes,
and Edward Araujo Júnior

Introduction

Because of the wide variety of clinical presentations associated with fetal growth restriction (FGR), the exact definition and best management of this condition are elusive. In clinical practice, a fetal weight estimation below the 10th percentile remains the most commonly accepted condition for identifying fetuses with FGR [1]. However, not all fetuses whose estimated weight is below the 10th percentile are true growth-restricted fetuses. In a significant percentage of these pregnancies, there are no placental insufficiency and low neonatal morbidity; these fetuses are classified as small for gestational age (SGA) [2]. However, monitoring these fetuses is as important as monitoring true growth-restricted fetuses because up to 23% of SGA fetuses are admitted to neonatal intensive care units [3].

The importance of early detection of fetuses that are SGA or experiencing FGR can be seen in the association between these conditions and high rates of adverse perinatal outcomes [4]. Clinical evaluation appears to be an adequate tool for

A. B. Peixoto (✉)
Discipline of Fetal Medicine, Department of Obstetrics, Paulista School of Medicine, Federal University of São Paulo (EPM-UNIFESP), São Paulo, SP, Brazil

Discipline of Obstetrics and Gynecology, University of Uberaba (UNIUBE), Uberaba, MG, Brazil

Department of Obstetrics and Gynecology, Federal University of Triângulo Mineiro (UFTM), Uberaba, MG, Brazil

L. M. Lopes
Department of Obstetrics and Gynaecology, Schulich School of Medicine and Dentistry, University of Western Ontario, London, ON, Canada

E. Araujo Júnior
Discipline of Fetal Medicine, Department of Obstetrics, Paulista School of Medicine, Federal University of São Paulo (EPM-UNIFESP), São Paulo, SP, Brazil

L. M. M. Nardozza et al. (eds.), *Fetal Growth Restriction*,
https://doi.org/10.1007/978-3-030-00051-6_8

screening FGR in low-risk populations because there is no clear evidence that serial ultrasound improves perinatal outcomes compared with clinical evaluation [5, 6]. This surveillance is performed based on maternal clinical history, symphysis-fundal height (SFH), obstetric ultrasonography, or a combination of the latter two [4].

In low-risk populations, healthcare professionals have achieved more success in detecting FGR using third-trimester ultrasonography than measurements of the uterine height (40–80% vs. 16%) [7–9]. However, when obstetric ultrasonography is not available and the last menstrual period (LMP) is not known, SFH measurement is an important tool for estimating the gestational age [10] and fetal weight [11]. Although this procedure has not yet been tested for cost-effectiveness, SFH measurement can be used as a screening tool to refer patients with decreased SFH for obstetric ultrasonography, when applicable [12].

In this chapter, we will address the clinical diagnosis of FGR based on SFH measurement as a screening tool.

Clinical Identification of Fetal Growth Restriction

Calculating Gestational Age

The precise determination of the gestational age is crucial for the diagnosis of FGR to establish obstetric guidelines and care strategies because the classification of the fetal weight as normal or abnormal is established using reference curves that compare it to the gestational age [13]. Several methods can be used throughout pregnancy to calculate the gestational age. The most commonly used tools in clinical practice are date of LMP, SFH measurement, and ultrasonography.

Until recently, date of LMP was the most commonly used method to estimate the gestational age; however, this method is not reliable because several issues can interfere with its validity [14–17]. For this reason, ultrasound is currently the method of choice for calculating the gestational age [18]. According to the International Society of Ultrasound in Obstetrics and Gynecology, this calculation should be performed based on the measurement of the crown-rump length, preferably at a gestational age between 10 and 13 + 6 weeks [19]. Even in the absence of first-trimester ultrasonography, ultrasound performed at 24 weeks is more accurate in determining the gestational age than LMP [20, 21].

A very common problem in developing countries is that pregnant women lack access to ultrasound exams to calculate the gestational age [22]. In addition, not all women are sure of their LMP or have irregular menstrual cycles, which decreases LMP reliability. SFH measurement is a widely available method that is simple to perform and is routinely used in almost every prenatal setting in the world. Although Neilson [23] concluded in a review that there is insufficient evidence to assess the use of SFH measurement during prenatal care, this may be the only piece of data collected and reported on prenatal cards in most underdeveloped countries that is indicative of gestational age [22]. In this context, White et al. [22] developed and compared the accuracy and power of three formulae used to calculate the gestational age based on SFH measurement. The authors produced an Excel spreadsheet that used the most predictive mathematical model to estimate the gestational age. The model requires a minimum of three SFH input values with their respective dates of measurement and can be accessed for free at the website http://www.tropmedres.ac/gestational-age.

Measuring Symphysis-Fundal Height

SFH should be measured in low-risk pregnancies using a nonelastic measuring tape and by the same healthcare professional. When SFH is measured, the pregnant woman must lie on her back on a firm surface and must have an empty bladder [12] (Figs. 8.1 and 8.2). To obtain this measurement, we start from the upper edge of the pubic symphysis (fixed point) to the fundus of the uterus (variable point), holding the tape using the cubital edge of the hand according to the technique described by Belizán et al. [24]. Although the name of the procedure is "symphysis-fundal height," some authors argue that the measurement should begin at the fundus of the uterus so that both hands are available for palpation. From the fundus of the uterus, the tape runs along the longitudinal axis of the uterus to the top of the pubic symphysis [12].

SFH measurement should be obtained as soon as the fetal viability limit is reached (24–26-week gestation) to monitor fetal growth [20, 25]. SFH measurements should be taken during the prenatal visit every 2 weeks, preferably by the same examiner, to assess the fetal growth. Measuring SFH at intervals shorter than 15 days is not recommended because the increase in fetal growth is less than the error of measurement [25].

SFH measurement is not indicated for all pregnancies; these exceptions require fetal biometry using ultrasound technology (Table 8.1). Pregnancies that do not benefit from SFH typically fall into the following categories [25]: (1) measurement of fundal height unsuitable because of conditions such as fibroids or high maternal body mass index (BMI); (2) pregnancy risk and considered high risk and requiring serial ultrasonography owing to aspects such as history of SGA, history of pre-eclampsia, or multiple pregnancy; and (3) pregnancies with positive results on screening tests, such as first-trimester serologic markers or second-trimester uterine artery Doppler.

Once SFH is measured, the obtained value should preferably be plotted on a customized chart of uterine height throughout pregnancy to determine whether the value is appropriate for the gestational age [26]. We should avoid the rule that "1 week of gestation equals 1 cm of the uterine fundus" because SFH values vary between populations and change over time, thus requiring graphic representation.

A prospective study was recently conducted in eight countries (INTERGROWTH 21st) to determine international SFH standards derived from healthy pregnancies with good maternal and perinatal outcomes [27]. The reference curves are available free of charge at the following website: https://intergrowth21.tghn.org/site_media/media/medialibrary/2017/04/04_SFH.pdf. We use these reference values in our department when monitoring low-risk pregnant women.

Once the SFH measurement is plotted upon the chart, the findings will be considered abnormal whenever the measurement is below the 10th percentile for gestational age. Longitudinal evaluation of SFH measurements also helps identify

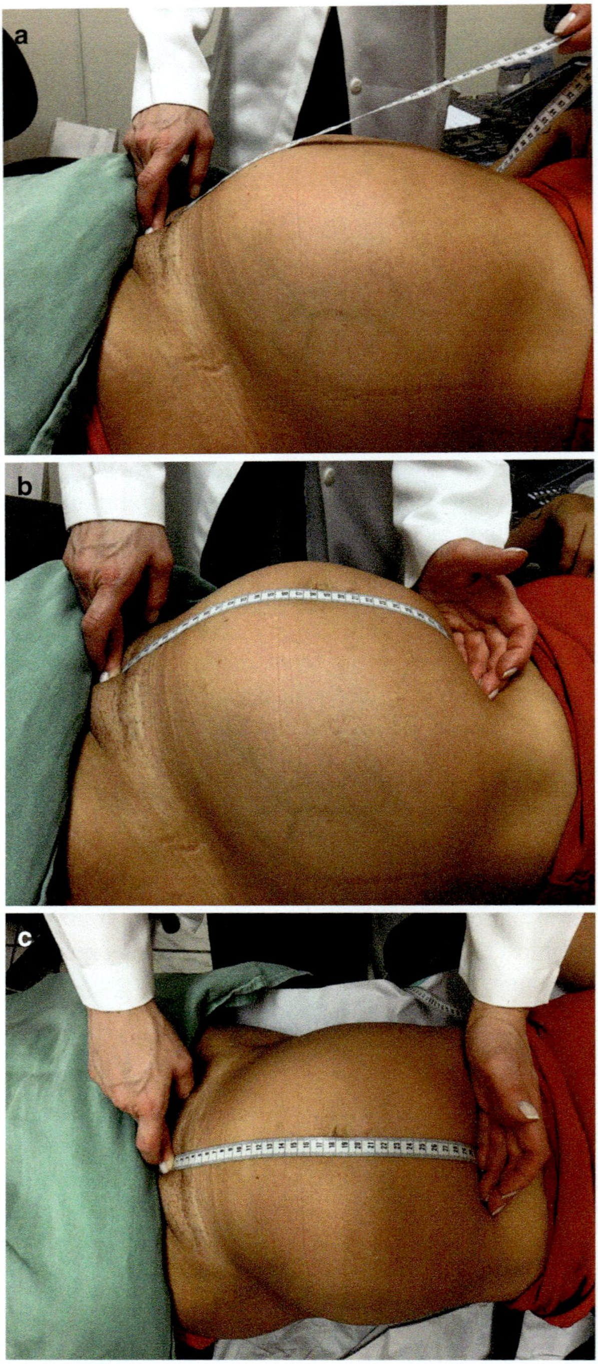

Fig. 8.1 Method of symphysis-fundal height measurement following the symphysis-fundus technique. (**a**) Identification of the upper edge of the pubic symphysis; (**b** and **c**) use of the cubital edge of the hand to hold the tape to the fundus of the uterus

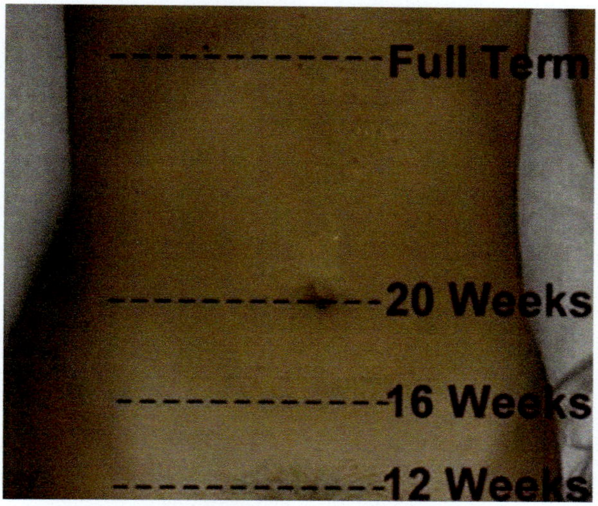

Fig. 8.2 Symphysis-fundal height measurement according to different gestational ages

Table 8.1 Recommendations for symphysis-fundal height (SFH) measurements and serial ultrasound in screening for fetal growth restriction (FGR)

Measurement of SFH	Low-risk pregnancies
	Start gestational age of 24–26 weeks
	Two-week interval
	Same examiner
Serial ultrasound	*Unable to measure SFH*
	Large fibroids
	BMI >35 kg/m^2
	Idiopathic polyhydramnios
	Increased risk of FGR
	Multiple pregnancy
	History of FGR
	Fetal death in prior pregnancy
	Chronic arterial hypertension
	History of preeclampsia
	Thrombophilia
	Autoimmune diseases
	Kidney disease
	Diabetes prior to pregnancy
	Maternal age >40 years
	Use of alcohol or illicit drugs
	Levels of PAPP-A <0.4 MoM
	Mean PI of uterine arteries >95th percentile

BMI body mass index, *PI* pulsatility index, *PAPP-A* pregnancy-associated plasma protein A

low-risk patients with probable fetal growth abnormalities. Fetal growth is considered abnormal when measurements reveal static growth, slow growth, or excessive growth (Fig. 8.3) [12]. In the presence of any of these findings, the patient should be referred for obstetric ultrasonography (Fig. 8.4) [25].

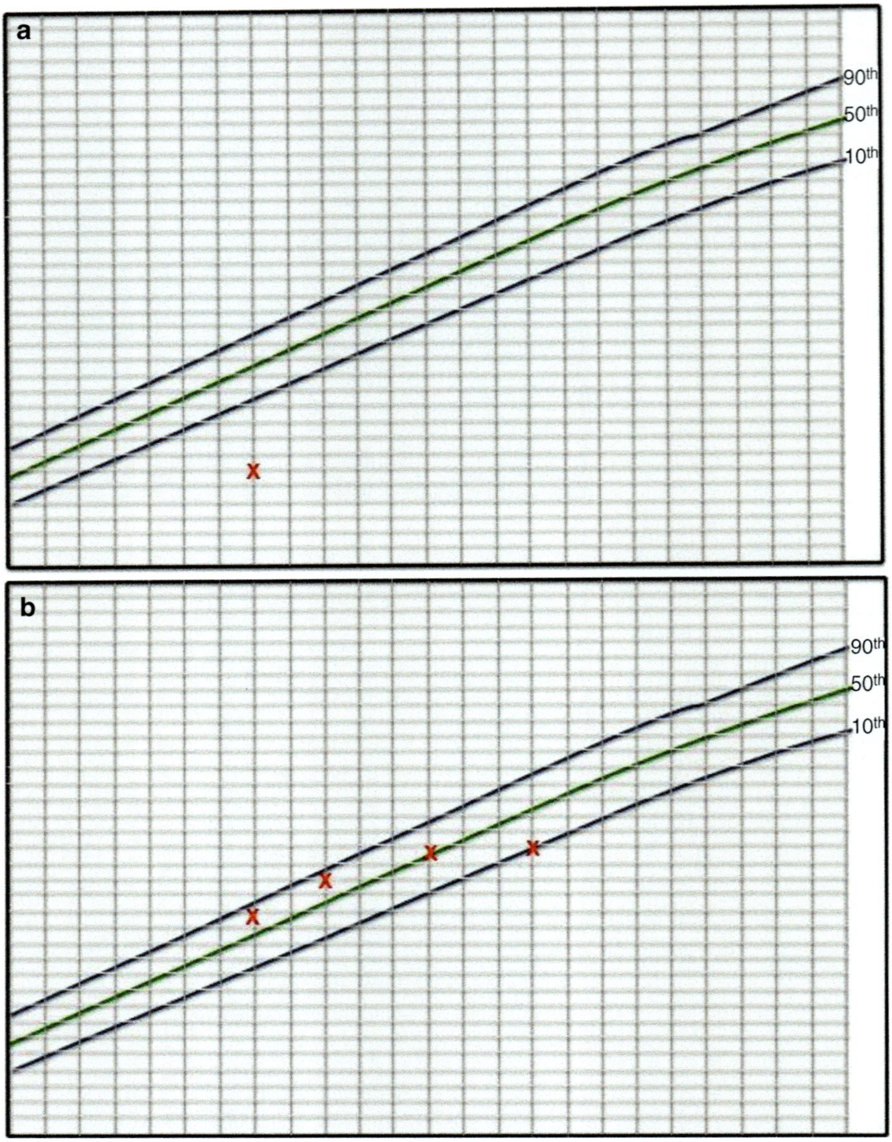

Fig. 8.3 Abnormal patterns in symphysis-fundal height measurement. (**a**) First measurement below the 10th percentile; (**b**) longitudinal evaluation suggesting static growth; (**c**) longitudinal evaluation suggesting slow growth; (**d**) longitudinal evaluation suggesting accelerated growth

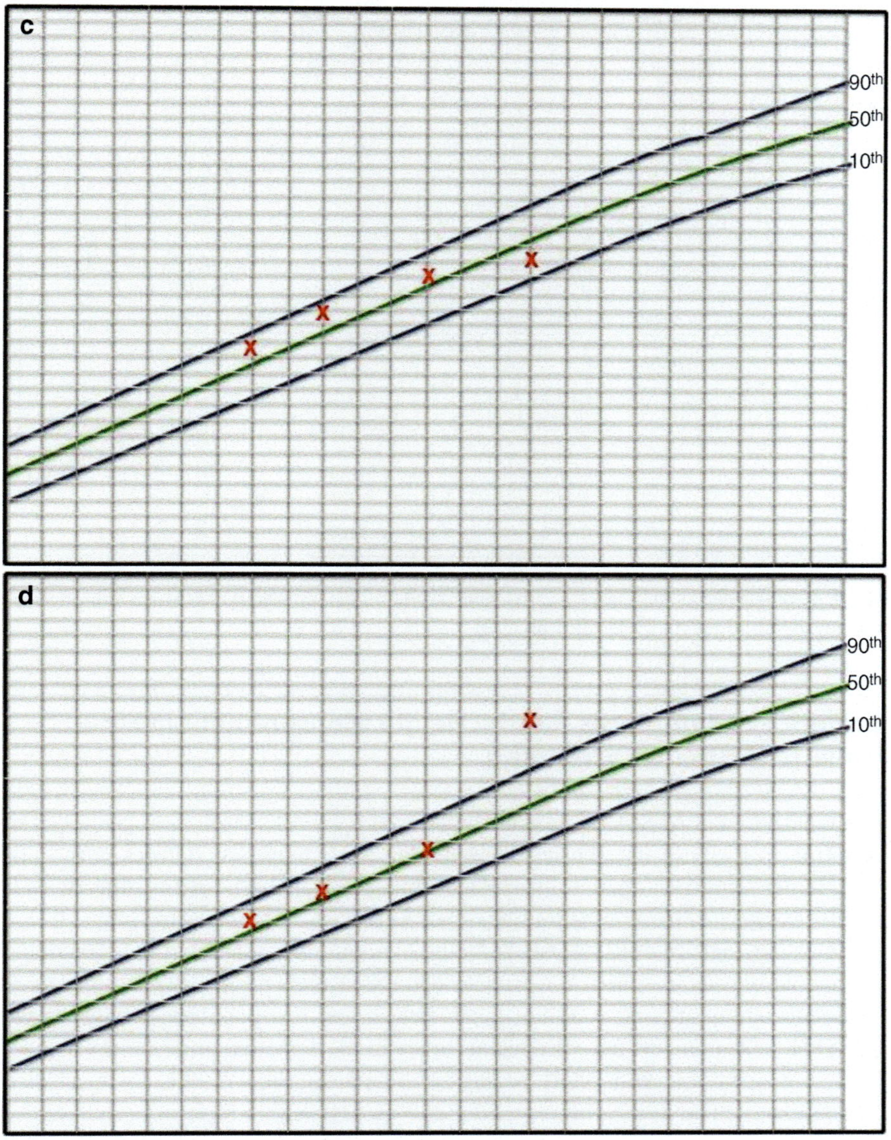

Fig. 8.3 (continued)

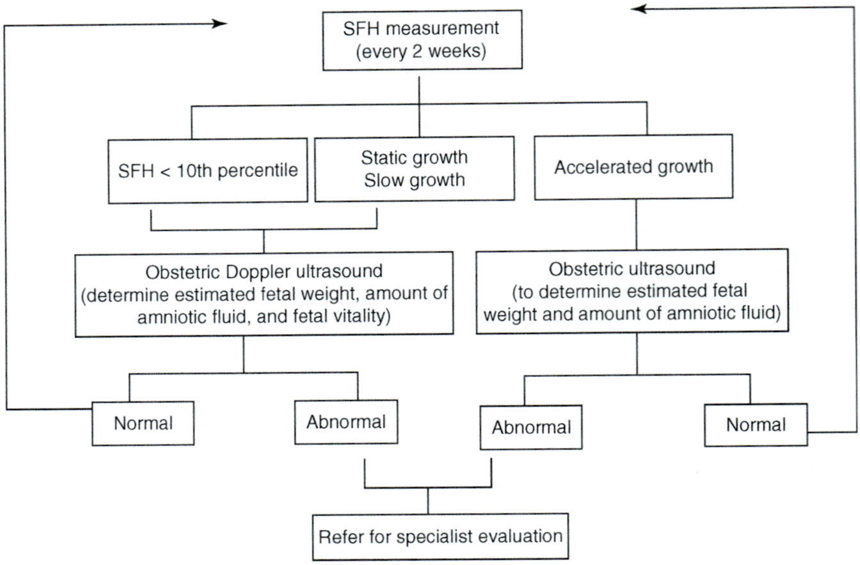

Fig. 8.4 Flowchart of fetal growth restriction (FGR) screening in low-risk patients through the symphysis-fundal height (SFH) measurement

Evidence of Symphysis-Fundal Height Measurement in Fetal Growth Restriction Screening

The measurement of SFH is recommended every 2 weeks starting at 24 weeks of gestation to increase the chances of detecting SGA fetuses or fetuses with FGR [25]. To date, however, there is insufficient evidence from high-quality clinical trials to fully assess the effect of the routine use of SFH measurement during prenatal care on pregnancy outcomes [28]. Data from the literature is inconsistent in terms of the methodology used, the inclusion criteria, and the results [12, 24, 29].

Cohort and case-control studies conducted in low-risk populations have shown that SFH measurements have limited accuracy in the detection of newborns that are SGA and newborns with FGR (<2nd or 3rd percentile) [7, 30]. In unselected populations, sensitivity (S) increases to 32–44% [31, 32]. In high-risk populations, S was 37% among SGA neonates and 53% among FGR cases (<2nd or 3rd percentile) [30].

Martinelli et al. [33], in their evaluation of the use of SFH measurement to diagnose FGR in a high-risk population wherein they used the known curves of uterine height evolution from their own practice as the standard [34], obtained an a S of 78%, a specificity (SPC) of 77.1%, a positive predictive value (PPV) of 47.6%, and a negative predictive value (NPV) of 92.9%, considering a measurement of the uterine height below the 10th percentile. Using 5th percentile as the limit, the results were S = 64%, SPC = 89.9%, PPV = 62.7%, and NPV = 90.4% for FGR diagnosis.

A meta-analysis evaluated the accuracy of SFH measurement in detecting SGA and low-birth-weight fetuses [35]. The analysis included 26 articles (*n* = 16, 750), which mainly included hospital patients. In the case of SGA detection, S and SPC were 58% and 73%, respectively, whereas in case of low-birth-weight detection, S and SPC were 72% and 73%, respectively. The authors concluded that the SFH measurement is unsuitable able for screening for SGA and low-birth-weight fetuses; however, the results of this review may be biased because it included studies across a broad range of ethnic groups, clinical contexts, and spectrums of diseases. Despite a mix of such diverse cases, the study did not evaluate the effect of these factors on pooled estimates, thus making it difficult to interpret the findings in the context of low-risk pregnancies.

Maternal obesity, anomalous fetal presentation, large fibromas, polyhydramnios, and fetal head engagement contribute to a decrease in the PPV of SFH measurements and are also associated with significant intra- and interobserver variation [12]. However, serial SFH measurement can improve PPV [36].

Pay et al. [37] found that the quality of the estimates of low birth weight and SGA is low in early pregnancy but increases as the pregnancy reaches full term. Important but fewer intuitive results are that the detection rate of SGA does not improve with serial SFH measurement because these changes are commonly considered to be signs of an increased risk of SGA. However, increasing or decreasing trends in SFH measurements did not contribute to the predictive capacity beyond what was already obtained using the most recent SFH measurement.

Haragan et al. [38] compared SFH and fetal abdominal circumference measurements using a portable ultrasonography device to predict FGR or large for gestational age fetuses. They found that portable ultrasound produced S and SPC higher than SFH measurements for the detection of FGR (100% vs. 42.86% and 92.62% vs. 85.24%, respectively).

The impact of SFH measurements on perinatal outcomes is unclear. A systematic review found only one study of 1639 women that demonstrated that SFH measurement did not improve any of the perinatal outcomes evaluated [23]. To date, there are no clinical trials comparing customized SFH charts with non-customized SFH charts or their effectiveness in identifying adverse perinatal outcomes [24]. However, observational studies suggest that customized SFH charts improve the detection of low birth weight [26].

Conclusion

SFH may be the first parameter to alert healthcare providers to suspect SGA fetuses and FGR; however, its use in the prenatal routine should be restricted to the surveillance of low-risk and unselected pregnancies. SFH is useful in prenatal care in places with limited access to ultrasonography and in cases in which primary care is provided by nursing professionals to ensure the identification of signs that suggest SGA fetuses or FGR.

References

1. Battaglia FC, Lubchenco LO. A practical classification of newborn infants by weight and gestational age. J Pediatr. 1976;71:159–63.
2. Figueras F, Gratacos E. An integrated approach to fetal growth restriction. Best Pract Res Clin Obstet Gynaecol. 2017;38:48–58.
3. McCowan LM, Harding JE, Roberts AB, Barker SE, Ford C, Stewart AW. A pilot randomized controlled trial of two regimens of fetal surveillance for small-for-gestational-age fetuses with normal results of umbilical artery Doppler velocimetry. Am J Obstet Gynecol. 2000;182:81–6.
4. Gaziano EP, Knox N, Ferrera B, Brandt DG, Calvin SE, Knox GE. Is it time to reassess the risk for the growth-retarded fetus with normal Doppler velocimetry of the umbilical artery? Am J Obstet Gynecol. 1994;170:734–43.
5. Harkness UF, Mari G. Diagnosis and management of intrauterine growth restriction. Clin Perinatol. 2004;31:743–64.
6. Duff GB. A randomized controlled trial in a hospital population of ultrasound measurement screening for the small for dates baby. Aust N Z J Obstet Gynaecol. 1993;33:374–8.
7. Kean LH, Liu DT. Antenatal care as a screening tool for the detection of small for gestational age babies in the low risk population. J Obstet Gynaecol. 1996;16:77–82.
8. Lindqvist PG, Molin J. Does antenatal identification of small-for-gestational age fetuses significantly improve their outcome? Ultrasound Obstet Gynecol. 2005;25:258–64.
9. Souka AP, Papastefanou I, Pilalis A, Michalitsi V, Kassanos D. Performance of third-trimester ultrasound for prediction of small-for-gestational-age neonates and evaluation of contingency screening policies. Ultrasound Obstet Gynecol. 2012;39:535–42.
10. Rondo PH, Maia Filho NL, Valverde KK. Symphysis–fundal height and size at birth. Int J Gynaecol Obstet. 2003;81:53–4.
11. Mongelli M, Gardosi J. Estimation of fetal weight by symphysis–fundus height measurement. Int J Gynaecol Obstet. 2004;85:50–1.
12. Morse K, Williams A, Gardosi J. Fetal growth screening by fundal height measurement. Best Pract Res Clin Obstet Gynaecol. 2009;23:809–18.
13. Matias A, Tiago P, Montenegro N. Calculation of gestational age. Methods and problems. Acta Medica Port. 2002;15:17–21.
14. Hall MH, Carr-Hill RA, Fraser C, Campbell D, Samphier ML. The extent and antecedents of uncertain gestation. Br J Obstet Gynaecol. 1985;92:445–51.
15. Persson PH, Kullander S. Long-term experience of general ultrasound screening in pregnancy. Am J Obstet Gynecol. 1983;146:942–7.
16. Geirsson RT, Busby-Earle RM. Certain dates may not provide a reliable estimate of gestational age. Br J Obstet Gynaecol. 1991;98:108–9.
17. Chiazze L Jr, Brayer FT, Macisco JJ Jr, Parker MP, Duffy BJ. The length and variability of the human menstrual cycle. JAMA. 1968;203:377–80.
18. Committee on Obstetric Practice. Committee opinion no. 688: management of suboptimally dated pregnancies. Obstet Gynecol. 2017;129:e29–32.
19. Salomon LJ, Alfirevic Z, Bilardo CM, Chalouhi GE, Ghi T, Kagan KO, et al. ISUOG practice guidelines: performance of first-trimester fetal ultrasound scan. Ultrasound Obstet Gynecol. 2013;41:102–13.
20. National Collaborating Centre for Women's and Children's Health (UK). Antenatal care: routine care for the healthy pregnant woman. London: RCOG Press; 2008.
21. Nakling J, Buhaug H, Backe B. The biologic error in gestational length related to the use of the first day of last menstrual period as a proxy for the start of pregnancy. Early Hum Dev. 2005;81:833–9.
22. White LJ, Lee SJ, Stepniewska K, Simpson JA, Dwell SL, Arunjerdja R, et al. Estimation of gestational age from fundal height: a solution for resource-poor settings. J R Soc Interface. 2012;9:503–10.

23. Neilson JP. Symphysis-fundal height measurement in pregnancy. Cochrane Database Syst Rev. 2000;2:CD000944.
24. Belizán JM, Villar J, Nardin JC, Malamud J, De Vicurna LS. Diagnosis of intrauterine growth retardation by a simple clinical method: measurement of uterine height. Am J Obstet Gynecol. 1978;131:643–6.
25. Royal College of Obstetricians & Gynaecologists. Small-for-gestational age fetus, investigation and management. RCOG Green Top Guideline 2013; No. 31.
26. Gardosi J, Francis A. Controlled trial of fundal height measurement plotted on customised antenatal growth charts. Br J Obstet Gynaecol. 1999;106:309–17.
27. Papageorghiou AT, Ohuma EO, Gravett MG, Hirst J, da Silveira MF, Lambert A, et al. International standards for symphysis-fundal height based on serial measurements from the Fetal Growth Longitudinal Study of the INTERGROWTH-21st Project: prospective cohort study in eight countries. BMJ. 2016;355:i5662.
28. Robert Peter J, Ho JJ, Valliapan J, Sivasangari S. Symphysial fundal height (SFH) measurement in pregnancy for detecting abnormal fetal growth. Cochrane Database Syst Rev. 2012;7:CD008136.
29. Quaranta P, Currell R, Redman CW, Robinson JS. Prediction of small-for-dates infants by measurement of symphysial-fundal-height. Br J Obstet Gynaecol. 1981;88:115–9.
30. Bais JM, Eskes M, Pel M, Bonsel GJ, Bleker OP. Effectiveness of detection of intrauterine growth retardation by abdominal palpation as screening test in a low risk population: an observational study. Eur J Obstet Gynecol Reprod Biol. 2004;116:164–9.
31. Hall MH, Chng PK, MacGillivray I. Is routine antenatal care worthwhile? Lancet. 1980;2:78–80.
32. Rosenberg K, Grant JM, Hepburn M. Antenatal detection of growth retardation: actual practice in a large maternity hospital. Br J Obstet Gynaecol. 1982;9:12–5.
33. Martinelli S, Bittar RE, Zugaib M. Prediction of fetal growth restriction by measurement of uterine height. Rev Bras Ginecol Obstet. 2004;26:383–9.
34. Martinelli S, Bittar RE, Zugaib M. Proposal of a New Uterine Height Growth Curve for Pregnancies between 20 and 42 Weeks. Rev Bras Ginecol Obstet. 2001;23:235–41.
35. Goto E. Prediction of low birthweight and small for gestational age from symphysis-fundal height mainly in developing countries: a meta-analysis. J Epidemiol Community Health. 2013;67:999–1005.
36. Bailey SM, Sarmandal P, Grant JM. A comparison of three methods of assessing inter–observer variation applied to measurements of symphysis–fundus height. Br J Obstet Gynaecol. 1989;96:1266–71.
37. Pay A, Frøen JF, Staff AC, Jacobsson B, Gjessing HK. Prediction of small-for-gestational-age status by symphysis-fundus height: a registry-based population cohort study. BJOG. 2016;123:1167–73.
38. Haragan AF, Hulsey TC, Hawk AF, Newman RB, Chang EY. Diagnostic accuracy of fundal height and handheld ultrasound-measured abdominal circumference to screen for fetal growth abnormalities. Am J Obstet Gynecol. 2015;212:820.e1–8.

Ultrasonography Diagnosis

9

Nicola Fratelli, Cristina Zanardini, and Federico Prefumo

Introduction

Fetal growth is a dynamic process determined by a combination of genetic, intrauterine, and environmental influences. Fetal growth restriction (FGR) is defined as the failure of a fetus to meet its growth potential as a consequence of impaired placental function [1]. Accurate dating of pregnancy is essential to assess fetal size, and ultrasound measurement of the embryo or fetus in the first trimester (up to and including 13 + 6 weeks of gestation) is the most accurate method to establish or confirm gestational age and is vital for determining the appropriateness of fetal growth later in pregnancy. Guidelines are available for estimating the due date based on ultrasonography and the last menstrual period in pregnancy; however, when pregnancy results from assisted reproductive technology (ART), the ART-derived gestational age should be used to assign the estimated due date (EDD). For instance, the EDD for a pregnancy that resulted from in vitro fertilization should be assigned using the date of the conception or in case of frozen embryo the date of transfer corrected by the age of the embryo [2].

When gray-scale ultrasonography alone is used to screen for fetal growth restriction, different approaches are put in place to identify those fetuses who fail to achieve their own individual growth potential; these include: (1) sonographic fetal weight estimation, (2) customized growth charts, (3) use of serial ultrasound evaluations to assess fetal growth, and (4) assessment of fetal body proportions.

N. Fratelli · C. Zanardini · F. Prefumo (✉)
Department of Obstetrics and Gynaecology,
ASST Spedali Civili di Brescia, University of Brescia,
Brescia, Italy

L. M. M. Nardozza et al. (eds.), *Fetal Growth Restriction*,
https://doi.org/10.1007/978-3-030-00051-6_9

Sonographic Fetal Weight Estimation

Assessment of fetal growth with a onetime measurement is standard clinical practice, despite recognition that a single measurement can only indicate size, not growth. The most accurate method to determine fetal size is to estimate the fetal weight. For this purpose, the fetal biometric measurements commonly used are biparietal diameter (BPD), head circumference (HC), abdominal circumference (AC), and femur length (FL). These biometric measurements can be combined into an estimated fetal weight (EFW) using various formulae to provide a more straightforward and clinically relevant estimate of fetal growth. A number of different formulas for estimating EFW from ultrasound measurements have been described. Nonetheless, the 1985 model published by Hadlock et al. [3] remains one of the most accurate and widely employed [4].

The most commonly adopted screening approach is through ultrasonography as it allows to assess the deviation of the fetal size from a reference population defining empirically as small for gestational age (SGA) those fetuses with an estimated fetal weight (EFW) below the 10th percentile for gestation. However, the majority of SGA fetuses are constitutionally small and healthy rather than growth restricted and are at low risk for adverse perinatal outcome [5]. This approach is further limited by the fact that it may overlook those fetuses with impaired growth and an increased risk of adverse outcome in which abdominal circumference and EFW remain above the 10th percentile for gestation [6]. Thus, additional measures to identify failure to achieve individual growth potential are needed to establish the diagnosis of FGR, and in clinical practice, the definition of FGR is often based on a combination of measures of fetal size and abnormal Doppler studies [1]. Severe SGA fetuses however have unfavorable long-term outcome even in the absence of abnormal functional parameters; therefore a recent consensus identifies AC or EFW <3rd percentile for gestation, in the absence of congenital anomalies, as stand-alone biometric parameters that allow the diagnosis of FGR [1]. Growth charts should be based on EFW rather than actual birth weight as the latter is unavailable for obstetric decision-making in the antenatal and intrapartum periods. In routine practice, the EFW is often compared with the distribution of birth weight. However, it should really be compared to an adequate and specific reference range. EFW estimates should not be plotted on newborn birth weight charts, since these include a large proportion of FGR fetuses delivered early in gestation and, therefore, a diagnosis of FGR could be missed [7]. Salomon et al. highlighted this important discrepancy between birth weight and EFW at the same gestational age in fetuses that eventually are delivered preterm [8]. They reported that EFW and birth weight charts tend to merge toward the end of pregnancy, which supports the evidence that EFW at term provides a good estimate of the actual birth weight [9].

There are many published fetal growth charts available, and the choice of chart used also requires careful consideration as several potentially confusing terms and concepts associated with fetal size and growth are reported in the literature. The distinction between fetal growth "standards" and fetal growth "references" is one of the main issues. Descriptive fetal growth charts that have been developed based on populations of fetuses from normal and complicated pregnancies are called "references," whereas prescriptive growth charts are called "standards" [10]. Prescriptive charts describe growth under optimal conditions, i.e., they provide ranges for what should be expected when women are healthy and arise from normal pregnant populations. The main difference, put in simple words, is that fetal growth "references" describe how fetuses are growing, while fetal growth "standards" describe how a fetus should grow [7]. The NICHD fetal growth study [11], WHO [12], and Intergrowth-21st [13] percentiles for international use are three examples of prescriptive growth charts ("standard"). An area of controversy is whether a single growth reference is representative of growth, regardless of ethnic or geographical origin: Intergrowth-21st studies introduced standards for fetal growth and birth weight based on the concept of "one size fits all"; the NICHD fetal growth study [11] also used the expression "standard" but acknowledged variation and established ethnic-specific curves; finally, the WHO fetal growth study also acknowledged that variation across populations exists [12]. Intergrowth-21st [13] made the assumption that there would be no differences internationally among countries or racial/ethnic groups in fetal growth when conditions were optimal, and they found differences in crown-rump length and head circumference among countries but interpreted the differences as not meaningful and presented a pooled standard. The WHO Multicentre Growth Reference Study [12] was designed to create a pooled reference, although they evaluated for and presented country differences, along with discussion of the implications. The NICHD study [11] was designed to assess whether racial-/ethnic-specific fetal growth standards were needed, in recognition of the fact that fetal size is commonly estimated from dimensions (head circumference, abdominal circumference, and femur length) in which there are known differences in children and adults of differing racial/ethnic groups. A pooled standard would be derived if no racial/ethnic differences were found. Highly statistically significant racial/ethnic differences in fetal growth were found resulting in the publication of racial-/ethnic-specific-derived standards. Despite all three studies including low-risk status women, the percentiles for fetal dimensions and estimated fetal weight varied among the studies [14]. When applying these standards to a clinical population, it is important to be aware that different percentages of SGA fetuses will be identified. Also, it may be necessary to use more restrictive cutoff points, such as the 2.5th percentile for SGA fetuses. Ideally, a comparison of diagnostic accuracy, or misclassification rates, of small-for-gestational-age and large-for-gestational-age fetuses in relation to morbidity and mortality using different criteria is necessary to make recommendations and remains an important data gap [14]. In clinical practice identification of the appropriate percentile cutoffs in relation to neonatal morbidity and mortality is needed in local populations, depending on which fetal growth chart is used.

Customized Growth Charts

Differences in fetal growth have been shown between countries and between individual maternal characteristics such as height, weight, and parity [11–13]. Customized charts adjust for constitutional or physiologic variation and exclude pathologic factors that affect growth, thereby defining an optimized standard that represents the growth potential of each individual fetus [15, 16]. In the customized model, the variables for adjustment are derived from birth weights of normally formed term fetuses delivered after uncomplicated pregnancies. The model adjusts for the physiologic but not pathologic variables and results in a constant that represents an expected optimal birth weight at the end of an uncomplicated pregnancy. Maternal characteristics are entered into a software program (GROW; Gestation Network; Birmingham, UK, www.gestation.net) to calculate an individually adjusted term optimal weight for 40.0 weeks (280 days) of gestation. This predicted weight endpoint is then combined with a standard proportionality function [16] to provide a gestation-related optimal weight (GROW) curve. The standard Hadlock EFW curve [17] was used and converted it from a fetal weight-by-gestation curve to a percent of term weight-by-gestational age curve, with the Hadlock 40-week weight assigned 100%. This allows any term optimal weight to be substituted for 100%, thereby specifying the expected weight for gestational age trajectory (GROW curve) up to that predicted endpoint. The normal range around the GROW curve is derived from the standard error of the multiple regression model and the term optimal weight that together give a coefficient of variation (CV) of 11%; the 90th and 10th percentile limits are then reached by 1.28 CV or 14% of the term optimal weight [16]. The use of a fetal, rather than a neonatal, weight-based standard helps to highlight the association between fetal growth restriction and preterm birth because the standard is derived from normal term pregnancies; the prevalence of SGA in preterm babies tends to be hidden by the use of a neonatal curve that is derived from preterm birth weights that are abnormal by definition [8]. For antenatal surveillance, customized GROW charts are produced at the beginning of pregnancy, once the expected date of delivery is confirmed by the ultrasound dating scan. The chart is either printed out at the beginning of pregnancy or can be displayed electronically. A global version of the GROW percentile calculator was recently released and includes coefficients for over 100 ethnic or country of origin groups [18]. Although Gardosi et al. [19] reported that, in England, regions with a high uptake of an accreditation program in customized fetal growth experienced a significant reduction in stillbirths when compared with areas in which uptake was low, a recent systematic review of the published data performed in order to assess if customized models can better detect fetal growth disturbances associated with adverse perinatal outcomes concluded that customized charts are not better than population charts in identifying pathologically small fetuses at higher risk [20]. Therefore, prospective randomized controlled trials are required to determine whether applying customized models would reduce the occurrence of perinatal death and other severe complications. Other approaches to generating customized growth charts involved including paternal characteristics in the model, as well as using quantile regression analysis for a more accurate centile calculation [21, 22]. Also these approaches require however a prospective assessment of clinical validity.

Use of Serial Ultrasound Evaluations to Assess Fetal Growth

As fetal growth is a dynamic process, and its assessment requires at least two observations separated in time, an intuitive approach to improve the diagnosis of FGR is the use of serial ultrasound evaluations. In infants it has been shown that growth velocity is more predictive of size later in life than any single measurement of infant size; however, the best approach to interpret the information obtained from serial measurements of the same fetus remains unclear [23]. Serial ultrasound evaluations can be interpreted as fetal growth velocity, conditional percentiles, projection-based methods, or individualized growth assessment (IGA).

Fetal growth velocity can be defined as the change in fetal size between two points during gestation [23]. This approach can be applied to the change in either a specific fetal biometric index (e.g., AC) or in EFW and is usually expressed as the change in absolute value of the biometric index per time unit (e.g., mm/wk or g/d) or as the change in z-score (i.e., the value of the biometric index normalized for gestational age) per time unit. The methodology used to generate growth velocity standards can be broadly divided into two types. The first and most commonly used ("average growth velocity") is based on the assumption that fetal growth is linear throughout the time interval studied. After the measurement of fetal size on two time points along gestation, the average growth velocity is calculated by dividing the difference in fetal size by the time interval between these two points. In the case of >2 sets of measurements, the average growth velocity can be calculated using linear regression [23]. The second methodological approach for the calculation of fetal growth velocity ("instantaneous growth velocity") describes the change of the individual biometry as a function of gestational age [24]. This approach may be more accurate for the generation of growth velocity standards since, in contrast to the average growth velocity approach, it is not limited by the assumption that fetal growth is linear within a given time interval [23].

Conditional centiles are an alternative method for defining fetal growth potential. EFW percentile is calculated taking into account the previous weight estimation of the same fetus earlier in pregnancy. With this approach the EFW calculated during the first scan (conditioning scan) is used to adjust the standard growth curve to the expected growth trajectory of the individual fetus, and the EFW percentile at the time of the subsequent scan is determined based on this new adjusted curve. This method is discussed in detail elsewhere in the book [25].

Projection-based methods use linear mixed-effects models to predict EFW at a later point in gestation based on two or more observations of EFW. A projected EFW below a fixed cutoff, usually 5th or 10th percentile for gestational age, suggests fetal growth restriction [23, 26].

Individualized growth assessment relies on the interpretation of third trimester fetal size assessments on the basis of the degree to which they deviate from the expected growth curve of the same individual fetus; this curve is based on two sonographic assessments performed <26 weeks of gestation, presumably prior to the onset of any pathologic factor that may affect fetal growth [27].

When growth restriction is suspected, serial ultrasound scans can be used to assess fetal growth. However, even if serial AC measurements are used in clinical practice, there is no clear definition of what constitutes normal fetal growth and which fetal biometric parameters should be evaluated. Given that repeated measurements in a short time interval are highly inaccurate, the International Society of Ultrasound in Obstetrics and Gynecology (ISUOG) recommends that serial growth scans are optimally performed at least 3 weeks from a previous scan when indicated [28].

All the approaches described in this paragraph are used to quantify any decrease in EFW associated with adverse perinatal outcome [29] and might be useful in high-risk pregnancies where they appear to improve the detection of FGR at increased risk of adverse perinatal outcomes, decreasing the risk of falsely diagnosing healthy constitutionally SGA fetuses as growth restricted [23]. However further studies are needed to quantify the predictive accuracy of these tools, to determine the optimal timing of the conditioning ultrasound, the optimal time interval between scans, and the overall cost-effectiveness of the screening program. Ideally these approaches should be validated in different populations using perinatal death and other severe complications as clinically relevant outcomes [23].

Assessment of Fetal Body Proportions

It has been suggested that because of the brain-sparing phenomenon, fetal AC would be the first biometric index to be affected in cases of placental insufficiency, leading to the assumption that growth-restricted fetuses with small AC in relation to another reference biometric index that is unaffected by fetal malnutrition (asymmetric pattern) are more likely to be the result of placental insufficiency and are at higher risk of adverse perinatal outcome [30]. Fetal body proportions used to assess fetal asymmetry are based on a ratio between AC and a reference biometric index assumed to be less sensitive to placental insufficiency. The most commonly used ratio is the HC/AC ratio, as fetal HC is only minimally affected by placental insufficiency or by external pressure. The median HC/AC ratio in early pregnancy is about 1.2 and decreases along gestation, being about 1.0 at term [23]. Although abnormal ratios are associated with SGA at birth and with adverse perinatal outcomes, the literature shows that HC/AC has a lower predictive accuracy than other more specific measures of placental function, such as maternal and fetal Doppler evaluation [23]. Moreover it has been traditionally assumed that assessment of fetal body proportions may provide information on the etiology of FGR, so that fetal causes of FGR such as chromosomal abnormalities were thought to be associated with early-onset symmetric pattern, while placental insufficiency was considered to be associated with late-onset asymmetric pattern. However, it seems that the timing of insult is more important than the etiology of FGR in determining fetal growth pattern, with early insults (placental or fetal) resulting in symmetric patterns, while insults taking place later in pregnancy result in asymmetric patterns [23]. Further studies are needed to determine whether the assessment of fetal body proportion can contribute to the diagnosis of late FGR, where umbilical artery Doppler is typically normal, improving the diagnosis of FGR and adverse perinatal outcome.

Timing of Ultrasound Assessment

The routine use of late ultrasound (after 24 weeks) in low-risk or unselected pregnancies is not associated with significant variations in the incidence of perinatal mortality (8 studies, $n = 30.675$; RR 1.01; 95% CI, 0.67–1.54), preterm birth before 37 weeks (2 studies, $n = 17.151$; RR 0.96; 95% CI, 0.85–1.08), induction of labor (6 studies, $n = 22.663$; RR 0.93; 95% CI, 0.81–1.07), or caesarean section (6 studies, $n = 27.461$; RR 1.03; 95% CI, 0.92–1.15) [31]. Due to this lack of efficacy, most guidelines do not recommend routine assessment of fetal growth by ultrasound in the third trimester of pregnancy, suggesting to prescribe it only in the presence of clinical indications. In recent years, there has been a large debate in the international literature on the possibility of reducing term mortality through a more effective recognition of FGR cases [32]. However, in countries like Italy and France where a routine ultrasound examination is offered within the national health system at 28–32 weeks, such strategy seems to be able to identify less than 30% of fetuses destined to be term SGA newborns [33, 34]. Recent studies of high methodological quality suggest instead a greater sensitivity of ultrasound examinations performed at 35–37 weeks [35, 36], but the eventual effect of this approach on pregnancy outcomes has yet to be demonstrated with a high level of evidence.

Conclusion

To conclude, it must be highlighted that fetal growth is a dynamic process. Fetal growth restriction refers to a fetus that has failed to reach its biological growth potential because of placental dysfunction. However FGR has considerable overlap with SGA even if it is more difficult to define in practice, as not all FGR infants have a birth weight <10th centile. Suboptimal fetal growth is important as placental insufficiency is a major contributor to the pathophysiology in SGA pregnancies and contributes to the adverse perinatal outcome. The best ultrasound approach to identify failure to achieve individual growth has yet to be determined. Ideally, such approach should be validated in different populations against perinatal death and other clinically relevant outcomes.

References

1. Gordijn SJ, Beune IM, Thilaganathan B, Papageorghiou A, Baschat AA, Baker PN, et al. Consensus definition of fetal growth restriction: a Delphi procedure. Ultrasound Obstet Gynecol. 2016;48:333–9.
2. ACOG Committee opinion no. 700: Methods for estimating the due date. Obstet Gynecol. 2017;129:e150–4.

3. Hadlock FP, Harrist RB, Sharman RS, Deter RL, Park SK. Estimation of fetal weight with the use of head, body, and femur measurements – a prospective study. Am J Obstet Gynecol. 1985;151:333–7.
4. Hammami A, Mazer Zumaeta A, Syngelaki A, Akolekar R, Nicolaides KH. Ultrasonographic estimation of fetal weight: development of new model and assessment of performance of previous models. Ultrasound Obstet Gynecol. 2018;52:35–43.
5. Beune IM, Bloomfield FH, Ganzevoort W, Embleton ND, Rozance PJ, van Wassenaer-Leemhuis AG, et al. Consensus based definition of growth restriction in the newborn. J Pediatr. 2018;196:71–76.
6. Iliodromiti S, Mackay DF, Smith GC, Pell JP, Sattar N, Lawlor DA, et al. Customised and noncustomised birth weight centiles and prediction of stillbirth and infant mortality and morbidity: a cohort study of 979,912 term singleton pregnancies in Scotland. PLoS Med. 2017;14:e1002228.
7. O'Gorman N, Salomon LJ. Fetal biometry to assess the size and growth of the fetus. Best Pract Res Clin Obstet Gynaecol. 2018;49:3–15.
8. Salomon LJ, Bernard JP, Ville Y. Estimation of fetal weight: reference range at 20–36 weeks' gestation and comparison with actual birth-weight reference range. Ultrasound Obstet Gynecol. 2007;29:550–5.
9. Chauhan SP, Hendrix NW, Magann EF, Morrison JC, Scardo JA, Berghella V. A review of sonographic estimate of fetal weight: vagaries of accuracy. J Matern Fetal Neonatal Med. 2005;18:211–20.
10. Ioannou C, Talbot K, Ohuma E, Sarris I, Villar J, Conde-Agudelo A, et al. Systematic review of methodology used in ultrasound studies aimed at creating charts of fetal size. BJOG. 2012;119:1425–39.
11. Buck Louis GM, Grewal J, Albert PS, Sciscione A, Wing DA, Grobman WA, et al. Racial/ethnic standards for fetal growth: the NICHD Fetal Growth Studies. Am J Obstet Gynecol. 2015;213:449.e441.
12. Kiserud T, Piaggio G, Carroli G, Widmer M, Carvalho J, Neerup Jensen L, et al. The World Health Organization fetal growth charts: a multinational longitudinal study of ultrasound biometric measurements and estimated fetal weight. PLoS Med. 2017;14:e1002220.
13. Stirnemann J, Villar J, Salomon LJ, Ohuma E, Ruyan P, Altman DG, et al. International estimated fetal weight standards of the INTERGROWTH-21(st) Project. Ultrasound Obstet Gynecol. 2017;49:478–86.
14. Grantz KL, Hediger ML, Liu D, Buck Louis GM. Fetal growth standards: the NICHD fetal growth study approach in context with INTERGROWTH-21st and the World Health Organization Multicentre Growth Reference Study. Am J Obstet Gynecol. 2018;218:S641–S655.e628.
15. Gardosi J, Chang A, Kalyan B, Sahota D, Symonds EM. Customised antenatal growth charts. Lancet. 1992;339:283–7.
16. Gardosi J, Mongelli M, Wilcox M, Chang A. An adjustable fetal weight standard. Ultrasound Obstet Gynecol. 1995;6:168–74.
17. Hadlock FP, Harrist RB, Martinez-Poyer J. In utero analysis of fetal growth: a sonographic weight standard. Radiology. 1991;181:129–33.
18. Gardosi J, Francis A, Turner S, Williams M. Customized growth charts: rationale, validation and clinical benefits. Am J Obstet Gynecol. 2018;218:S609–18.
19. Gardosi J, Madurasinghe V, Williams M, Malik A, Francis A. Maternal and fetal risk factors for stillbirth: population based study. BMJ. 2013;346:f108.
20. Chiossi G, Pedroza C, Costantine MM, Truong VT, Gargano G, Saade GR. Customized vs. population-based growth charts to identify neonates at risk of adverse outcome: systematic review and Bayesian meta-analysis of observational studies. Ultrasound Obstet Gynecol. 2017;50:156–66.
21. Ghi T, Cariello L, Rizzo L, Ferrazzi E, Periti E, Prefumo F, et al. Customized fetal growth charts for parents' characteristics, race, and parity by quantile regression analysis: a cross-sectional multicenter Italian study. J Ultrasound Med. 2016;35:83–92.

22. Ghi T, Prefumo F, Fichera A, Lanna M, Periti E, Persico N, et al. Development of customized fetal growth charts in twins. Am J Obstet Gynecol. 2017;216:514.e511–7.
23. Hiersch L, Melamed N. Fetal growth velocity and body proportion in the assessment of growth. Am J Obstet Gynecol. 2018;218:S700–11. e701
24. Deter RL, Harrist RB. Growth standards for anatomic measurements and growth rates derived from longitudinal studies of normal fetal growth. J Clin Ultrasound. 1992;20:381–8.
25. Deter RL, Rossavik IK, Harrist RB, Hadlock FP. Mathematic modeling of fetal growth: development of individual growth curve standards. Obstet Gynecol. 1986;68:156–61.
26. Tarca AL, Hernandez-Andrade E, Ahn H, Garcia M, Xu Z, Korzeniewski SJ, Set a. Single and serial fetal biometry to detect preterm and term small- and large-for-gestational-age neonates: a longitudinal cohort study. PLoS One. 2016;11:e0164161.
27. Deter RL. Individualized growth assessment: evaluation of growth using each fetus as its own control. Semin Perinatol. 2004;28:23–32.
28. Salomon LJ, Alfirevic Z, Berghella V, Bilardo C, Hernandez-Andrade E, Johnsen SL, et al. Practice guidelines for performance of the routine mid-trimester fetal ultrasound scan. Ultrasound Obstet Gynecol. 2011;37:116–26.
29. Stratton JF, Scanaill SN, Stuart B, Turner MJ. Are babies of normal birth weight who fail to reach their growth potential as diagnosed by ultrasound at increased risk? Ultrasound Obstet Gynecol. 1995;5:114–8.
30. Breeze AC, Lees CC. Prediction and perinatal outcomes of fetal growth restriction. Semin Fetal Neonatal Med. 2007;12:383–97.
31. Bricker L, Medley N, Pratt JJ. Routine ultrasound in late pregnancy (after 24 weeks' gestation). Cochrane Database Syst Rev. 2015;6:CD001451.
32. Gardosi J, Giddings S, Clifford S, Wood L, Francis A. Association between reduced stillbirth rates in England and regional uptake of accreditation training in customised fetal growth assessment. BMJ Open. 2013;3:e003942.
33. Fratelli N, Valcamonico A, Prefumo F, Pagani G, Guarneri T, Frusca T. Effects of antenatal recognition and follow-up on perinatal outcomes in small-for-gestational age infants delivered after 36 weeks. Acta Obstet Gynecol Scand. 2013;92:223–9.
34. Monier I, Blondel B, Ego A, Kaminiski M, Goffinet F, Zeitlin J. Poor effectiveness of antenatal detection of fetal growth restriction and consequences for obstetric management and neonatal outcomes: a French national study. BJOG. 2015;122:518–27.
35. Sovio U, White IR, Dacey A, Pasupathy D, Smith GCS. Screening for fetal growth restriction with universal third trimester ultrasonography in nulliparous women in the Pregnancy Outcome Prediction (POP) study: a prospective cohort study. Lancet. 2015;386:2089–97.
36. Roma E, Arnau A, Berdala R, Bergos C, Montesinos J, Figueras F. Ultrasound screening for fetal growth restriction at 36 vs 32 weeks' gestation: a randomized trial (ROUTE). Ultrasound Obstet Gynecol. 2015;46:391–7.

Doppler Diagnosis

10

Andrea Dall'Asta, Tullio Ghi, and Tiziana Frusca

Introduction

Fetal growth restriction (FGR) is a disorder affecting the fetal development and an acknowledged risk factor for poor neonatal condition at birth and impaired neurodevelopment and diseases such as hypertension, metabolic syndrome, and obesity in the adulthood [1–6].

FGR may be secondary to a number of other conditions which include congenital anomalies or genetic syndromes, intrauterine infections, and drug or substance misuse; however, most cases of FGR occur as a consequence of placental insufficiency leading to fetal hypoxia [7]. Currently, it is not possible to reverse the progressive nature of FGR; therefore, timed delivery remains the only effective intervention [7, 8].

FGR is currently subclassified into two entities, namely, early FGR and late FGR, which differ in terms of clinical manifestations, association with hypertension, Doppler features and patterns of deterioration, and severity of the placental dysfunction [7, 9–11] other than for the gestational age at diagnosis, which is conventionally set at or below 32 weeks for early FGR and beyond 32 weeks for late-onset FGR. As a general rule, early FGR is defined by fetal smallness and abnormal umbilical artery (UA) pulsatility index (PI) and shows a 60–70% association with hypertensive disorder or the pregnancy; on the other hand, late FGR is most commonly characterized by normal UA Doppler and only rarely co-existent with gestational hypertension or preeclampsia [7, 9].

Fetal adaptation to chronic placental insufficiency and hypoxia leads to the preferential diversion of the fetal cardiac output in favor of the left ventricle, which is ultimately responsible for the redirection of the fetal blood flow to the brain and the heart [12–14]. When fetal hypoxia worsens, adaptive mechanisms result in abnormal arterial and venous flow [15].

A. Dall'Asta · T. Ghi · T. Frusca (✉)
Department of Medicine and Surgery, Obstetrics and Gynecology Unit, University of Parma, Parma, Italy

L. M. M. Nardozza et al. (eds.), *Fetal Growth Restriction*,
https://doi.org/10.1007/978-3-030-00051-6_10

Fetal smallness is not a synonym of FGR as fetuses whose estimated fetal weight is below the 10th percentile for the given gestation may be constitutionally small but healthy and not necessarily growth restricted. These are defined as small for gestational age (SGA) fetuses. On the other hand, available evidence has suggested that an estimated fetal weight >10th percentile does not necessarily denote normal fetal growth, particularly at late gestation [16–19]. Therefore, FGR should be referred to fetuses with pathological smallness caused by an underlying functional problem, and hence a definition including not only a biometric cutoff but also Doppler indices of feto-placental function is currently agreed in most fetal medicine units [9, 16, 20, 21].

As stated by the Society for Maternal and Fetal Medicine, antenatal detection of FGR can improve outcomes by allowing selection of appropriate fetal surveillance and optimizing the timing of delivery [3].

Doppler ultrasound has become an essential tool in maternal and fetal medicine and particularly in the diagnosis and the surveillance of the growth-restricted fetus. Abnormalities of placental and fetal blood flows are a prominent feature of FGR caused by underlying placental dysfunction. In this chapter, we synthesize and assess the evidence-based role of the umbilical artery (UA), middle cerebral artery (MCA), ductus venosus (DV), and fetal cardiac Doppler in the diagnosis and monitoring of non-anomalous singleton fetuses with FGR of suspected placental origin.

Pathophysiology of Fetal Growth Restriction of Placental Origin

FGR is a complex process of adaptation of the growing fetus to the restricted metabolic supply of the placenta, unable to negotiate the full requirements of fetal genetic potential [20]. Each metabolic pathway, organ, and function reshapes a strategy to cope with this deprived environment [14].

Doppler assessment of the FGR fetus relies on the evaluation of the fetal well-being by examining hypoxemia-triggered compensatory signs in the fetal circulation. Available data suggest that there are in fact various patterns of Doppler deterioration occurring in a truly sequential manner, meaning that an initial abnormal Doppler finding is followed by another and another over time [22, 23]. In 2008, Turan et al. described "mild placental dysfunction," "progressive placental dysfunction," and "severe early-onset placental dysfunction" as three different patterns of Doppler deterioration in FGR [23]. These presumed sequences and their potential to anticipate fetal deterioration form the basis for Doppler diagnosis and surveillance in FGR. According to the most common of them (i.e., "progressive placental dysfunction"), which occurred in almost 50% of all cases, placental insufficiency results in increased resistance of the feto-placental unit and in compensatory hemodynamic changes which include blood flow redistribution toward essential fetal organs (brain, heart, and adrenal glands) at the expense of other organ systems [14, 23, 24]. This phenomenon is attributed to a "brain sparing" adaptive response of the cerebral blood vessels to the local effects of fetal hypoxemia with or without hypercapnia and is due to their autoregulatory capability to vasodilate in the event of reduced perfusion. As a result, decreased resistance to blood flow is found in the MCA.

These initial - "early" - changes are followed by elevations in venous Doppler indices. Abnormal DV Doppler waveforms either may be related to the vasodilatation of the isthmus of the DV, which is dependent on local mediators such as nitric oxide or prostaglandins [25], or may reflect an increased pressure in the right atrium as a result of the relative inability of the cardiac systolic function to overcome the increased peripheral resistance and the metabolic needs of the myocardium [26]. Therefore, DV flow abnormalities are regarded as "late" Doppler abnormalities which indicate that the adaptive mechanisms are overwhelmed and impending decompensation resulting in metabolic acidemia and cerebral hypoxia will shortly result in pathological fetal heart rate patterns and stillbirth [27–29].

It is important to note that the velocity of the Doppler deterioration as a sign of fetal adaptation to placental insufficiency varies depending on the gestational age [14]. This latter parameter is of paramount importance when considering the monitoring frequency, the administration of antenatal steroids and delivery [23].

Targets for Doppler Examination in the Fetus

Umbilical Artery

Umbilical artery Doppler allows the assessment of the resistance to blood perfusion of the feto-placental unit. Umbilical arteries are paired vessels carrying blood mostly pumped in the descending aorta by the right ventricle through the ductus arteriosus which obliterate after birth. The flow features of the umbilical artery can be assessed in a noninvasive qualitative manner using continuous or pulsed-wave Doppler ultrasound [30]. There is a significant difference in the impedance of the umbilical cord [31] – and therefore in the Doppler indices – at the fetal end, in the free loop, and at the placental end, being such impedance highest at the fetal end. Reference ranges for umbilical artery Doppler indices at these sites have been published [32, 33]. In clinical practice, Doppler waveforms of the umbilical artery can be obtained from any segment along the umbilical cord [3]; however, according to the International Guidelines, measurements of the Doppler indices of the umbilical artery should be made in a free cord loop in singletons [34]. Again, International Guidelines state that in multiple pregnancies and/or when comparing repeated measurements longitudinally, recordings from fixed sites, i.e., fetal end, placental end, or intra-abdominal portion, may be more reliable [34].

As a general rule for all Doppler measurements, the angle of correction is not necessary when measuring the PI; however, the angle of insonation should be <30 degrees, ideally as close to 0 degrees as possible. Additionally, Doppler indices should be obtained in the absence of fetal breathing and when the waveform is uniform [34].

Although there are other quantitative assessments of umbilical artery Doppler (e.g., resistance index) available, the systolic to diastolic (S/D) ratio and pulsatility index (PI) represent those most commonly used as they allow to manage most cases of suspected IUGR. Qualitatively, UA Doppler is assessed in terms of patterns of the end-diastolic flow (EDF), which is positive under normal circumstances; however, pathological increase of the vascular resistance caused by an obliteration of the placental vascular bed by over 50% progressively leads to absent EDF (AEDF) and reversed EDF (REDF) (Fig. 10.1).

Evaluation of placental function by UA Doppler has become a clinical standard to distinguish between SGA and FGR [7, 9, 16, 20]. Studies conducted on animal models and placental pathology have demonstrated that the obliteration of more than 50% of the placental vessels is required before absent or reversed end-diastolic velocities appear [35, 36]. On the other hand, small fetuses with normal UA Doppler are now considered as SGA or constitutionally small [16, 20, 21, 37, 38]. This may not be true for late-onset cases, in which a substantial proportion of cases with a normal UA have true FGR and are at risk of adverse perinatal outcome [39–42].

Umbilical artery Doppler is related to fetal acidemia [43] and is the only measure that provides both diagnostic and prognostic information for the management of FGR [44]. A Cochrane systematic review reported that the use of UA Doppler was associated with a reduction in perinatal deaths, inductions of labor, and cesarean deliveries [45]. According to the Royal College of Obstetricians and Gynecologists,

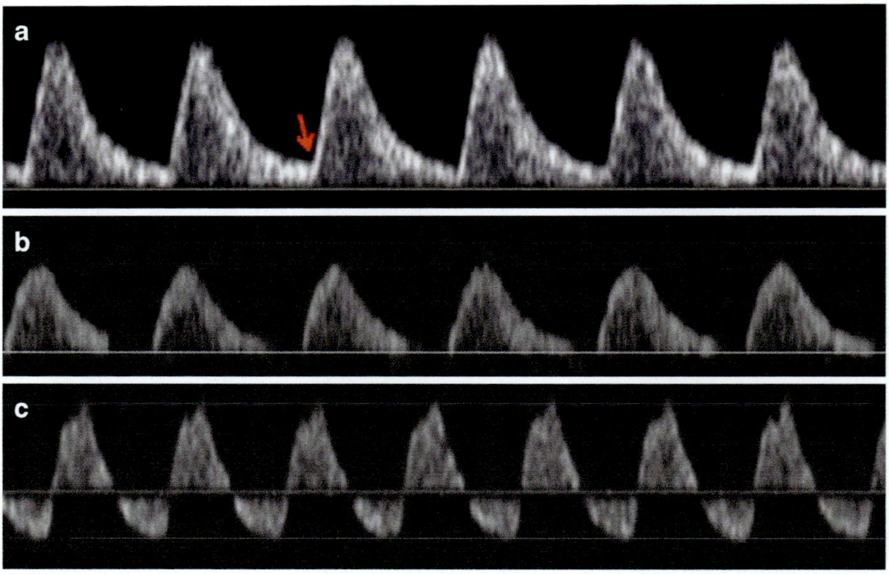

Fig. 10.1 Doppler assessment of the umbilical artery. (**a**) Umbilical artery Doppler showing high pulsatility index and positive end-diastolic flow (EDF, pointed by the arrow). (**b**) Umbilical artery Doppler with absent end-diastolic flow (AEDF). (**c**) Umbilical artery Doppler showing reverse end-diastolic flow (REDF)

the use of UA Doppler in a high-risk population reduces perinatal morbidity and mortality and should be the primary surveillance tool in the SGA fetus [46].

Umbilical artery flow identifies different degrees of impaired placental function. Absent end-diastolic flow (AEDF) and/or reversed end-diastolic flow (REDF), often considered a unique entity as absent/reversed end-diastolic flow (AREDF), indicate an important reduction of the function of the placenta. Longitudinal studies on high-risk pregnancies have shown that the transition from AEDF to REDF may be slow and gradual. AEDF can last for days and weeks before abnormal heart rate pattern or delivery [47], while REDF, which represents an extreme abnormality in waveform, has been related to a significant perinatal morbidity and mortality [47, 48] and to a higher incidence of long-term permanent neurologic damage compared to FGR fetuses with positive EDF [7, 49]. Absent or reversed EDF are mostly found in early FGR, and these patterns have been reported to be present on average 1 week before acute fetal deterioration. Up to 40% of fetuses with acidosis show this umbilical flow pattern [50]. Despite the fact that an association exists between the presence of REDF in the umbilical artery and adverse perinatal outcome (with a sensitivity and specificity of about 60%), it is not clear whether this association is confounded by prematurity [7]. Absent or reversed EDF in the umbilical artery is commonly associated with severe FGR with birthweight <3rd percentile for gestational age and oligohydramnios [3].

Middle Cerebral Artery

The middle cerebral arteries (MCAs) are two of the major branches of the circle of Willis and carry >80% of the cerebral circulation in the fetus [3, 34]. The MCAs are the most accessible cerebral vessels for ultrasound imaging in the fetus and can be sampled on an axial section of the brain including the thalami and the sphenoid bone wings [3, 34]. Color flow mapping should be used to identify the circle of Willis, and Doppler sampling should be performed at the proximal third of the MCA in order to obtain the best reproducibility [34, 51] (Fig. 10.2).

Under normal conditions, the cerebral circulation is characterized by high impedance and shows high PI with continuous forward flow present throughout the cardiac cycle [52]. A reduction of the PI of the MCA identifies a process of adaptation by vasodilatation which is known as the "brain sparing effect" and has been associated with adverse fetal and perinatal outcome and suboptimal neurodevelopment at 2 years of age not only in early severe FGR flagged by an abnormal umbilical arterial PI but also in late and term FGR fetuses with normal UA PI [42, 53–55]. Despite these associations, available data have shown that cerebral Doppler is not useful for the diagnosis and the management in early FGR [56]. As regards late FGR, a potential role of MCA Doppler for the differential diagnosis between SGA and late FGR has been demonstrated [57–60]. Nevertheless, MCA Doppler testing of suspected late FGR fetuses has not been evaluated in randomized trials, and to date no specific intervention has been shown to improve outcomes based on abnormal findings [3].

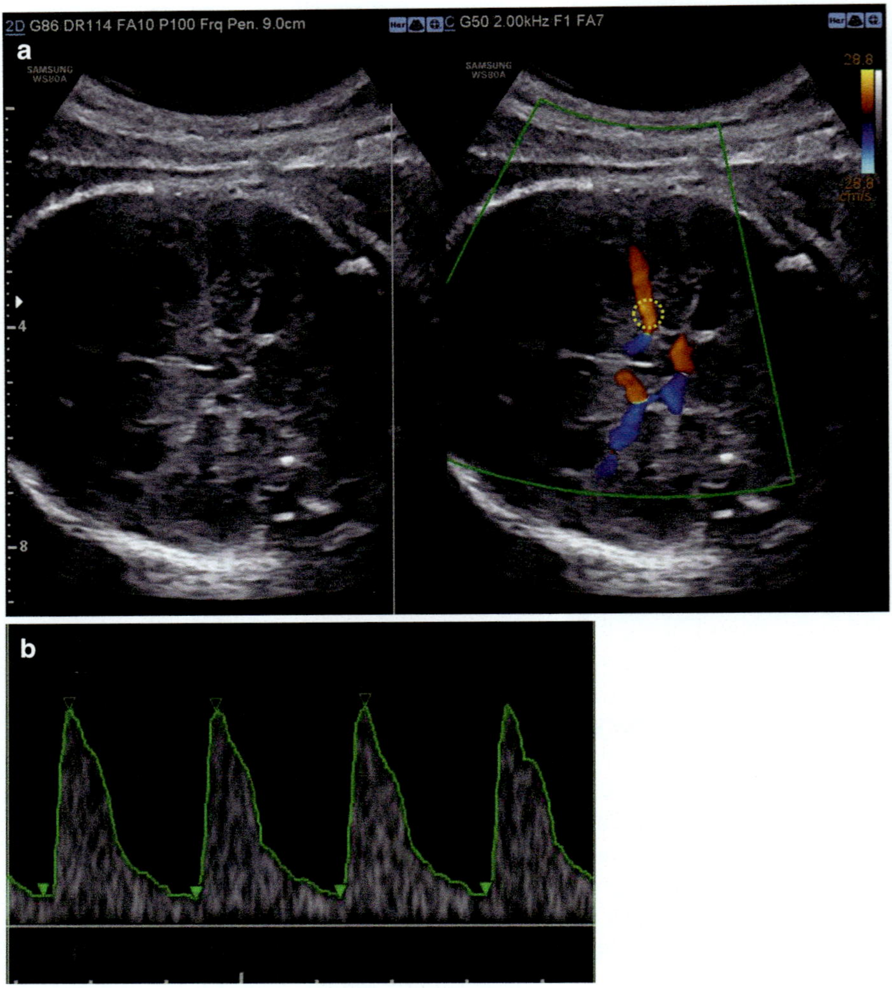

Fig. 10.2 Doppler assessment of the middle cerebral artery (MCA). (**a**) On gray-scale ultrasound, the MCA can be sampled on an axial section of the brain including the thalami and the sphenoid bone wings (left). Color flow mapping can identify the circle of Willis (right). Doppler sampling should be performed at the proximal third of the MCA (circled) in order to obtain the best reproducibility. (**b**) Normal MCA Doppler waveform showing low diastolic flow suggestive of high intracerebral resistance

MCA Doppler can be combined with the UA Doppler in the cerebroplacental ratio (CPR), also named as cerebro-umbilical (C-U) ratio; the umbilico-cerebral (U-C) ratio represents an inverted ratio of the same parameters and is suggested to be a better discriminator within the context of abnormal findings [56]. The cerebroplacental ratio (CPR) quantifies the redistribution of cardiac output by dividing the Doppler indices of the MCA with that of the UA. This ratio has been demonstrated to be more sensitive to hypoxia than its individual components on their own and to better correlate with adverse outcome in SGA/FGR fetuses [61, 62] but also in apparently normally grown fetuses close to term [17–19, 63, 64]. Recent data suggest that reduced CPR together with uterine artery (UtA) Doppler represents the parameters which allow a differential diagnosis between SGA and late FGR fetuses with normal UA Doppler [42, 57–60].

Ongoing and planned trials are likely to provide further insights into the actual role of the cerebral Doppler – on its own or paired with UA within the context of the CPR or the U-C ratio – in the management of late FGR, particularly clarifying whether anticipating delivery based on abnormal CPR findings may improve the neurodevelopmental outcome in the infanthood (http://www.truffle-study.org/research/).

Ductus Venosus

The ductus venosus (DV) is one of the three arterial-to-venous shunts existing in fetal life and is responsible for the diversion of well-oxygenated blood from the umbilical vein to the inferior vena cava and the right atrium, thus bypassing the intrahepatic vascular system. Anatomically the DV consists in a narrow inlet whose diameter may vary depending upon local mediators such as nitric oxide and prostaglandins, thus determining a variation in the percentage of blood shunted through the DV. Under normal circumstances, the DV diverts a percentage of venous blood ranging between 30% at midgestation and 15% at term pregnancy; however, FGR is associated with increased ductus venosus (DV) shunting. Among the precordial vessels available for Doppler assessment in FGR fetuses (the others are represented by the inferior vena cava and the umbilical vein), the DV represents the most important one both for prognostic and diagnostic purposes in early FGR fetuses as demonstrated by the results of the TRUFFLE study [9, 65–69].

The DV can be visualized both with gray-scale ultrasound and with color or power Doppler either in a midsagittal or a transverse section of the fetal abdomen as a narrow vessel arising from the umbilical vein and a vertical oblique course to the inferior vena cava just below the diaphragm. Color flow mapping at its isthmic portion demonstrates the high velocity with "aliasing" at the narrow entrance of the DV and indicates the standard sampling site for Doppler measurements [3, 34].

Continuous forward flow throughout the cardiac cycle is seen in the normal fetus [3, 34, 72]. The correct sampling of the DV most commonly determines a biphasic waveform constituted by the "S" component, which represents the first increase in venous forward velocities as a result of the ventricular systole; the "D" component, which represents the second peak of velocity occurring during the passive ventricular filling of the ventricular diastole of the cardiac cycle; and finally the "A" component representing the late ventricular filling dependent on the atrial contraction which occurs in the late diastole of the cardiac cycle [3, 34] (Fig. 10.3). Rarely, non-pulsating recordings may be seen in healthy fetuses [34]. The DV Doppler can be assessed quantitatively by means of the DV PI, which is low under normal circumstances and increases as a result of the vasodilatation of the isthmus of the DV

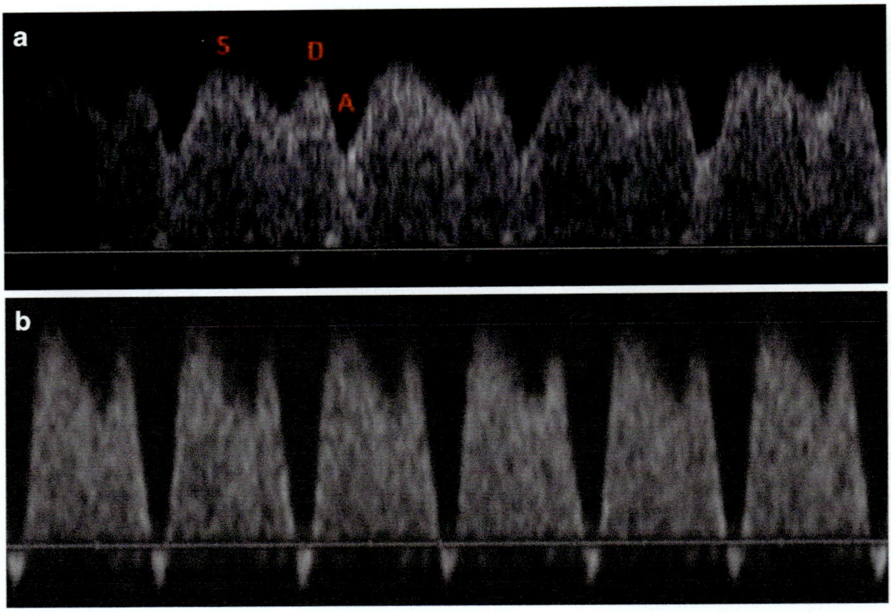

Fig. 10.3 Doppler assessment of the ductus venosus (DV). (**a**) DV showing biphasic waveform characterized by an "S" component, which corresponds to the ventricular systole; a "D" component, which represents the second peak of velocity occurring during the passive ventricular filling of the ventricular diastole of the cardiac cycle; and a late diastole "A" component corresponding to the late ventricular filling dependent on the atrial contraction. In (**b**) reversed "A-" wave at 30 weeks

and of cardiac dysfunction both in terms of increased preload and afterload resistance. Qualitative evaluation of the DV Doppler includes the assessment of the "A" component of the waveform which in the case of decreased, absent, or reversed flow represents myocardial impairment and increased ventricular end-diastolic pressure resulting from an increase in right ventricular afterload. This abnormal waveform in the ductus venosus has been documented in FGR fetuses and linked to increased neonatal mortality rate [71, 72]. A semiquantitative evaluation of the DV Doppler has also been suggested; however, there is no evidence-based data supporting its usefulness for the management of early or late FGR fetuses [73].

There is no available data on DV Doppler in late FGR fetuses. As regards early FGR, evidence from the Trial of Randomized Umbilical and Fetal Flow in Europe (TRUFFLE study) has shown the crucial role of DV Doppler for the management of preterm growth-restricted fetuses before 32 weeks of gestation [9, 65–69]. In contrast to the alterations of the UA and the MCA Doppler, which represent early signs of impaired placental function, DV flow waveforms become abnormal only in advanced stages of fetal compromise [27, 74, 75]. It has been shown that the PI of the DV is related to acidemia at cordocentesis [28] and low pH at birth, being the DV PI inversely related to the UA pH at birth [76]. Absence or reversal of the DV "A-wave" represent signs of late adaptation to chronic hypoxia and impending decompensation similar to the REDF in the umbilical artery. In 2001, Hecher et al.

described the time sequence of changes in fetal monitoring variables in early FGR and demonstrated that DV Doppler and short-term variation (STV) of fetal heart rate, which can be measured by means of computerized cardiotocography (cCTG), are important indicators for the optimal timing of delivery before 32 weeks of gestation [27]. More recent data have shown high specificity of the absence or reversal of the DV A-wave for the prediction of low UA pH at birth [24] and significant association with perinatal death regardless of the gestational age at delivery [76]. These findings were confirmed by the results of the TRUFFLE study [9, 65–69].

Cardiac Function in Fetal Growth Restriction: Rationale for the Doppler Investigation of the Fetal Heart

During fetal life, the right and the left ventricles work in parallel and have independent outputs, with a right ventricular dominance [13]. As a result of the "early" changes described by the most common pattern of Doppler deterioration occurring in FGR fetuses, which we have detailed, increased umbilical resistance leads to an increase in the right ventricular afterload. Conversely, the onset of the "brain sparing" effect leads to a reduction in left ventricular afterload leading to a preferential shift of the cardiac output to the left ventricle and hence to the brain and to the coronary vessels arising from the ascending aorta.

Other than the "brain sparing effect," additional evidence has shown an increase in the coronary flow in FGR fetuses which was called the "heart-sparing effect" [77]. Such increased blood supply, together with the intrinsic mechanisms responsible for the autoregulation of the coronary flow - which are dependent upon the relative concentrations of oxygen and carbon dioxide, hydrogen ions, potassium, lactate, adenosine, and other metabolites and are activated in cases of chronic hypoxia such as FGR [77] - seem to explain why the coronary vessels can be imaged at earlier gestation in FGR fetuses compared to normally grown ones [78]. Nevertheless, no quantitative comparisons of the coronary flow between FGR and normal fetuses have been undertaken, and no prospective evaluation of the coronary flow in FGR and its correlation with Doppler and infant outcomes has been performed.

Following cerebral – and cardiac – redistribution, no further blood shifting occurs; however, a longitudinal reduction in the cardiac output occurs as a result of worsening hypoxia which leads to a progressive increase both of the left and the right ventricular afterload as well as an increased venous return from the superior vena cava secondary to the "brain sparing" process. These ultimately increase the filling pressure of the right atrium and lead to the Doppler abnormalities of the DV [25, 26]. Such scenario of progressive systolic and diastolic overload in fact represents a continuum of abnormal filling and emptying pressures which need to be overcome by the fetal heart of the growth-restricted fetus, and it seems reasonable to hypothesize that different steps of cardiac overload are responsible for the three different phenotypes of morphological remodeling of the fetal heart in FGR which have been very recently described [79].

Based on these assumptions, the analysis of fetal cardiac function in FGR might provide important information on the hemodynamic status and the cardiovascular adaptation of the fetus and help in the differential diagnosis between FGR and SGA [80]. A broad range of US techniques have been applied for evaluation of fetal cardiac function, and several fetal myocardial functional parameters have been evaluated and suggested as potentially useful within the context of fetal smallness. Nevertheless, their use in early and late FGR is not supported by any clinical evidence, and today none of them leads to changes in the perinatal management compared to the "conventional" assessment of peripheral arteries and the venous system [81].

Doppler of the Aortic Isthmus

The aortic isthmus (AoI) is the segment of the aorta located between the origin of the left subclavian artery and the connection of the ductus arteriosus to the descending aorta. The AoI is the only arterial connection between the right ventricle, which supplies mainly the systemic and placental circulations, and the left ventricle, which supplies essentially the cerebral vascular network [8, 82]; therefore, its blood flow pattern reflects the balance between ventricular outputs and the relative difference in vascular impedance in either vascular system. The rationale for the Doppler assessment of the AoI is represented by the fact that during diastole, when the aortic and pulmonary valves are closed, the direction of blood flow in the AoI solely reflects the differences between the downstream impedances of the right (mainly placental vascular resistance) and left (mainly cerebral vascular resistance) ventricles [8].

The AoI can be visualized using gray-scale (B-mode) ultrasound either on the longitudinal view of the aortic arch or on the cross-sectional view of the upper thorax at the level of the three-vessel/trachea views [83, 84] (Fig. 10.4). Once the vascular segment is identified, pulsed-wave Doppler velocimetry can be performed after the adjustment of the size of the sample gate according to the size of the AoI, which is dependent upon gestational age [85].

Antenatal Doppler study of the AoI includes the quantitative assessment of the peak systolic (PSV), end-diastolic (EDV), and time-averaged maximum (TAMXV) velocities through the AoI itself; the semiquantitative evaluation of the PI and/or of the isthmic flow index (IFI), which was devised in order to include the amount and direction of blood flow and is computed as (PSV + EDV)/PSV [86]; and the qualitative description of antegrade or retrograde flow [87–90]. Under normal conditions, AoI velocity waveforms show antegrade flow during systole and diastole because the placental resistances are lower than those present in the fetal upper body. The normal waveform of the AoI is characterized by a quick systolic upstroke (short acceleration time) with mean peak systolic velocities ranging between 30 and 100 cm/s followed by a more gradual deceleration of the velocity and a narrow incisura at the end of systole, which is usually absent before 20 weeks of gestation. Retrograde flow during diastole or net blood flow

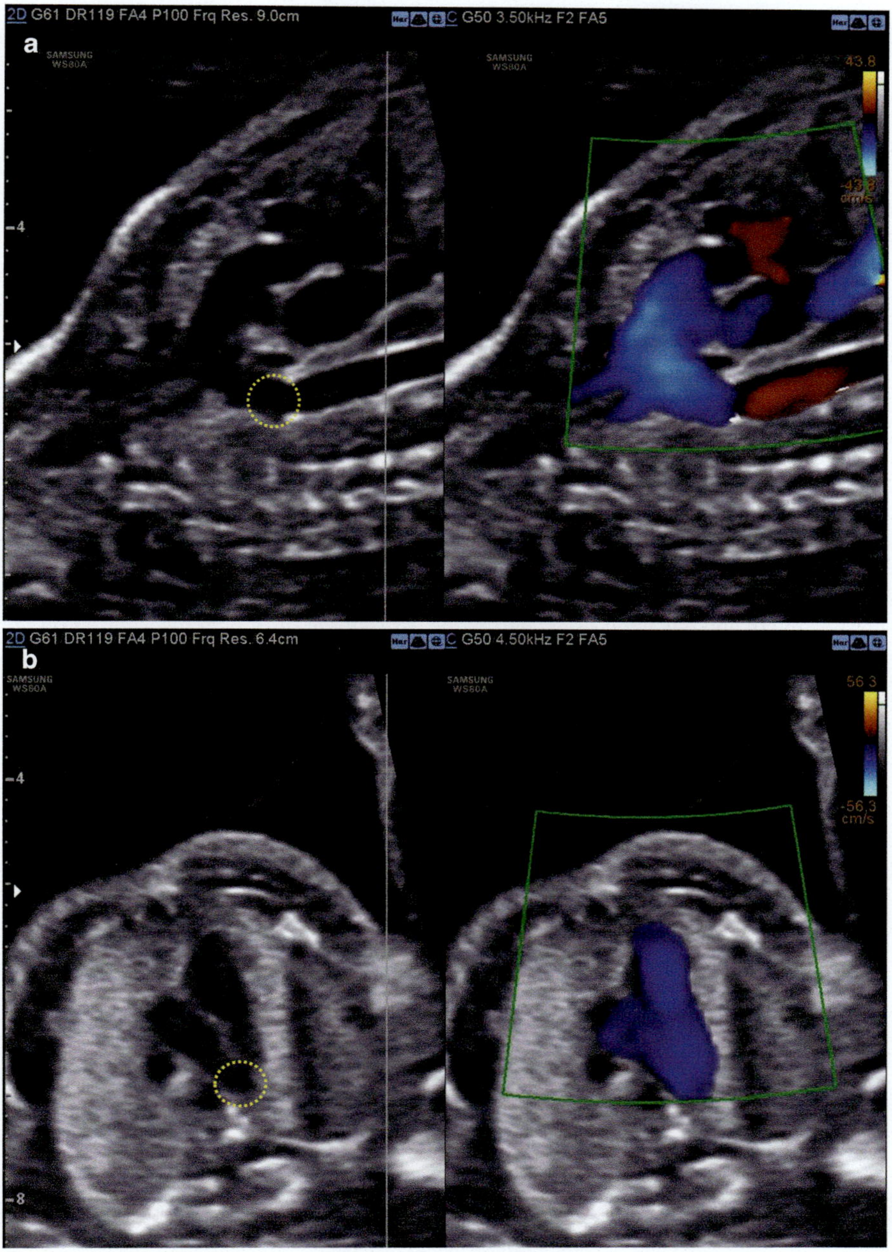

Fig. 10.4 Gray-scale (B-mode) and color Doppler imaging of the aortic isthmus (circled) on the longitudinal view of the aortic arch (**a**) and on the cross-sectional view of the upper thorax at the level of the three-vessel/trachea view (**b**)

reversal is always abnormal and can be observed in the case of chronic placental insufficiency associated with increased peripheral resistance and vasodilatation of the cerebral circulation.

As before mentioned, in the absence of randomized or prospective data, there is no role for the Doppler of the AoI for the diagnosis and the monitoring of early or late FGR. Even though from a pathophysiology point of view it is reasonable to hypothesize a relationship between the Doppler indices through the AoI and UA and DV Doppler features as a consequence of the changes in peripheral and cerebral resistances, controversial results have emerged from the studies evaluating such correlations [82, 89, 91, 92]. Regarding postnatal assessment, available data suggest an association between adverse perinatal outcome and neurodevelopmental deficits and abnormal Doppler recordings in the AoI in terms of predominant reversed diastolic blood flow and IFI <0.70 with net reversed diastolic flow through the AoI [82], even though this relationship has shown a low sensitivity [93].

E/A Ratio

Doppler ultrasound allows the evaluation of the diastolic component of the fetal cardiac cycle and has been suggested in the assessment of FGR fetuses based on the assumption that increased afterload and chronic hypoxia ultimately lead to increased preload and impairment of the diastolic function in the case of advanced fetal compromise.

The E/A ratio is one of the parameters suggested for the evaluation of the cardiac diastolic function in the fetus. It is defined by the ratio between the E (early or passive) velocity, which is measured during the early passive ventricular filling and is related to the process of myocardial relaxation and negative pressure applied by the ventricles, and the A (atrial, active, or late) velocity, which represents the active ventricular filling during atrial contraction.

The E/A ratio can be measured by evaluating the transmitral or the transtricuspidal waveforms obtained with pulsed-wave Doppler and continuous wave Doppler. Recordings are obtained at the level of the four-chamber view of the fetal heart, in which the Doppler sample gate is located just below either atrioventricular valve, where a biphasic waveform is usually displayed in the normal fetus (Fig. 10.5). It is recommended to keep the Doppler sample gate between 2 and 3 mm in order to avoid contamination with artifacts from wall motion and from the outflow tracts. The biphasic nature of the E/A waveform is lost if the Doppler gate is located too deep within the ventricle. There are some mild differences between both sides of the heart which are constantly observed in all normal pregnancies as the right E and A waveforms have higher velocities and their ratio is slightly lower than that of the left side [94]. Recordings must be performed in the absence of fetal breathing and without maternal and fetal movements.

Uncomplicated pregnancies show a progressive increase of the E/A ratio across gestation [95]. Conversely, in SGA fetuses the E/A ratio does not increase, and its values are significantly lower than in normal fetuses. A reduced E/A ratio indicates

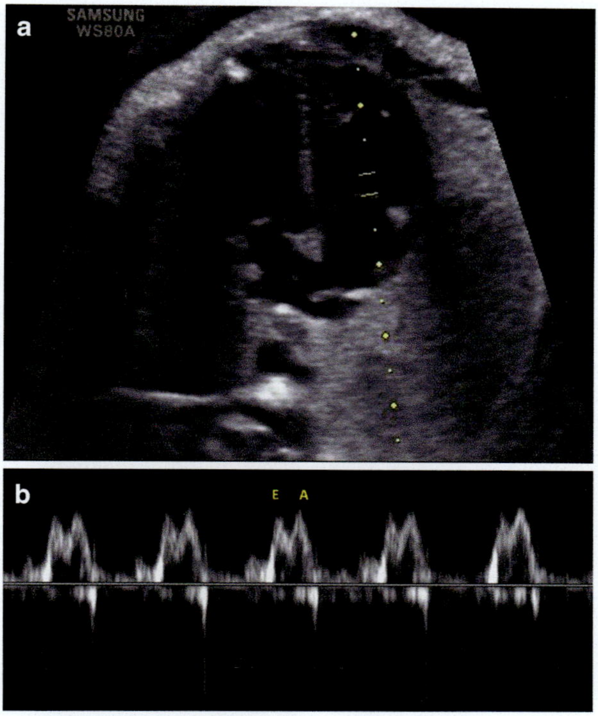

Fig. 10.5 Pulsed-wave Doppler assessment of the E/A ratio at the level of the tricuspid valve. (**a**) Four-chamber view of the fetal heart, in which the Doppler sample gate is located just below the tricuspid valve. (**b**) Biphasic waveform which is displayed in the normal fetus, representing the passive ventricular filling in early diastole (E component) and the active ventricular filling ("A," atrial, active, or late component) which occurs during atrial contraction

that the process of ventricular filling depends more on the atrial contraction than on the negative pressure during relaxation. The two main conditions affecting the ratios - i.e. chronic hypoxia and cardiac overload - might affect the relaxation process, thus reducing the E/A ratios. On a small cohort of FGR fetuses, Figueras et al. reported lower E/A ratios in both atrioventricular valves compared to normally grown fetuses with early deterioration of the right E/A ratio [96]. More recent data suggested that there is a "continuum" in the deterioration of the E/A ratio, with monophasic diastolic waves associated with abnormalities in all prenatal cardiac parameters in fetuses with severe FGR who eventually died or developed neurological damage [97]. However, this observation was not confirmed in prospective studies; therefore, to date there is no clinical role for the E/A ratio in the diagnosis and management of FGR fetuses.

Myocardial Performance Index

The myocardial performance index (MPI) – also named as Tei index – is a parameter that reflects both systolic and diastolic functions as the sum of the isovolumetric contraction time (ICT) and isovolumetric relaxation time (IRT) divided by the ejection time (EJT): (ICT + IRT)/EJT [98].

The MPI can be measured either with pulsed-wave (PW) or tissue Doppler technique. From a cross-sectional view of the fetal thorax, recordings must be performed from the four-chamber view of the heart with an apical projection and an angle of insonation below 20°. Using PW Doppler, a sample gate of about 3–4 mm needs to be placed to include both the lateral wall of the ascending aorta and the mitral valve where the clicks corresponding to the opening and closing of the two valves can be clearly visualized [99]. This allows the sampling of the E/A and of the aortic ejection waveforms. The isovolumetric contraction time (ICT), ejection time (ET), and isovolumetric relaxation time (IRT) can be calculated using the clicks of the mitral and aortic valves as landmarks as shown in Fig. 10.6. Briefly, the isovolumetric contraction time (ICT, ms) represents the time from closure of the mitral valve to the opening of the aortic valve; the isovolumetric relaxation time (IRT, ms) represents the time from closure of the aortic valve to the opening of mitral valve; the ejection time (ET, ms) or systolic time interval represents the time from opening of the aortic valve to its closure. Using Tissue Doppler technique, the MPI can be measured by placing a 2–3 mm pulsed-wave gate in the basal part of the left and right ventricular free walls (at the level of the mitral and tricuspid valve annulus, respectively). Peak annular velocities need to be measured during early diastole (E), atrial contraction (A), and systole (S) and provide the same waveform landmarks used with PW

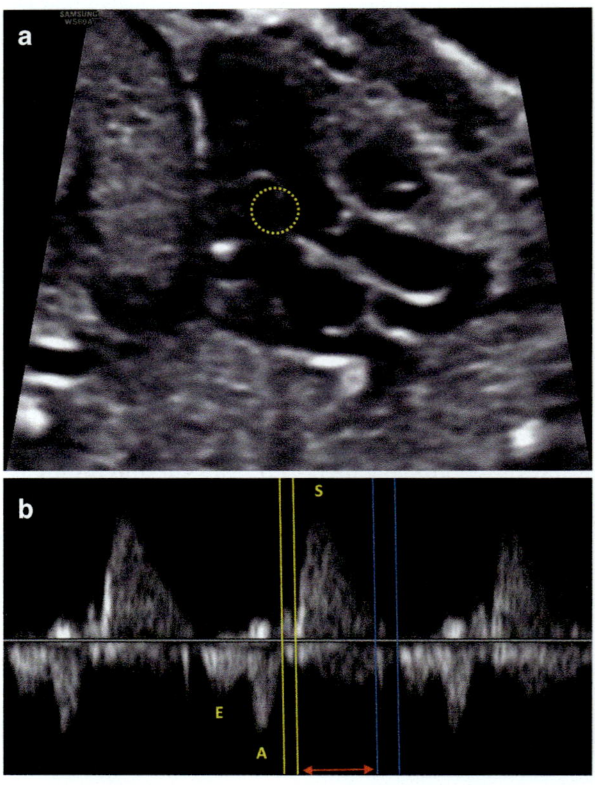

Fig. 10.6 Pulsed-wave Doppler assessment of the myocardial performance index (MPI). (**a**) Recordings must be performed from the four-chamber view of the heart with an apical projection of the heart; the sample gate needs to be placed to include both the lateral wall of the ascending aorta in order to sample the E/A and the aortic ejection (S) waveforms (circled in yellow). (**b**) The isovolumetric contraction time (ICT) (comprised between the yellow lines), ejection time (ET) (red arrow), and isovolumetric relaxation time (IRT) (comprised between the blue lines) are calculated using the clicks of the mitral and aortic valves as landmarks

Doppler. Using either technique, measurements of all the components need to be obtained from the same cardiac cycle.

A significantly higher MPI in FGR compared to appropriately grown fetuses was demonstrated by Hassan et al. [100]. Raised MPI is seen in the early stages of cardiac adaptation to FGR, presumably secondary to hypoxia, and remains elevated throughout the different stages of deterioration in FGR deterioration, similarly to the AoI and DV PI. Available evidence from longitudinal studies has demonstrated that an abnormal increase of the MPI can be detected prior to the UA Doppler becoming abnormal [93] and showing absent or reversed end-diastolic blood flow [101].

The finding of increased MPI has been suggested as a potential discriminator between FGR and SGA in fetuses showing reduced biometry but normal Doppler [102, 103]. Hernandez-Andrade et al. suggested that the combination of these parameters might be useful for defining the monitoring strategy and the optimal time of delivery [104]; however, there is no evidence-based strategy including the MPI among the parameters for the monitoring of FGR fetuses.

Maternal Doppler and Fetal Growth Restriction

Doppler Examination of the Uterine Arteries

Uterine arteries are paired vessels responsible for the blood supply of the uterus in the nonpregnant state and of the uterus and the feto-placental unit during pregnancy. These vessels, whose impedance is physiologically elevated with low diastolic flow in the nonpregnant state, undergo major anatomic and functional adaptation during pregnancy as a result of the trophoblastic invasion of the maternal spiral arterioles – named as "remodeling" – in the first half of gestation. Under normal conditions, a sharp decrease in uterine artery (UtA) impedance to flow occurs as placental implantation progresses, which is reflected by the increased flow in diastole and disappearance of the notch present in the nonpregnant UtA [105, 106]. The "remodeling" of the spiral arteries is usually completed by 24 weeks, and indeed less prominent changes in UtA Doppler occur in the third trimester.

While absolute velocities have been of little or no clinical importance, semiquantitative (PI) and qualitative assessment of the velocity waveforms is commonly evaluated. Qualitatively, the persistence of the protodiastolic "notch" of the a uterine artery Doppler waveform in the late second and third trimesters has been used to identify abnormal uterine circulation in pregnancy (Fig. 10.7) [71, 107]. Caution, however, should be used against relying solely on the presence of a notch in the uterine artery Doppler waveform to define an abnormal uterine circulation as clinicians should consider also the semiquantitative measurement of the PI, with a value >95th percentile for gestational age considered abnormal [108].

Different techniques for the assessment of the UtA Doppler have been described for the first vs the second and third trimesters [34]; however, FGR of placental origin manifests as early as the second trimester. From this gestation, UtA can be

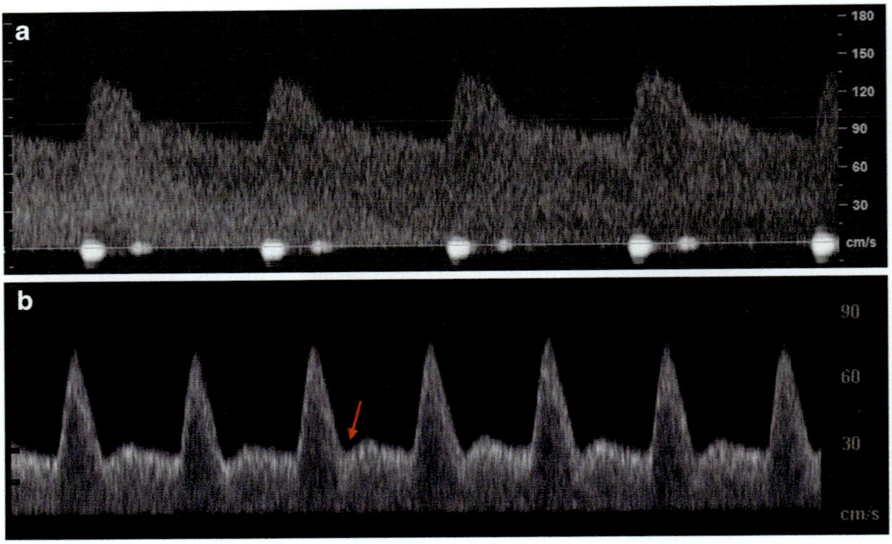

Fig. 10.7 Doppler assessment of the uterine artery Doppler. (**a**) Normal waveform showing high diastolic flow and absent notch. (**b**) Abnormal waveform showing low diastolic flow with notching (arrow)

visualized either transabdominally or transvaginally. Different reference ranges have been published for each approach [109, 110]; however, given its high accuracy and reproducibility, the transabdominal approach is performed unless a transvaginal scan is deemed as necessary for other reasons [111]. Transabdominally, the probe needs to be placed longitudinally in the lower lateral quadrant of the abdomen, angled medially. The UtA can be demonstrated by color Doppler velocimetry as it originates from the anterior division of the hypogastric artery and just before it enters the uterus at the uterine-cervical junction. Pulsed Doppler velocimetry of the uterine artery should be obtained 1 cm downstream from the crossover point between the UtA and the hypogastric artery and before the UtA divides into the uterine and cervical branches [3, 34]. In a small proportion of cases the uterine artery branches before the intersection of the external iliac artery and the sample volume should be placed on the artery just before the bifurcation of the uterine artery.

Abnormal UtA Doppler best identifies the severe early-onset complications of impaired placentation. The systematic review and meta-analysis conducted by Cnossen et al. in 2008 further demonstrated the role of UtA Doppler ultrasonography as a predictor of FGR, particularly when performed in the second trimester and particularly for early FGR [107]. It is important to note that there is a continuum of Doppler abnormality of the UtA ranging from mild increase of the PI above the 95th percentile for the gestation to severe abnormality of the PI with bilateral protodiastolic notching, which seems to impact on the likelihood of complications during the index pregnancy.

There is also evidence that a high impedance to flow in the uterine arteries during the third trimester is associated with an increased risk of adverse perinatal events regardless of fetal size in pregnancies with normal UA Doppler [113–115], thus supporting the concept that abnormally raised UtA PI in the third trimester may help in discriminating between SGA and late FGR, as discussed later in this chapter [57, 58, 116].

Maternal Hemodynamics and Fetal Growth Restriction

Placental perfusion and function are among the determinants of the intrauterine growth of the fetus, the remaining being represented by the intrinsic growth potential of the fetus. In the last decade, great interest has arisen toward maternal cardiovascular function in order to understand how placental perfusion is sustained under normal circumstances [117, 118] and which are the features of suboptimal hemodynamic adaptation to the pregnancy. This research field, which traditionally relies on dedicated cardiology evaluation by means of echocardiography, has been further implemented with the advent of novel semiautomated devices such as the ultrasound cardiac output monitor (USCOM) [119–121], which allows the measurements of the cardiac systolic parameters by means of pulsed-wave Doppler.

Normal pregnancy is characterized by a longitudinal increase of the cardiac output (CO) which is coupled with a reduction of the systemic vascular resistance (SVR). According to the historical pathophysiology theory, hypertensive disorders of the pregnancy (HDP) are secondary to impaired placental function as a result of suboptimal remodeling of the spiral arteries, which precludes the reduction of the resistance of the uterine circulation, which is characterized by high resistance in the nonpregnant state and in early pregnancy, into a low resistance circulation. Such abnormality of the implantation process can also explain FGR within the context of HDP [122, 123]. Nevertheless, available evidence has shown that placental pathology does not invariably demonstrate the obliteration of the placental villi in preeclampsia, particularly at late gestation [124], and fetal size is not invariably small in preeclampsia [125].

As early as 2008, Valensise et al., within a cohort of women identified at risk of HDP based on abnormal midtrimester uterine artery Doppler, demonstrated the existence of two different hemodynamic patterns in the context of preeclampsia, the former, which was eventually defined as "early" preeclampsia, being associated with reduced CO, increased systemic vascular resistance SVR, and small fetal size, and the latter, named as "late preeclampsia," showing the opposite hemodynamic pattern and associated with normal size or large fetuses [126]. This hypothesis of the existence of two phenotypes of preeclampsia associated with specular incidence of FGR and large for gestational age has been further supported Verlohren et al. [127].

Other authors have suggested that placenta should not be considered in isolation without regard to the fact that its function is dependent on the perfusion by the maternal circulation [128]. Low CO and high SVR represent the hemodynamic surrogates of abnormal cardiovascular adaptation to the pregnancy with placental underperfusion, and it is not surprising that both of them have been related to FGR

[129]. Very recently Ferrazzi et al. suggested that the presence or the absence of FGR may represent a better discriminator than gestational age at onset of the two different phenotypes of preeclampsia, the "early preeclampsia" one being associated with FGR and the "late preeclampsia" one being related with normal or increased fetal size [130]. It is important to point out that all the above represent research findings with no acknowledged role in the diagnosis or in the management of FGR; however, these data suggest that the assessment of the maternal cardiovascular function during pregnancy may become a reliable tool for a pathophysiology approach for the diagnosis and the treatment of conditions of abnormal placental function such as HDP and FGR.

How to Diagnose Early and Late Fetal Growth Restriction

A prerequisite for the correct diagnosis of FGR is accurate dating of the pregnancy, ideally in the first trimester [131]. Furthermore, based on the assumption that fetal size is influenced by ethnicity, sex, parity, maternal size, and genetic factors, antenatal growth charts customized for maternal characteristics have been developed in order to improve the detection of abnormalities of the fetal growth [132–136]. Such approach has recently been challenged by the results from the Intergrowth study, which has shown that fetal growth patterns do not seem to be influenced by ethnic factors in healthy pregnancies under optimal environmental conditions [137]. Additionally, the quantitative comparison of the published fetal growth charts shows minimal differences which are unlikely to be of clinical impact. There is currently no evidence that routine use of customized growth charts can improve the detection and clinical outcomes in early FGR, in which the underlying severe placental dysfunction is almost invariably associated with fetal smallness and Doppler abnormalities. On the other hand, some authors suggest that a customized approach may improve the detection of third trimester SGA fetuses with normal UA Doppler but at risk of perinatal complications, although this is not widely agreed and does not represent the standard of care [132, 133, 135].

Multiple definitions of FGR have been suggested over the decades by national and international societies which have been summarized in Table 10.1 [20]. As it can be noted, most of them do not distinguish between early and late FGR; however, current thinking on the natural history of FGR differentiates these two types of FGR in terms of biochemical, histological, and clinical features and not only in terms of gestational age at diagnosis, which is conventionally set at or below 32 weeks for early FGR and beyond 32 weeks for late-onset FGR.

An EFW <10th percentile is acknowledged as the best clinical surrogate of FGR [138]. However, it is important to point out that EFW below the 10th centile for the gestation, albeit being diagnostic for fetal smallness, does not necessarily implies FGR, particularly when detected beyond 32 weeks [20, 21]. According to the criteria recently agreed through a Delphi procedure by a panel of International Fetal Medicine experts, early FGR is defined either by severe fetal smallness (EFW or AC <3rd centile) or "late" UA Doppler abnormalities (AEDF, REDF) taken in isolation or by a combination of fetal smallness and UA PI above the 95th percentile for

Table 10.1 Fetal growth restriction definition in recent literature

Institution/author	FGR definition
Baschat et al. 2007	Combination of small fetal abdominal circumference (AC) with elevated umbilical artery Doppler blood flow resistance
Cochrane 2013	Failure to reach the growth potential
DIGITAT 2012	Estimated fetal weight or an abdominal circumference below the 10th centile for gestational age
ACOG 2013	Fetuses with an estimated fetal weight that is less than the 10th percentile for gestational age
RCOG 2013	Small for gestational age (SGA) refers to an infant born with a birthweight less than the 10th centile Fetal growth restriction (FGR) is not synonymous with SGA
SOGC 2013	Intrauterine growth restriction refers to a fetus with an estimated fetal weight <10th percentile on ultrasound that, because of a pathologic process, has not attained its biologically determined growth potential
PORTO 2013	EFW <5th percentile and umbilical artery PI >95th percentile
TRUFFLE 2013	AC <10th percentile and umbilical artery PI >95th percentile

Reproduced from Dall'Asta et al. [20]
EFW estimated fetal weight, *PI* pulsatility index

gestation or UtA PI above the 95th percentile for the gestation detected before 32 weeks [16]. Such definition – which includes not only a biometric cut off but also Doppler indices of feto-placental function and is currently endorsed by most Fetal Medicine specialists [9, 16, 142] – summarizes the current understanding on the pathogenesis of FGR, which consists in pathological smallness caused by an underlying functional problem.

Late FGR is more common but less severe with absent or mild placental abnormalities. UA Doppler may be normal and cannot be relied for its diagnosis, however late growth restricted fetuses may react with decreased MCA impedance in response to hypoxemia. The recently agreed diagnostic criteria for late FGR include either severe fetal smallness detected beyond 32 weeks (EFW or AC <3rd percentile for gestational age) or two out of three among (1) EFW or AC <10th percentile for gestation, (2) longitudinal reduction of the fetal growth in terms of EFW or AC reduced by over two quartiles compared to those measured in the second trimester, and (3) CPR below the 5th percentile for the gestation or UA PI above the 95th percentile for gestational age [16]. As before mentioned, it is uncertain whether such growth assessment should be performed using population-based [136], customized [132–135], or universal fetal growth charts [137]. Additionally, there is great uncertainty as regards which is the optimal screening strategy – either universal or selective or contingent assessment of the fetal growth [140–142] – and which is the optimal gestational time frame for the evaluation of the fetal growth at late gestation. Recently published randomized data have shown that the universal screening of the fetal growth can identify up to three times higher number of late FGR fetuses [141] and that screening at 36 weeks performs better than the screening at 32 weeks [143]. Finally, it is important to note that beyond 32 weeks, an EFW or an AC >10th percentile for the gestational age does not necessarily exclude late FGR. Several groups have demonstrated that even apparently normally grown third trimester fetuses with reduced CPR are at increased risk of perinatal complications, thus suggesting that a reduced CPR per se may represent a Doppler sign of misdiagnosed placental insufficiency and failure to reach the growth potential [17–19, 63, 144].

Doppler Ultrasound and Management of Early Fetal Growth Restriction

The Trial Randomizing Umbilical and Fetal Flow in Europe (TRUFFLE) is the only randomized controlled trial which has evaluated and demonstrated the effectiveness of a standardized monitoring and delivery protocol for early FGR fetuses.

Based on the assumption that cCTG and DV represent those parameters which safely allow to delay delivery before fetal compromise occurs, the TRUFFLE protocol has demonstrated that the 2-year neurodevelopmental outcome of surviving early FGR fetuses is significantly better among those delivered based on late DV changes [9, 65–67, 69], even though no differences were noted among the three randomization arms of the TRUFFLE as regards the primary outcome – i.e., survival without neurodevelopmental impairment. DV has been demonstrated to be the most important Doppler parameter in the prediction of the short-term risk of intrauterine death (IUD) in early FGR [44]. Absent or reversed DV A-wave has been associated with increased risk of IUD (40–70%), and late-stage acidemia independently forms gestational age at delivery and shortly precedes spontaneous decelerations at CTG monitoring. DV PI above the 95th centile has also been related to a high risk of adverse outcome, although at lesser extent than that of reversed or absent DV A-wave [65]. Similarly, STV becomes abnormal in the case of advanced fetal deterioration [76], providing information similar to those of late DV changes for the short-term prediction of IUD. Although the optimal cutoff value of the STV for delivery has yet to be clarified, it is important to point out that, between 26 and 32 weeks, expectant management is accepted as long as either the DV or the STV is abnormal but not if both are abnormal [9, 65]. The lower cCTG-STV cutoff was chosen assuming the STV lowest cutoff clinically appropriate given the high chance of hypoxemia/acidemia below that. The presence of spontaneous, repetitive fetal heart rate decelerations or maternal indications should trigger delivery independently of DV and cCTG-STV evaluation.

The concept that perinatal outcomes in FGR fetuses are not negatively affected by expectant management is not novel, as it was also reported in a former randomized trial on FGR [145]. Nevertheless, the inclusion criteria in the GRIT study were not as strict as those of the TRUFFLE study, and the decision on how to monitor and when to deliver FGR fetuses was not standardized.

Safety nets for delivery within the late DV group of the TRUFFLE cohort included, other than absent or reversed "A-" wave of the DV, also STV <2.6 msec below 29 weeks and <3.0 msec between 29 and 32 weeks, spontaneous decelerations at CTG, UA REDF between 30 and 32 weeks, UA AEDF between 32 and 34 weeks, or UA PI >95th centile beyond 34 weeks. Umbilical artery Doppler per se is therefore not informative as to when delivery should be undertaken, unless the gestation is above 30 weeks [9, 65–67].

Within the TRUFFLE protocol, and particularly in the late DV group, safety nets accounted for a significant amount of indications for delivery, both in the primary [9, 65] and in a recently published secondary analysis of the datasets [69]. A subanalysis of babies delivered <32 weeks' gestation, in other words those whose management was strictly defined by the protocol, showed that more than one third delivered based on safety net criteria and another one third for other fetal or maternal reasons. Hence, in clinical practice, a significant proportion of fetuses will be delivered because of cCTG-STV abnormalities, even before DV changes occur. However, overall data from the TRUFFLE trial and its subanalyses have shown a better outcome by the integrated use of both DV and cCTG-STV [9, 65–67].

Beyond 32 weeks of gestation, the timing of delivery should no longer rely on DV and STV but should be based on UA Doppler. More specifically, delivery should be undertaken if AEDF between 32 and 34 weeks and if UA PI >95th centile when the gestation is above 34 weeks.

According to the TRUFFLE protocol, there is no role for the MCA Doppler or CPR in the management of early FGR fetuses. A secondary analysis of the datasets from the TRUFFLE cohort could not demonstrate any impact of the MCA PI measured close to delivery and its change over time on neonatal and 2-year neurodevelopmental outcome, thus concluding that gestational age at delivery remains the most important factor in determining neonatal survival without adverse outcome and, together with birthweight, infant outcome [56].

As regards the timing for fetal monitoring, a secondary analysis of the TRUFFLE cohort has shown that it is not possible to predict the occurrence of abnormal STV or A-wave indicating delivery, concluding that STV should be monitored at least on a daily basis [146]. On the other hand, fetal Doppler can be measured twice a week or on alternate days in the case of advanced fetal compromise.

Within the TRUFFLE protocol, there is no role for the biophysical profile and conventional CTG in the monitoring of early FGR fetuses. Similarly, the evaluation of uterine artery Doppler is not recommended given the lack of data supporting its usefulness in the management of early FGR [42, 147]. Furthermore, there is no data as regards the decision for inpatient versus outpatient management of FGR fetuses. Most cases of isolated FGR are monitored in an outpatient setting even though the decision for inpatient monitoring can be taken on a subjective basis. Of note, 60–70% of cases of early FGR are associated with hypertensive complications of the pregnancy [9]. In such cases, particularly in the case of PE, admission seems advisable despite the lack of clinical evidence.

Doppler Ultrasound and Management of Late Fetal Growth Restriction

Given its relatively high frequency, late FGR is estimated to be responsible for over 50% of cases of IUD and misdiagnosed in most of them. Differently from early FGR, for which an evidence-based protocol for diagnosis, monitoring, and timing of delivery exists, there is no prospective nor randomized trial which has led to an evidence-based approach for the management of late FGR.

The Prospective Observational Trial to Optimize Pediatric Health in Intrauterine Growth Restriction (PORTO) study demonstrated that EFW <3rd centile for gestation is associated with adverse perinatal outcomes regardless of UA, MCA, and other Doppler parameters, thus showing that EFW <3rd centile represents an indicator of severity of the restriction of the fetal growth [139].

The CPR was first described for the monitoring of FGR fetuses [61] and is currently considered an early sign of placental chronic hypoxia, hence among the discriminators between constitutionally small fetuses and growth-restricted ones [16, 57–59]. However, its actual clinical significance is yet to be determined as it has not been clarified whether abnormally reduced CPR represents an adaptive mechanism or an indicator of ongoing functional compromise [148, 149]. Available data suggest that late FGR fetuses with low CPR are at increased risk of IUD and of obstetrics intervention due to intrapartum distress and neonatal morbidity regardless of birthweight [42, 150] and also of adverse neurodevelopmental outcomes [54]. Therefore, even though the CPR is currently widely used for the monitoring of FGR fetuses beyond 32 weeks, it is uncertain whether delivery based on reduced CPR is beneficial [148].

As regards maternal Doppler, abnormalities of the UtA PI in the third trimester have been associated with SGA and with an increased risk of adverse perinatal outcomes including stillbirth, obstetric intervention due to fetal distress, and neonatal acidemia [58]. Computerized CTG also represents a primary tool for the monitoring of late FGR fetuses; however, it has not been clarified which STV cutoff should be considered indicative of fetal acidemia and lead to the decision to expedite delivery before term.

In conclusion, albeit in the absence of grade A evidence and guidelines, available data suggest that an EFW <3rd centile and abnormalities of the CPR and of the UtA PI are to be considered risk factors for severity of adverse perinatal outcomes and perinatal death in late FGR [58]. Therefore, in the presence of such abnormal findings, we suggest close Doppler and cCTG monitoring – i.e., twice weekly between 32 and 37 weeks – and delivery at 37 weeks.

A randomized study is needed in order to overcome such uncertainty as regards the optimal monitoring strategy and timing of delivery of late FGR. In these fetuses, the risk of IUD or perinatal death is low. On the other hand, late preterm and early-term delivery are risk factors for mild but relevant neonatal complications which may impact on short-term and potentially also on long-term outcome and neurodevelopment [151, 152]. Therefore, we believe that the implementation of a protocol for the antenatal management of late FGR to be tested within a randomized trial will need a joint risk-benefit assessment by obstetricians and neonatologists. The ongoing trial by the TRUFFLE group and the planned TRUFFLE 2 randomized controlled study are likely to provide further insights into the actual role of the cerebral Doppler – on its own or paired with UA within the CPR – in the management of late-onset FGR and particularly to clarify whether anticipating delivery based on abnormal CPR is beneficial for the short- and long-term health of the late FGR fetus (http://www.truffle-study.org/research/).

Conclusion

- UA Doppler is related to fetal acidemia and provides both diagnostic and prognostic information for the management of FGR. The use of UA Doppler in a high-risk population reduces perinatal morbidity and mortality and is considered the primary surveillance tool in small fetuses. UA AEDF or REDF is mostly found in early FGR and has been reported to be present on average 1 week before acute fetal deterioration.
- Cerebral Doppler is not useful for the diagnosis and the management in early FGR. A potential role of MCA Doppler for the differential diagnosis between SGA and late FGR has been demonstrated; nevertheless MCA Doppler testing of suspected late FGR fetuses has not been evaluated in randomized trials, and to date no specific intervention has been shown to improve outcomes based on abnormal findings.
- The CPR has shown a good correlation with adverse outcome in FGR but also in apparently normally grown fetuses close to term and has been suggested for the differential diagnosis between SGA and FGR fetuses with normal UA Doppler.
- DV flow waveforms become abnormal only in advanced stages of fetal compromise, and the DV PI is inversely related to cord pH at birth. Evidence from the TRUFFLE has shown the crucial role of DV Doppler for the management of preterm growth-restricted fetuses before 32 weeks of gestation. There is no available data on DV Doppler in late FGR fetuses.
- The "heart-sparing effect" is the result of intrinsic mechanisms responsible for the autoregulation of the coronary flow which are activated in cases of chronic hypoxia – such as FGR – and leads to an increased blood supply to the fetal heart. No role of the "heart-sparing effect" for the diagnosis or the management of early or late FGR has been demonstrated to date.
- Doppler of the aortic isthmus, myocardial performance index, and E/A ratio represent Doppler cardiac parameters which have been studied in the context of FGR. There is no evidence-based role for any of them for the management or the diagnosis of early or late FGR.
- Abnormal UtA Doppler best identifies the severe early-onset complications of impaired placentation, particularly when performed in the second trimester and particularly for early FGR. There is also evidence that a high impedance to flow in the uterine arteries during the third trimester is associated with an increased risk of adverse perinatal events regardless of fetal size in pregnancies with normal umbilical artery Doppler, thus supporting the concept that raised UtA PI in the third trimester may help in discriminating between SGA and late FGR.
- There is no evidence-based role for Doppler assessment of the maternal cardiac function for the diagnosis or the management of FGR.

- According to the randomized evidence from the TRUFFLE study, beyond 32 weeks, the timing of delivery should be decided either based on late DV changes or safety net criteria, which include STV <2.6 ms below 29 weeks and <3.0 ms between 29 and 32 weeks, spontaneous decelerations at CTG, UA REDF between 30 and 32 weeks, UA AEDF between 32 and 34 weeks, or UA PI >95th centile beyond 34 weeks. Umbilical artery Doppler per se is not informative as to when delivery should be undertaken unless the gestation is above 30 weeks.
- Albeit in the absence of grade A evidence and guidelines for late FGR, available data suggest that an EFW <3rd centile and abnormalities of the CPR and of the UtA PI are to be considered independent indicators of severity of adverse perinatal outcomes and perinatal death in late FGR. These parameters should be taken into account when considering the option of delivery in late FGR.

References

1. Mcintire DD, Bloom SL, Casey BM, Leveno KJ. Birth weight in relation to morbidity and mortality among newborn infants. N Engl J Med. 1999;340:1234–8.
2. Garite TJ, Combs CA, Maurel K, Das A, Huls K, Porreco R, et al. A multicenter prospective study of neonatal outcomes at less than 32 weeks associated with indications for maternal admission and delivery. Am J Obstet Gynecol. 2017;217:72.e1–9.
3. Society for Maternal-Fetal Medicine Publications Committee, Berkley E, Chauhan SP, Abuhamad A. Doppler assessment of the fetus with intrauterine growth restriction. Am J Obstet Gynecol. 2012;206:300–8.
4. Yanney M, Marlow N. Paediatric consequences of fetal growth restriction. Semin Fetal Neonatal Med. 2004;9:411–8.
5. Marlow N, Wolke D, Bracewell MA, Samara M, The Epicure Study Group. Neurologic and developmental disability at six years of age after extremely preterm birth. N Engl J Med. 2005;352:9–19.
6. Low J, Handley M, Burke S, Peters RD, Pater EA, Killen HL, et al. Association of intrauterine growth retardation and learning deficits at age 9 to it years. Am J Obstet Gynecol. 1992;162:1499–505.
7. Figueras F, Gardosi J. Intrauterine growth restriction: new concepts in antenatal surveillance, diagnosis, and management. Am J Obstet Gynecol. 2011;204:288–300.
8. Kennelly MM, Farah N, Turner MJ, Stuart B. Aortic isthmus Doppler velocimetry: role in assessment of preterm fetal growth restriction. Prenat Diagn. 2010;30:395–401.
9. Lees C, Marlow N, Arabin B, Bilardo CM, Brezinka C, Derks JB, et al. Perinatal morbidity and mortality in early-onset fetal growth restriction: cohort outcomes of the trial of randomized umbilical and fetal flow in Europe (TRUFFLE). Ultrasound Obstet Gynecol. 2013;42:400–8.
10. Gardosi J, Chang A, Kalyan B, Sahota D, Symonds EM. Customised antenatal growth charts. Lancet. 1992;339:283–7.
11. Gardosi J, Giddings S, Buller S, Southam M, Williams M. Preventing stillbirths through improved antenatal recognition of pregnancies at risk due to fetal growth restriction. Public Health. 2014;128:698–702.
12. Van den Wijngaard JA, Groenenberg IA, Wladimiroff JW, Hop WC. Cerebral Doppler ultrasound of the human fetus. Br J Obstet Gynaecol. 1989;96:845–9.
13. Rizzo G, Arduini D, Romanini C. Doppler echocardiographic assessment of fetal cardiac function. Ultrasound Obstet Gynecol. 1992;2:434–45.

14. Stampalija T, Casati D, Monasta L, Sassi R, Rivolta MW, Muggiasca ML, et al. Brain sparing effect in growth-restricted fetuses is associated with decreased cardiac acceleration and deceleration capacities: a case-control study. BJOG. 2016;123:1947–54.
15. Hecher K, Campbell S, Doyle P, Harrington K, Nicolaides K. Assessment of fetal compromise by Doppler ultrasound investigation of the fetal circulation, arterial, intracardiac, and venous blood flow velocity studies. Circulation. 1995;91:129–38.
16. Gordijn SJ, Beune IM, Thilaganathan B, Papageorghiou A, Baschat AA, Baker PN, et al. Consensus definition of fetal growth restriction: a Delphi procedure. Ultrasound Obstet Gynecol. 2016;48:333–9.
17. Khalil A, Morales-Rosello J, Khan N, Nath M, Agarwal P, Bhide A, et al. Is cerebroplacental ratio a marker of impaired fetal growth velocity and adverse pregnancy outcome? Am J Obstet Gynecol. 2017;216:606.e1–606.e10.
18. Khalil A, Thilaganathan B. Role of uteroplacental and fetal Doppler in identifying fetal growth restriction at term. Best Pract Res Clin Obstet Gynaecol. 2017;38:38–47.
19. Morales-Roselló J, Khalil A, Morlando M, Papageorghiou A, Bhide A, Thilaganathan B. Changes in fetal Doppler indices as a marker of failure to reach growth potential at term. Ultrasound Obstet Gynecol. 2014;43:303–10.
20. Dall'Asta A, Brunelli V, Prefumo F, Frusca T, Lees CC. Early onset fetal growth restriction. Matern Health Neonatol Perinatol. 2017;3:2.
21. Dall'Asta A, Lees C. Early second-trimester fetal growth restriction and adverse perinatal outcomes. Obstet Gynecol. 2018;131:739–40.
22. Unterscheider J, Daly S, Geary MP, Kennelly MM, McAuliffe FM, O'Donoghue K, et al. Predictable progressive Doppler deterioration in IUGR: does it really exist? Am J Obstet Gynecol. 2013;209:539.e1–7.
23. Turan OM, Turan S, Gungor S, Berg C, Moyano D, Gembruch U, et al. Progression of Doppler abnormalities in intrauterine growth restriction. Ultrasound Obstet Gynecol. 2008;32:160–7.
24. Baschat AA, Güclü S, Kush ML, Gembruch U, Weiner CP, Harman CR. Venous Doppler in the prediction of acid-base status of growth-restricted fetuses with elevated placental blood flow resistance. Am J Obstet Gynecol. 2004;191:277–84.
25. Ferrazzi E, Bellotti M, Galan H, Pennati G, Bozzo M, Rigano S, et al. Doppler investigation in intrauterine growth restriction – from qualitative indices to flow measurements: a review of the experience of a collaborative group. Ann N Y Acad Sci. 2001;943:316–25.
26. Kiserud T, Kessler J, Ebbing C, Rasmussen S. Ductus venosus shunting in growth-restricted foetuses and the effect of umbilical circulatory compromise. Ultrasound Obstet Gynecol. 2006;28:143–9.
27. Hecher K, Bilardo CM, Stigter RH, Ville Y, Hackelöer BJ, Kok HJ, et al. Monitoring of fetuses with intrauterine growth restriction: a longitudinal study. Ultrasound Obstet Gynecol. 2001;18:564–70.
28. Hecher K, Snijders R, Campbell S, Nicolaides K. Fetal venous, intracardiac, and arterial blood flow measurements in intrauterine growth retardation; relationship with fetal blood gases. Am J Obstet Gynecol. 1995;173:10–5.
29. Rizzo G, Capponi A, Arduini D, Romanini C. The value of fetal arterial, cardiac and venous flows in predicting pH and blood gases measured in umbilical blood at cordocentesis in growth retarded fetuses. Br J Obstet Gyanecol. 1995;102:963–9.
30. Kingdom JC, Burrell SJ, Kaufmann P. Pathology and clinical implications of abnormal umbilical artery Doppler waveforms. Ultrasound Obstet Gynecol. 1997;9:271–86.
31. Khare M, Paul S, Konje J. Variation in Doppler indices along the length of the cord from the intraabdominal to the placental insertion. Acta Obstet Gynecol Scand. 2006;85:922–8.
32. Acharya G, Wilsgaard T, Berntsen G, Maltau J, Kiserud T. Reference ranges for serial measurements of blood velocity and pulsatility index at the intra-abdominal portion, and fetal and placental ends of the umbilical artery. Ultrasound Obstet Gynecol. 2005;26:162–9.
33. Acharya G, Wilsgaard T, Berntsen G, Maltau J, Kiserud T. Reference ranges for serial measurements of umbilical artery Doppler indices in the second half of pregnancy. Am J Obstet Gynecol. 2005;192:937–44.

34. Bhide A, Acharya G, Bilardo CM, Brezinka C, Cafici D, Hernandez-Andrade E, et al. ISUOG practice guidelines: use of Doppler ultrasonography in obstetrics. Ultrasound Obstet Gynecol. 2013;41:233–9.
35. Morrow RJ, Adamson SL, Bull SB, Ritchie JW. Effect of placental embolization on the umbilical arterial velocity waveform in fetal sheep. Am J Obstet Gynecol. 1989;161:1055–60.
36. Thompson RS, Trudinger BJ. Doppler waveform pulsatility index and resistance, pressure and flow in the umbilical placental circulation: an investigation using a mathematical model. Ultrasound Med Biol. 1990;16:449–58.
37. Soothill PW, Bobrow CS, Holmes R. Small for gestational age is not a diagnosis. Ultrasound Obstet Gynecol. 1999;13:225–8.
38. Bobrow CS, Soothill PW. Fetal growth velocity: a cautionary tale. Lancet. 1999;353:1460.
39. McCowan LM, Harding JE, Stewart AW. Umbilical artery Doppler studies in small for gestational age babies reflect disease severity. BJOG. 2000;107:916–25.
40. Figueras F, Eixarch E, Gratacos E, Gardosi J. Predictiveness of antenatal umbilical artery Doppler for adverse pregnancy outcome in small-for-gestational-age babies according to customised birthweight centiles: population based study. BJOG. 2008;115:590–4.
41. Doctor BA, O'Riordan MA, Kirchner HL, Shah D, Hack M. Perinatal correlates and neonatal outcomes of small for gestational age infants born at term gestation. Am J Obstet Gynecol. 2001;185:652–9.
42. Severi FM, Bocchi C, Visentin A, Falco P, Cobellis L, Florio P, et al. Uterine and fetal cerebral Doppler predict the outcome of third-trimester small-for-gestational age fetuses with normal umbilical artery Doppler. Ultrasound Obstet Gynecol. 2002;19:225–8.
43. Pardi G, Cetin I, Marconi AM, Lanfranchi A, Bozzetti P, Ferrazzi E, et al. Diagnostic value of blood sampling in fetuses with growth retardation. N Engl J Med. 1993;328:692–6.
44. Figueras F, Gratacos E. Update on the diagnosis and classification of fetal growth restriction and proposal of a stage-based management protocol. Fetal Diagn Ther. 2014;36:86–98.
45. Alfirevic Z, Stampalija T, Gyte GM. Fetal and umbilical Doppler ultrasound in high-risk pregnancies. Cochrane Database Syst Rev. 2013;11:CD007529.
46. RCOG Green Top Guidline No. 31. The investigation and management of the small-for-gestational age fetus. January 2014.
47. Arduini D, Rizzo G, Romanini C. The development of abnormal heart rate patterns after absent end-diastolic velocity in umbilical artery: analysis of risk factors. Am J Obstet Gynecol. 1993;168:43–50.
48. Brar H, Platt L. Reverse end diastolic flow velocity on umbilical artery velocimetry in high pregnancies: an ominous finding with adverse pregnancy outcome. Am J Obstet Gynecol. 1988;159:559–61.
49. Valcamonico A, Danti L, Frusca T, Soregaroli M, Zucca S, Abrami F, et al. Absent end diastolic velocity in umbilical artery: risk of neonatal morbidity and brain damage. Am J Obstet Gynecol. 1994;170:796–801.
50. Ferrazzi E, Bozzo M, Rigano S, Bellotti M, Morabito A, Pardi G, et al. Temporal sequence of abnormal Doppler changes in the peripheral and central circulatory systems of the severely growth-restricted fetus. Ultrasound Obstet Gynecol. 2002;19:140–6.
51. Mari G, Abuhamad AZ, Cosmi E, Segata M, Altaye M, Akiyama M. Middle cerebral artery peak systolic velocity: technique and variability. J Ultrasound Med. 2005;24:425–30.
52. Mari G, Deter RL. Middle cerebral artery flow velocity waveforms in normal and small for gestational age fetuses. Am J Obstet Gynecol. 1992;166:1262–70.
53. Hernandez-Andrade E, Stampalija T, Figueras F. Cerebral blood flow studies in the diagnosis and management of intrauterine growth restriction. Curr Opin Obstet Gynecol. 2013;25:138–44.
54. Meher S, Hernandez-Andrade E, Basheer SN, Lees C. Impact of cerebral redistribution on neurodevelopmental outcome in small-for-gestational-age or growth-restricted babies: a systematic review. Ultrasound Obstet Gynecol. 2015;46:398–404.

55. Eixarch E, Meler E, Iraola A, Illa M, Crispi F, Hernandez-Andrade E, et al. Neurodevelopmental outcome in 2-year-old infants who were small-for-gestational age term fetuses with cerebral blood flow redistribution. Ultrasound Obstet Gynecol. 2008;32:894–9.
56. Stampalija T, Arabin B, Wolf H, Bilardo CM, Lees C, TRUFFLE investigators. Is middle cerebral artery Doppler related to neonatal and 2-year infant outcome in early fetal growth restriction. Am J Obstet Gynecol. 2017;216:521.e1–13.
57. Parra-Saavedra M, Simeone S, Triunfo S, Crovetto F, Botet F, Nadal A, et al. Correlation between histological signs of placental underperfusion and perinatal morbidity in late-onset small-for-gestational-age fetuses. Ultrasound Obstet Gynecol. 2015;45:149–55.
58. Figueras F, Savchev S, Triunfo S, Crovetto F, Gratacos E. An integrated model with classification criteria to predict small-for-gestational-age fetuses at risk of adverse perinatal outcome. Ultrasound Obstet Gynecol. 2015;45:279–85.
59. Triunfo S, Crispi F, Gratacos E, Figueras F. Prediction of delivery of small-for-gestational-age neonates and adverse perinatal outcome by fetoplacental Doppler at 37 weeks' gestation. Ultrasound Obstet Gynecol. 2017;49:364–71.
60. Cruz-Martínez R, Figueras F, Hernandez-Andrade E, Oros D, Gratacos E. Fetal brain Doppler to predict cesarean delivery for nonreassuring fetal status in term small-for-gestational-age fetuses. Obstet Gynecol. 2011;117:618–26.
61. Gramellini D, Folli MC, Raboni S, Vadora E, Merialdi A. Cerebral-umbilical Doppler ratio as a predictor of adverse perinatal outcome. Obstet Gynecol. 1992;79:416–20.
62. Baschat AA, Gembruch U. The cerebroplacental Doppler ratio revisited. Ultrasound Obstet Gynecol. 2003;21:124–7.
63. Prior T, Mullins E, Bennett P, Kumar S. Prediction of intrapartum fetal compromise using the cerebro-umbilical ratio: a prospective observational study. Am J Obstet Gynecol. 2013;208:124.e1–6.
64. Kiserud T. Physiology of the fetal circulation. Semin Fetal Neonatal Med. 2005;10:493–503.
65. Lees CC, Marlow N, van Wassenaer-Leemhuis A, Arabin B, Bilardo CM, Brezinka C, et al. 2 year neurodevelopmental and intermediate perinatal outcomes in infants with very preterm fetal growth restriction (TRUFFLE): a randomised trial. Lancet. 2015;385:2162–72.
66. Bilardo CM, Hecher K, Visser GH, Papageorghiou AT, Marlow N, Thilaganathan B, et al. Severe fetal growth restriction at 26–32 weeks: key messages from the TRUFFLE study. Ultrasound Obstet Gynecol. 2017;50:285–90.
67. Frusca T, Todros T, Lees C, Bilardo CM, TRUFFLE Investigators. Outcome in early-onset fetal growth restriction is best combining computerized fetal heart rate analysis with ductus venosus Doppler: insights from the Trial of Umbilical and Fetal Flow in Europe. Am J Obstet Gynecol. 2018;218:S783–9.
68. Ganzevoort W, Mensing Van Charante N, Thilaganathan B, Prefumo F, Arabin B, Bilardo CM, et al. How to monitor pregnancies complicated by fetal growth restriction and delivery before 32 weeks: post-hoc analysis of TRUFFLE study. Ultrasound Obstet Gynecol. 2017;49:769–77.
69. Visser GH, Bilardo CM, Derks JB, Ferrazzi E, Fratelli N, Frusca T, et al. Fetal monitoring indications for delivery and 2-year outcome in 310 infants with fetal growth restriction delivered before 32 weeks' gestation in the TRUFFLE study. Ultrasound Obstet Gynecol. 2017;50:347–52.
70. Baschat AA, Turan OM, Turan S. Ductus venosus blood-flow patterns: more than meets the eye? Ultrasound Obstet Gynecol. 2012;39:598–9.
71. Baschat AA, Hecher K. Fetal growth restriction due to placental disease. Semin Perinatol. 2004;28:67–80.
72. Baschat AA. Fetal responses to placental insufficiency: an update. BJOG. 2004;111:1031–41.
73. Turan OM, Turan S, Sanapo L, Rosenbloom JI, Baschat AA. Semiquantitative classification of ductus venosus blood flow patterns. Ultrasound Obstet Gynecol. 2014;43:508–14.
74. Cosmi E, Ambrosini G, D'Antona D, Saccardi C, Mari G. Doppler, cardiotocography, and biophysical profile changes in growth-restricted fetuses. Obstet Gynecol. 2005;106:1240–5.

75. Baschat AA, Gembruch U, Harmann CR. The sequence of changes in Doppler and biophysical parameters as severe fetal growth restriction worsens. Ultrasound Obstet Gynecol. 2001;18:571–7.
76. Schwarze A, Gembruch U, Krapp M, Katalinic A, Germer U, Axt-Fliedner R. Qualitative venous Doppler flow waveform analysis in preterm intrauterine growth-restricted fetuses with ARED flow in the umbilical artery – correlation with short-term outcome. Ultrasound Obstet Gynecol. 2005;25:573–9.
77. Chaoui R. The fetal 'heart-sparing effect' detected by the assessment of coronary blood flow: a further ominous sign of fetal compromise. Ultrasound Obstet Gynecol. 1996;7:5–9.
78. Baschat AA, Gembruch U, Reiss I, Gortner L, Diedrich K. Demonstration of fetal coronary blood flow by Doppler ultrasound in relation to arterial and venous flow velocity waveforms and perinatal outcome – the 'heart-sparing effect'. Ultrasound Obstet Gynecol. 1997;9:162–72.
79. Crispi F, Figueras F, Cruz-Lemini M, Bartrons J, Bijnens B, Gratacos E. Cardiovascular programming in children born small for gestational age and relationship with prenatal signs of severity. Am J Obstet Gynecol. 2012;207:121.e1–9.
80. Hernandez-Andrade E, Benavides-Serralde JA, Cruz-Martinez R, Welsh A, Mancilla-Ramirez J. Evaluation of conventional Doppler fetal cardiac function parameters: E/A ratios, outflow tracts, and myocardial performance index. Fetal Diagn Ther. 2012;32:22–9.
81. Cruz-Martinez R, Figueras F, Benavides-Serralde A, Crispi F, Hernandez-Andrade E, Gratacos E. Sequence of changes in myocardial performance index in relation to aortic isthmus and ductus venosus Doppler in fetuses with early-onset intrauterine growth restriction. Ultrasound Obstet Gynecol. 2011;38:179–84.
82. Del Río M, Martínez JM, Figueras F, Bennasar M, Olivella A, Palacio M, et al. Doppler assessment of the aortic isthmus and perinatal outcome in preterm fetuses with severe intrauterine growth restriction. Ultrasound Obstet Gynecol. 2008;31:41–7.
83. Del Río M, Martinez JM, Figueras F, Bennasar M, Palacio M, Gomez O, et al. Doppler assessment of fetal aortic isthmus blood flow in two different sonographic planes during the second half of gestation. Ultrasound Obstet Gynecol. 2005;26:170–4.
84. Rizzo G, Capponi A, Vendola M, Pietrolucci ME, Arduini D. Relationship between aortic isthmus and ductus venosus velocity waveforms in severe growth restricted fetuses. Prenat Diagn. 2008;28:1042–7.
85. Acharya G. Technical aspects of aortic isthmus Doppler velocimetry in human fetuses. Ultrasound Obstet Gynecol. 2009;33:628–33.
86. Ruskamp J, Fouron JC, Gosselin J, Raboisson MJ, Infante-Rivard C, Proulx F. Reference values for an index of fetal aortic isthmus blood flow during the second half of pregnancy. Ultrasound Obstet Gynecol. 2003;21:441–4.
87. Bonnin P, Fouron JC, Teyssier G, Sonesson SE, Skoll A. Quantitative assessment of circulatory changes in the fetal aortic isthmus during progressive increase of resistance to umbilical blood flow. Circulation. 1993;88:216–22.
88. Fouron JC. The unrecognized physiological and clinical significance of the fetal aortic isthmus. Ultrasound Obstet Gynecol. 2003;22:441–7.
89. Makikallio K, Jouppila P, Rasanen J. Retrograde net blood flow in the aortic isthmus in relation to human fetal arterial and venous circulations. Ultrasound Obstet Gynecol. 2002;19:147–52.
90. Makikallio K, Jouppila P, Rasanen J. Retrograde aortic isthmus net blood flow and human fetal cardiac function in placental insufficiency. Ultrasound Obstet Gynecol. 2003;22:351–7.
91. Jouppila P, Kirkinen P. Increased vascular resistance in the descending aorta of the human fetus in hypoxia. Br J Obstet Gynaecol. 1984;91:853–6.
92. Arabin B, Siebert M, Jimenez E, Saling E. Obstetrical characteristics of a loss of end-diastolic velocities in the fetal aorta and/or umbilical artery using Doppler ultrasound. Gynecol Obstet Investig. 1988;25:173–80.
93. Fouron JC, Gosseli J, Raboisson MJ, Lamoureux J, Tison CA, Fouron C, et al. The relationship between an aortic isthmus blood flow velocity and the postnatal neurodevelopmental status of fetuses with placental circulatory insufficiency. Am J Obstet Gynecol. 2005;192:497–503.

94. Van der Mooren K, Barendregt LG, Wladimiroff JW. Fetal atrioventricular and outflow tract flow velocity waveforms during normal second half of pregnancy. Am J Obstet Gyencol. 1991;165:668–74.
95. Tulzer G, Khowsathit P, Gudmundsson S, Wood DC, Tian ZY, Schmitt K, et al. Diastolic function of the fetal heart during second and third trimester: a prospective longitudinal Doppler-echocardiographic study. Eur J Pediatr. 1994;153:151–4.
96. Figueras F, Puerto B, Martinez JM, Cararach V, Vanrell JA. Cardiac function monitoring of fetuses with growth restriction. Eur J Obstet Gynecol Reprod Biol. 2003;110:159–63.
97. Mäkikallio K, Räsänen J, Mäkikallio T, Vuolteenaho O, Huhta JC. Human fetal cardiovascular profile score and neonatal outcome in intrauterine growth restriction. Ultrasound Obstet Gynecol. 2008;31:48–54.
98. Tei C, Ling LH, Hodge DO, Bailey KR, Oh JK, Rodeheffer RJ, et al. New index of combined systolic and diastolic myocardial performance: a simple and reproducible measure of cardiac function – a study in normal and dilated cardiomyopathy. J Cardiol. 1995;26:357–66.
99. Van Mieghem T, Klaritsch P, Doné E, Gucciardo L, Lewi P, Verhaeghe J, et al. Assessment of fetal cardiac function before and after therapy for twin-to-twin transfusion syndrome. Am J Obstet Gynecol. 2009;200:400.e1–7.
100. Hassan WA, Brockelsby J, Alberry M, Fanelli T, Wladimiroff J, Lees CC. Cardiac function in early onset small for gestational age and growth restricted fetuses. Eur J Obstet Gynecol Reprod Biol. 2013;171:262–5.
101. Benavides-Serralde A, Scheier M, Cruz-Martinez R, Crispi F, Figueras F, Gratacos E, et al. Changes in central and peripheral circulation in intrauterine growth-restricted fetuses at different stages of umbilical artery flow deterioration: new fetal cardiac and brain parameters. Gynecol Obstet Investig. 2011;71:274–80.
102. Pérez-Cruz M, Cruz-Lemini M, Fernández MT, Parra JA, Bartrons J, Gómez-Roig MD, et al. Fetal cardiac function in late-onset intrauterine growth restriction vs small-for-gestational age, as defined by estimated fetal weight, cerebroplacental ratio and uterine artery Doppler. Ultrasound Obstet Gynecol. 2015;46:465–71.
103. Cruz-Martinez R, Figueras F, Hernandez-Andrade E, Oros D, Gratacos E. Changes in myocardial performance index and aortic isthmus and ductus venosus Doppler in term, small-for-gestational age fetuses with normal umbilical artery pulsatility index. Ultrasound Obstet Gynecol. 2011;38:400–5.
104. Hernandez-Andrade E, Crispi F, Benavides-Serralde JA, Plasencia W, Diesel HF, Eixarch E, et al. Contribution of the myocardial performance index and aortic isthmus blood flow index to predicting mortality in preterm growth-restricted fetuses. Ultrasound Obstet Gynecol. 2009;34:430–6.
105. Jurkovic D, Jauniaux E, Kurjak A, Hustin J, Campbell S, Nicolaides KH. Transvaginal color Doppler assessment of the uteroplacental circulation in early pregnancy. Obstet Gynecol. 1991;77:365–9.
106. Jauniaux E, Jurkovic D, Campbell S, Hustin J. Doppler ultrasonographic features of the developing placental circulation; correlation with anatomic findings. Am J Obstet Gynecol. 1992;166:585–7.
107. Cnossen JS, Morris RK, ter Riet G, Mol BW, van der Post JA, Coomarasamy A, et al. Use of uterine artery Doppler ultrasonography to predict pre-eclampsia and intrauterine growth restriction: a systematic review and bivariable meta-analysis. CMAJ. 2008;178:701–11.
108. Sciscione AC, Hayes EJ; Society for Maternal-Fetal Medicine. Uterine artery Doppler flow studies in obstetric practice. Am J Obstet Gynecol. 2009;201:121–6.
109. Gòmez O, Figueras F, Fernàndez S, Bennasar M, Martìnez JM, Puerto B, et al. Reference ranges for uterine artery mean pulsatility index at 11–41 weeks of gestation. Ultrasound Obstet Gynecol. 2008;32:128–32.
110. Papageorghiou AT, Yu CK, Bindra R, Pandis G, Nicolaides KH; Fetal Medicine Foundation Second Trimester Screening Group. Multicenter screening for pre-eclampsia and fetal growth restriction by transvaginal uterine artery Doppler at 23 weeks of gestation. Ultrasound Obstet Gynecol. 2001;18:441–9.

111. Ferreira AE, Mauad Filho F, Abreu PS, Mauad FM, Araujo Júnior E, Martins WP. Reproducibility of first- and second-trimester uterine artery pulsatility index measured by transvaginal and transabdominal ultrasound. Ultrasound Obstet Gynecol. 2015;46: 546–52.
112. Li N, Ghosh G, Gudmundsson S. Uterine artery Doppler in high-risk pregnancies at 23–24 gestational weeks is of value in predicting adverse outcome of pregnancy and selecting cases for more intense surveillance. Acta Obstet Gynecol Scand. 2014;93:1276–81.
113. Khalil AA, Morales-Rosello J, Elsaddig M, Khan N, Papageorghiou A, Bhide A, et al. The association between fetal Doppler and admission to neonatal unit at term. Am J Obstet Gynecol. 2015;213:57.e1–7.
114. Papageorghiou AT, Yu CK, Cicero S, Bower S, Nicolaides KH. Second-trimester uterine artery Doppler screening in unselected populations: a review. J Matern Fetal Neonatal Med. 2002;12:78–88.
115. Valiño N, Giunta G, Gallo DM, Akolekar R, Nicolaides KH. Uterine artery pulsatility index at 30–34 weeks' gestation in the prediction of adverse perinatal outcome. Ultrasound Obstet Gynecol. 2016;47:308–15.
116. Cruz-Martinez R, Savchev S, Cruz-Lemini M, Mendez A, Gratacos E, Figueras F. Clinical utility of third-trimester uterine artery Doppler in the prediction of brain hemodynamic deterioration and adverse perinatal outcome in small-for-gestational-age fetuses. Ultrasound Obstet Gynecol. 2015;45:273–8.
117. Flo K, Wilsgaard T, Vårtun A, Acharya G. A longitudinal study of the relationship between maternal cardiac output measured by impedance cardiography and uterine artery blood flow in the second half of pregnancy. BJOG Int J Obstet Gynaecol. 2010;117:837–44.
118. Ghi T, degli Esposti D, Montaguti E, Rosticci M, Tancredi S, Youssef A, et al. Maternal cardiac evaluation during uncomplicated twin pregnancy with emphasis on the diastolic function. Am J Obstet Gynecol. 2015;213:376.e1–8.
119. Valensise H, Tiralongo GM, Pisani I, Farsetti D, Lo Presti D, Gagliardi G, et al. Maternal hemodynamics early in labor: a possible link with obstetric risk? Ultrasound Obstet Gynecol. 2018;51:509–13.
120. Tiralongo GM, Pisani I, Vasapollo B, Khalil A, Thilaganathan B, Valensise H. Effect of a nitric oxide donor on maternal hemodynamics in fetal growth restriction. Ultrasound Obstet Gynecol. 2018;51:514–8.
121. Gagliardi G, Tiralongo GM, LoPresti D, Pisani I, Farsetti D, Vasapollo B, et al. Screening for pre-eclampsia in the first trimester: role of maternal hemodynamics and bioimpedance in non-obese patients. Ultrasound Obstet Gynecol. 2017;50:584–8.
122. Pijnenborg R, Vercruysse L, Hanssens M. The uterine spiral arteries in human pregnancy: facts and controversies. Placenta. 2006;27:939–58.
123. Steegers EA, von Dadelszen P, Duvekot JJ, Pijnenborg R. Pre-eclampsia. Lancet. 2010;376:631–44.
124. Mifsud W, Sebire NJ. Placental pathology in early-onset and late-onset fetal growth restriction. Fetal Diagn Ther. 2014;36:117–28.
125. Xiong X, Demianczuk NN, Saunders LD, Wang FL, Fraser WD. Impact of preeclampsia and gestational hypertension on birth weight by gestational age. Am J Epidemiol. 2002;155:203–9.
126. Valensise H, Vasapollo B, Gagliardi G, Novelli GP. Early and late preeclampsia: two different maternal hemodynamic states in the latent phase of the disease. Hypertension. 2008;52:873–80.
127. Verlohren S, Melchiorre K, Khalil A, Thilaganathan B. Uterine artery Doppler, birth weight and timing of onset of pre-eclampsia: providing insights into the dual etiology of late-onset pre-eclampsia. Ultrasound Obstet Gynecol. 2014;44:293–8.
128. Thilaganathan B. Pre-eclampsia is primarily a placental disorder: AGAINST: pre-eclampsia: the heart matters. BJOG. 2017;124:1763.
129. Stott D, Papastefanou I, Paraschiv D, Clark K, Kametas NA. Longitudinal maternal hemodynamics in pregnancies affected by fetal growth restriction. Ultrasound Obstet Gynecol. 2017;49:761–8.

130. Ferrazzi E, Stampalija T, Monasta L, Di Martino D, Vonck S, Gyselaers W. Maternal hemodynamics: a method to classify hypertensive disorders of pregnancy. Am J Obstet Gynecol. 2018;218:124.e1–124.e11.
131. Salomon LJ, Alfirevic Z, Bilardo CM, Chalouhi GE, Ghi T, Kagan KO, et al. ISUOG practice guidelines: performance of first-trimester fetal ultrasound scan. Ultrasound Obstet Gynecol. 2013;41:102–13.
132. Gardosi J, Clausson B, Francis A. The value of customised centiles in assessing perinatal mortality risk associated with parity and maternal size. BJOG. 2009;116:1356–63.
133. Odibo AO, Cahill AG, Odibo L, Roehl K, Macones GA. Prediction of intrauterine fetal death in small-for-gestational-age fetuses: impact of including ultrasound biometry in customized models. Ultrasound Obstet Gynecol. 2012;39:288–92.
134. Smith NA, Bukowski R, Thomas AM, Cantonwine D, Zera C, Robinson JN. Identification of pathologically small fetuses using customized, ultrasound and population-based growth norms. Ultrasound Obstet Gynecol. 2014;44:595–9.
135. Ghi T, Cariello L, Rizzo L, Ferrazzi E, Periti E, Prefumo F, et al. Customized fetal growth charts for parents' characteristics, race and parity by Quantile regression analysis: a cross-sectional multicenter Italian study. J Ultrasound Med. 2016;35:83–92.
136. Kiserud T, Piaggio G, Carroli G, Widmer M, Carvalho J, Neerup Jensen L, et al. The World Health Organization fetal growth charts: a multinational longitudinal study of ultrasound biometric measurements and estimated fetal weight. PLoS Med. 2017;14:e1002220.
137. Papageorghiou AT, Ohuma EO, Altman DG, Todros T, Cheikh Ismail L, Lambert A, et al. International standards for fetal growth based on serial ultrasound measurements: the Fetal Growth Longitudinal Study of the INTERGROWTH-21st Project. Lancet. 2014;384:869–79.
138. Miranda J, Rodriguez-Lopez M, Triunfo S, Sairanen M, Kouru H, Parra-Saavedra M, et al. Prediction of fetal growth restriction using estimated fetal weight vs a combined screening model in the third trimester. Ultrasound Obstet Gynecol. 2017;50:603–11.
139. Unterscheider J, Daly S, Geary MP, Kennelly MM, McAuliffe FM, O'Donoghue K, et al. Optimizing the definition of intrauterine growth restriction: the multicenter prospective PORTO Study. Am J Obstet Gynecol. 2013;208:290.e1–6.
140. Triunfo S, Crovetto F, Scazzocchio E, Parra-Saavedra M, Gratacos E, Figueras F. Contingent versus routine third-trimester screening for late fetal growth restriction. Ultrasound Obstet Gynecol. 2016;47:81–8.
141. Sovio U, White IR, Dacey A, Pasupathy D, Smith GCS. Screening for fetal growth restriction with universal third trimester ultrasonography in nulliparous women in the Pregnancy Outcome Prediction (POP) study: a prospective cohort study. Lancet. 2015;386:2089–97.
142. Bakalis S, Silva M, Akolekar R, Poon LC, Nicolaides KH. Prediction of small-for-gestational-age neonates: screening by fetal biometry at 30–34 weeks. Ultrasound Obstet Gynecol. 2015;45:551–8.
143. Roma E, Arnau A, Berdala R, Bergos C, Montesinos J, Figueras F. Ultrasound screening for fetal growth restriction at 36 vs 32 weeks' gestation: a randomized trial (ROUTE). Ultrasound Obstet Gynecol. 2015;46:391–7.
144. Dall'Asta A, Ghi T, Rizzo G, Cancemi A, Aloisio F, Arduini D, et al. Early labor cerebroplacental ratio assessment in uncomplicated term pregnancies and prediction of adverse perinatal outcomes: a prospective, multicentre study. Ultrasound Obstet Gynecol. 2018; https://doi.org/10.1002/uog.19113.
145. GRIT Study Group. A randomised trial of timed delivery for the compromised preterm fetus: short term outcomes and Bayesian interpretation. BJOG. 2003;110:27–32.
146. Wolf H, Arabin B, Lees CC, Oepkes D, Prefumo F, Thilaganathan B, et al. Longitudinal study of computerized cardiotocography in early fetal growth restriction. Ultrasound Obstet Gynecol. 2017;50:71–8.
147. Ghosh GS, Gudmundsson S. Uterine and umbilical artery Doppler are comparable in predicting perinatal outcome of growth-restricted fetuses. BJOG. 2009;116:424–30.
148. DeVore GR. The importance of the cerebroplacental ratio in the evaluation of fetal Well-being in SGA and AGA fetuses. Am J Obstet Gynecol. 2015;213:5–15.

149. Ghi T, Frusca T, Lees CC. Cerebroplacental ratio in fetal surveillance: an alert bell or a crash sound? Am J Obstet Gynecol. 2016;214:297–8.
150. Vergani P, Roncaglia N, Andreotti C, Arreghini A, Teruzzi M, Pezzullo JC, et al. Prognostic value of uterine artery Doppler velocimetry in growth-restricted fetuses delivered near term. Am J Obstet Gynecol. 2002;187:932–6.
151. Barker DJ, Osmond C, Golding J, Kuh D, Wadsworth ME. Growth in utero, blood pressure in childhood and adult life, and mortality from cardiovascular disease. BMJ. 1989;298:564–7.
152. Barker DJ. Fetal origins of coronary heart disease. BMJ. 1995;311:171–4.

Clinical Treatment

11

Luciano Marcondes Machado Nardozza,
Ana Carolina Rabachini Caetano,
and Ana Cristina Perez Zamarian

Introduction

Fetal growth restriction (FGR) is a complication in which the fetal weight is below the 10th percentile. It affects 5–10% of pregnancies [1] and is the second leading cause of perinatal mortality, responsible for approximately 30% of stillbirths and for increasing the frequency of premature births and intrapartum asphyxia. It is also associated with neonatal complications, including meconium aspiration, metabolic and blood disorders, cognitive dysfunction, and cerebral palsy [2]. Hypoxia/acidemia is estimated to be present in 30% of fetuses with growth restriction at birth [3]. Unfortunately, no effective therapy is currently available to reverse or at least interrupt the progressive course of placental insufficiency. Follow-up comprises optimizing care and appropriately timing childbirth and balancing the risks inherent in prematurity and those arising from acidemia with intrauterine permanence. While obstetric expectant management is adopted, fetal well-being is monitored through examinations such as ultrasound, antepartum cardiotocography, Doppler velocimetry, and fetal biophysical profile [4].

Within this context, the use of omega-3 (ω-3), vitamin D, sildenafil, statins, and nitric oxide has emerged as treatment options, in addition to bed rest and gene therapies, because of their ability to promote fetal development and growth.

L. M. M. Nardozza (✉) · A. C. R. Caetano · A. C. P. Zamarian
Discipline of Fetal Medicine, Department of Obstetrics, Paulista School of Medicine, Federal University of São Paulo (EPM-UNIFESP), São Paulo, SP, Brazil

L. M. M. Nardozza et al. (eds.), *Fetal Growth Restriction*,
https://doi.org/10.1007/978-3-030-00051-6_11

Omega-3

Omega-3 (ω-3) fatty acids (FAs) are polyunsaturated carboxylic acids with the first double bond at the third carbon atom. FAs are carboxylic acids (-COOH) containing an aliphatic chain, and they are produced by the breakdown of fat molecules. Therefore, FAs are organic compounds (their molecules contain carbon and hydrogen) and are classified as monounsaturated, polyunsaturated, and saturated FAs [5, 6]. Saturated FAs are compounds in which the carbon atoms are linked by single bonds; these are mainly found in animal products in the solid form. Unsaturated FAs contain carbons linked by one or more double bonds; these mainly exist in vegetables in the liquid form. Such FAs can be either monounsaturated (with one carbon–carbon double bond) or polyunsaturated. Omega (ω) is a classification of unsaturated FAs according to the position number of the carbon linked by the first double bond (3, 6, or 9), counting from the methyl radical (Fig. 11.1). Thus, we have the following ω FAs: (1) ω-3, alpha-linolenic acid, eicosapentaenoic acid (EPA), and docosahexaenoic acid (DHA); (2) ω-6, linoleic acid and arachidonic acid; and (3) ω-9, oleic acid.

Some FAs are termed "essential" because they cannot be synthesized by the body and must be obtained through the diet (ω-6/ω-3 = 5:1). Western diets and diets consumed in industrialized countries are rich in ω-6 polyunsaturated FAs (PUFAs) because of the consumption of vegetable oils and saturated fats and low in ω-3 PUFAs because of the low consumption of fish. Western diets have a ω-6/ω-3 ratio of approximately 10–20:1. Omega-3 (ω-3) and ω-6 FAs compete with each other for the Δ-6-desaturase enzyme, which is a common key enzyme for both metabolic pathways. Thus, each type of FA can interfere with the metabolism of the other and create nutritional implications. Omega-3 (ω-3) and ω-6 FAs are also precursors for eicosanoids, which are mediators of the lipid origin that modulate inflammatory and immune responses (Fig. 11.2).

These FAs influence cytokine production and the corresponding tissue response. In general, ω-3 FAs reduce systemic inflammatory response and ω-6 FAs increase it.

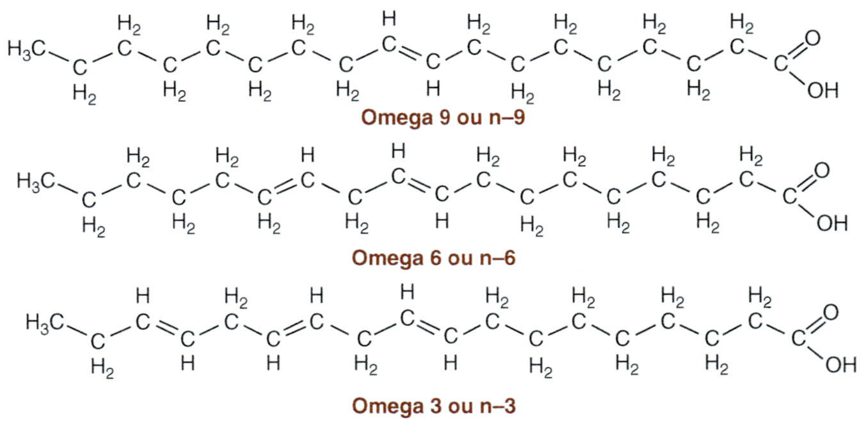

Fig. 11.1 Graphical representation of fatty acid nomenclature

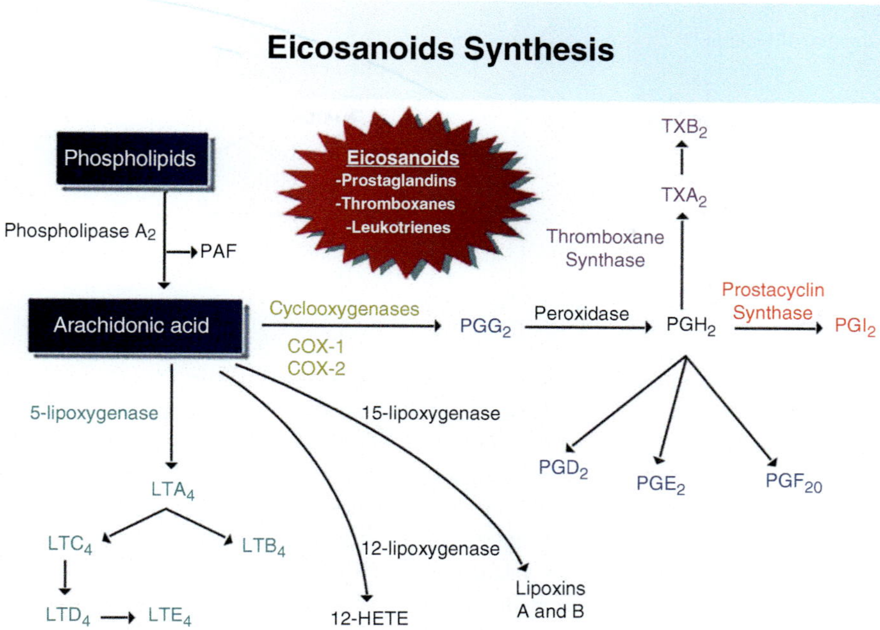

Fig. 11.2 Graphical representation of eicosanoid synthesis

Eicosanoids that result from the metabolism of ω-6 FAs are of the even-numbered series, 2-series prostaglandins, 4-series leukotrienes, and thromboxanes A2, and are important biochemical mediators involved in infection, inflammation, and tissue injury (↑PGE2). Eicosanoids of the odd-numbered series that result from the metabolism of ω-3 FAs, such as 3-series prostaglandins, 5-series leukotrienes, and thromboxanes A3, have a smaller inflammatory effect and a greater effect on the defense mechanism of the immune system (↓PGE2). Several benefits of ω-3 FAs have been described, including reducing triglyceride and LDL cholesterol levels, increasing HDL levels, playing an important role in allergies and inflammatory processes, increasing immune system protection, decreasing blood pressure and coronary artery diseases, rejuvenating skin, and improving depression and cognitive skills. Their use in obstetrics is controversial. Preterm labor prevention and intellectual development promotion have been reported [7–9]. Other researchers have reported that ω-3 supplementation does not influence the gestation period or fetal weight and have no effect on fetuses with growth restriction [10, 11]. Further studies must be conducted to demonstrate the real influence of ω-3 FAs on fetal growth and development.

Vitamin D

Vitamin D (Fig. 11.3), which promotes fetal development and growth, is an emerging treatment option for FGR. Vitamin D is a steroid that is involved in intestinal calcium absorption and calcium homeostasis regulation and is essential for the

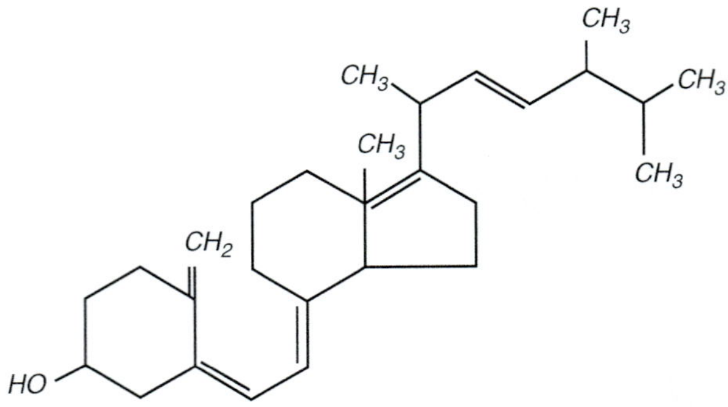

Fig. 11.3 Chemical structure of vitamin D

formation and maintenance of strong and healthy bones. Vitamin D deficiency can be caused by inadequate sun exposure, ineffective food intake, decreased absorption, abnormal metabolism, or resistance to vitamin D. Recently, several chronic diseases, such as cancer, hypertension, and osteoporosis, and several autoimmune diseases have been associated with vitamin D deficiency.

Humans have two sources of vitamin D: an exogenous source, provided by diet, in the forms of vitamin D_2 and D_3 and an endogenous source, in which cholecalciferol (D_3), which is the main source of vitamin D, is synthesized in the skin when ultraviolet B (UVB) radiation causes the photolysis of 7-dehydrocholesterol and its conversion to vitamin D_3. Exposure to sunlight or UVB radiation up to 18 IU/cm^2 in 3 h is sufficient. This process has two stages. The first stage occurs in the dermis and comprises the photoconversion of 7-dehydrocholesterol to previtamin D_3 or pre-cholecalciferol (Fig. 11.4). The second stage comprises a chemical isomerization that occurs depending on the body temperature, in which previtamin D slowly and progressively gets converted to vitamin D_3, which has a high affinity for vitamin D-binding protein (DBP), while previtamin D, which has a lower affinity, remains in the skin. When it reaches the skin capillary bed, vitamin D is bound to DBP and gets transported to the liver, where its metabolic transformation begins [12].

The two types of vitamin D undergo complex processing to become metabolically active. Initially, the prohormone undergoes 25th-carbon hydroxylation in the liver via the action of 25-vitamin D 1-hydroxylase (1-OHase), which is a part of an enzymatic system dependent on cytochrome P-450 (CYP27B), present in the liver microsomes and mitochondria. This reaction generates 25-hydroxyvitamin D [25(OH)D], which is the most abundant circulating form of vitamin D, with an average blood concentration of 20–50 ng/ml (50–125 nmol/L) and a half-life of approximately 3–4 weeks. Its pool in the bloodstream is estimated to be in dynamic equilibrium with the reserves of 25(OH)D (muscles and adipose tissue). This makes the blood concentration a reliable measurement of vitamin D in the body. Under normal conditions, the percentage of conversion to 25(OH)D is low, with an almost 50% distribution in the fat and muscle compartments. If vitamin D ingestion is excessive, then most of it gets fixed in fat tissues [12]. Because of its low biological activity, 25(OH)D is transported to the kidneys, where it undergoes a second hydroxylation, resulting in the active forms calcitriol (1,25-dihydroxyvitamin D

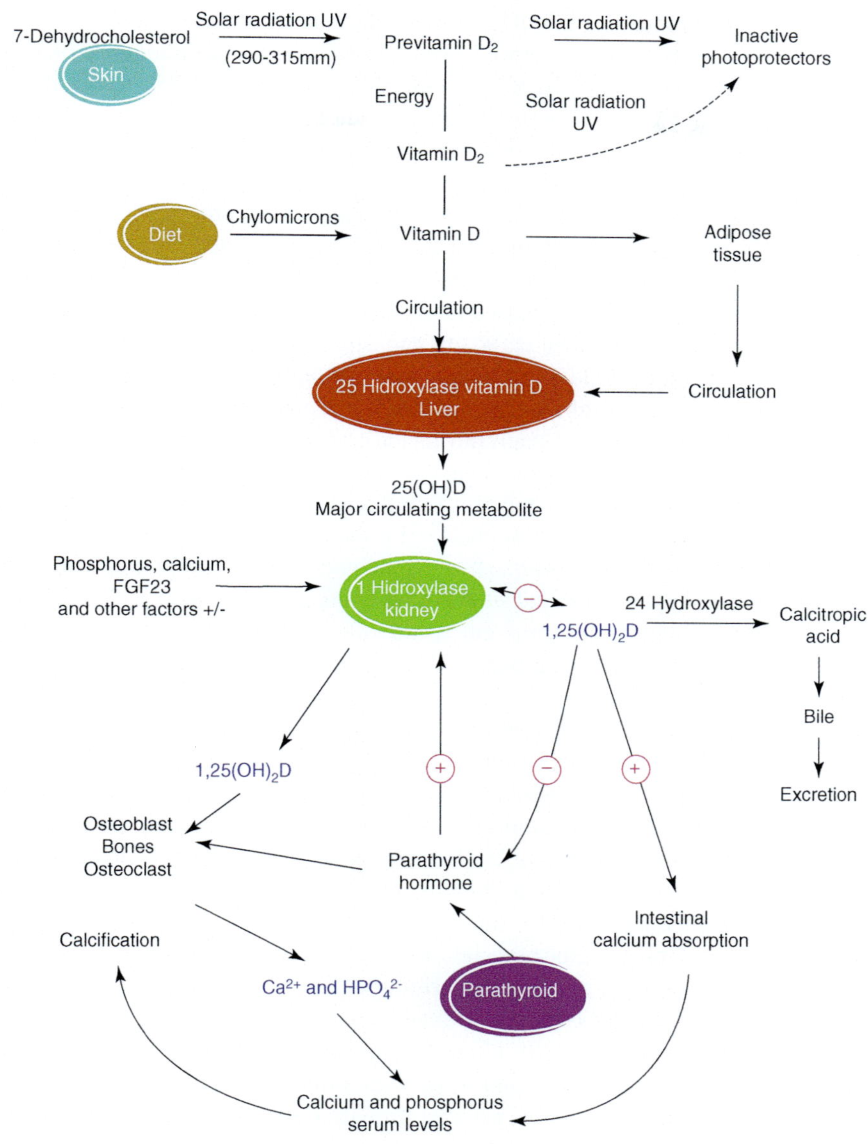

Fig. 11.4 Vitamin D synthesis, metabolism, and action regulating calcium and phosphorus levels and bone metabolism

[1,25$(OH)_2$D]) and calcitroic acid (24,25-dihydroxyvitamin D [24,25$(OH)_2$D]) via the action of 1-OHase enzymes and vitamin D-24-hydroxylase (24-OHase) present in the mitochondria of cells of the proximal convoluted tubule. DBP and 25(OH)D are filtered by the glomerulus and absorbed in the proximal tubule by low-density lipoprotein receptors, which control the capture of the 25(OH)D–DBP complex within the cells of the tube and the subsequent hydroxylation of 1,25$(OH)_2$D.

Several factors regulate 1,25(OH)2D levels, such as 1-OHase, the hydroxylation of which is activated by parathyroid hormone (PTH), and calcitonin, which is inhibited by the plasma levels of calcium, phosphorus, and 1,25$(OH)_2$D itself, whose half-life is 15 days. The blood concentration of phosphorus directly acts, without PTH intervention, and hypophosphatemia increases the production of 1,25$(OH)_2$D [12] (Fig. 11.4).

Recent studies have emphasized on the importance of the nontraditional roles of vitamin D in pregnancy and in the placenta and have reported an association of vitamin D deficiency in pregnancy with preeclampsia, insulin resistance, gestational diabetes, bacterial vaginosis, increased prematurity, and placental abruption, as well as FGR. Currently, nutrition in early life and other exogenous factors have been recognized to play a key role in the pathogenesis of and predisposition to diseases, which seem to go on to subsequent generations. Epigenetic changes establish a connection with the nutritional status during the critical periods of development and cause changes in gene expression that can lead to the development of disease phenotypes. However, whether vitamin D influences fetal growth, particularly in cases of growth restriction, remains unclear. Further, maternal vitamin D deficiency has been linked to numerous adverse health outcomes, but its association with FGR remains unclear. Population-based studies have confirmed that vitamin D deficiency is considered a public health problem worldwide, particularly in the developing countries, which affects all age groups and has more concerning effects on pregnant women.

In 2010, Bodnar et al. [13] tried to elucidate the association of maternal serum concentrations of 25-hydroxyvitamin D [25(OH)D] in early pregnancy with the risk of small-for-gestational-age (SGA) size and to explore the association between single-nucleotide maternal polymorphisms in the vitamin D receptor gene. Serum 25(OH)D was related to the risk of SGA among white mothers but not among black mothers. The findings suggest that vitamin D has a complex relationship with fetal growth that can vary according to ethnicity. In 2011, Robinson et al. [14] conducted a study aimed at identifying the association of vitamin D levels with the occurrence of SGA in patients with severe and early-onset preeclampsia. They found that vitamin D deficiency was associated with an increased risk of preeclampsia and its diagnosis in the severe and early clinical manifestations. Vitamin D levels were lower among patients with SGA and those with a diagnosis of severe, early-onset preeclampsia than among those without growth restriction. Thus, the authors suspected that vitamin D impacts fetal growth via placental mechanisms [14]. In 2013, Gernand et al. [15] confirmed the association of maternal vitamin D deficiency with FGR, but the mechanisms involved were unclear. They tested the hypothesis that maternal 25(OH)D was associated with an increased risk of placental insufficiency. The result was that the relationship between 25(OH)D and vascular damage was modified by the child's sex. No association was observed between maternal 25(OH)D and vascular disorder in mothers with female fetuses. Therefore, the findings suggested complex relationships among vitamin D, placental vascular damage, and birth weight, which differed according to the child's sex. Maternal vitamin D status may be beneficial for male and female descendants through different mechanisms. In 2014, Gernand et al. [16] examined the association of maternal serum concentrations of 25(OH)D with the risk of SGA newborns. The mean 25(OH)D concentration was lower in women with SGA newborns than in those with newborns with an adequate weight. Maternal obesity and ethnicity influenced this relationship. Maternal vitamin D status in the second trimester is associated with the risk of SGA in all women and in the subgroups of white and nonobese women.

In 2015, Khalessi et al. [17] found that maternal hypovitaminosis D harms fetal growth and causes adverse results in pregnancy, including FGR and low birth weight. The mean maternal vitamin D level was lower for newborns with low birth weight than for those with an adequate birth weight. All mothers of newborns with a head circumference of ≤33 cm also had vitamin D deficiency. In 2016, Miliku et al. [18] examined maternal vitamin D concentrations during pregnancy, fetal growth patterns, and the risk of adverse outcomes at birth and reported an association of low maternal 25(OH)D concentrations with FGR and with an increased risk of preterm birth and SGA size at birth. Further studies are needed to investigate the causality of these associations and the potential for public health interventions. In 2017, Wookey et al. [19] investigated whether DBP expression is altered in placental dysfunction associated with FGR. Their results showed significantly reduced placental DBP levels, which were strongly associated with idiopathic FGR. Thus, DBP may be a factor in unexplained placental dysfunction associated with idiopathic FGR and can potentially serve as a biomarker for this disease [19].

Sildenafil

Recently, one of the most widely studied treatments has been sildenafil, which is a phosphodiesterase type 5 inhibitor; it blocks the enzyme phosphodiesterase, preventing the degradation of cyclic guanosine monophosphate (cGMP) and potentializing the action of nitric oxide [20]. Maternal spiral arteries that have not undergone complete remodeling in the beginning of pregnancy present muscle layers that are still responsive to nitric oxide and can go through vasodilation, leading to an increased blood flow [21].

In November 2017, a meta-analysis by Paauw et al. [22] evaluated 24 studies on sildenafil and FGR published before November 2016. Of these, 22 were conducted using animal models, such as mice, rats, rabbits, sheep, and pigs, and the two studies with humans were randomized clinical trials. The meta-analysis found a significant increase in the fetal weight gain in the group that presented FGR and preeclampsia but not in the pregnancies without any complication. The maximum weight gain was approximately 10% [22]. Furthermore, it showed that differences between the studies, such as different medication dosages and administration methods, did not significantly influence the treatment effectiveness. However, a trend for a better effect was observed when the drug was orally and continuously administered and administered throughout the pregnancy [22]. Finally, the authors warned that few studies have evaluated the safety of using sildenafil during pregnancy because this medication crosses the placental barrier and may cause embryotoxicity at high doses. Further, adverse maternal effects such as intense headaches can occur.

A study including five placebo-controlled randomized multicenter clinical trials on the use of sildenafil and the prognosis for early-onset FGR (STRIDER) is in progress [23], encompassing Australia and New Zealand, the Netherlands, the United Kingdom, Ireland, and Canada. Pregnant women between 18 and 30 weeks with a diagnosis of early-onset, severe FGR are included. Each patient receives a 25 mg dose of sildenafil or a matching placebo thrice a day until 32 weeks of pregnancy. Although each center presents an autonomous clinical trial with a few differences expected between results, it is believed that the multicenter character of STRIDER may help elucidate the role of sildenafil on fetal growth and its safety and efficacy for use in clinical practice.

Nitric Oxide

Nitric oxide has been considered an important bioregulatory molecule acting on vascular tone [24]. It causes vasodilation, relaxes smooth muscle, and inhibits platelet aggregation and leukocyte adhesion. In pregnancies without any disease, uterine arteries increase the endothelial nitric oxide synthase activity and its protein expression, thereby improving uterine perfusion. This enzyme is also expressed in the placenta and the umbilical artery endothelium, where nitric oxide production contributes to a low resistance in fetal–placental circulation [24].

The exogenous administration of nitric oxide can present an important role in pregnancies with preeclampsia or FGR by increasing uteroplacental perfusion [25]. A randomized clinical trial, published in 2017, used nitroglycerin patches and placebo in pregnant women with FGR. The patches released 10 mg every 24 h and were used for 3 consecutive days. The result was decreased uterine and umbilical arteries resistance and pulsatility. Another study from the same year compared nitric oxide plus maternal plasma expansion with placebo in pregnant women with FGR. Glyceryl trinitrate transdermal patches releasing 5 mg every 24 h were used only 12 h a day to prevent tolerance. Fluid intake was increased to 2.5 l of water per day. After 2 weeks, a decrease in the systemic vascular resistance and an increase in the cardiac output were noticed in the group receiving the treatment. At birth, newborns from the medication group were at a greater weight percentile [26].

New technologies are being tested, such as using a vasodilator (SE175) that also releases nitric oxide combined with a peptide that would act only on the uterine and placental region, thereby minimizing tolerance and side effects. The group responsible for this research already has promising results in animals, with increased weight percentiles and decreased vascular resistance, showing that this may be a part of clinical practice in the coming years [27].

Bed Rest

Bed rest at the hospital or at home is widely prescribed for several obstetric complications, including preterm labor, hemorrhagic syndromes, multiple gestation, pregnancy hypertension, and FGR [28]. It is estimated that 700,000 patients are prescribed bed rest every year in the United States [29]. Patients with FGR are routinely advised to rest in an attempt to improve uteroplacental perfusion. Bed rest supposedly decreases the peripheral blood flow and inferior vena cava compression and improves the venous return and cardiac output, thereby increasing the uteroplacental circulation [30]. Furthermore, several patients are hospitalized for a stricter control of fetal well-being [28]. However, prolonged bed rest can be harmful to patients and may be associated with an increased risk of thromboembolism [31], muscle atrophy, constipation, and stress, as well as higher costs for the health system [30, 32].

A 2004 study with 104 high-risk patients in bed rest at a hospital showed maternal weekly weight gain to be less than the recommended gain and fetal weight at birth to be lower than the average weight (compared with newborns of the same gestational age, ethnicity, and sex). The study suggested that maternal weight loss associated with bed rest is related to a lower birth weight and an increased risk of FGR [29]. A Cochrane systematic review was conducted to evaluate the effects of bed rest in the hospital on patients with FGR. Only one study, with 107 patients, comparing hospital bed rest with outpatient management (with medical leave from work) was included in the review [33]. No statistically significant differences were observed in weight, gestational age at birth, and neonatal prognosis. The review concluded that there is not enough evidence for prescribing bed rest in the hospital for patients with FGR but pointed out that studies are too scarce to exclude any benefit with a reasonable degree of certainty. Although widely practiced, hospitalization for bed rest in FGR has no benefits proven by scientific evidence and is inconvenient to patients and their families, in addition to the increasing costs [28].

Maternal Gene Therapy with Vascular Endothelial Growth Factor (VEGF)

Inadequate trophoblast invasion results in an incomplete spiral artery remodeling and high-resistance, low-flow circulation [34, 35]. This mechanism leads to reduced placental perfusion, oxidative stress, and an imbalance between the angiogenic factors, such as VEGF and placental growth factor, and the anti-angiogenic factors, such as soluble fms-like tyrosine kinase-1 (sFIT-1) and soluble endoglin [36, 37]. A possible approach for the treatment of FGR would be increasing the VEGF levels in the uterine arteries, leading to vasodilation and an increase in angiogenesis. This can be accomplished by injecting the uterine arteries with adenovirus vectors coding for VEGF through interventional radiology, leading to a short-term increase in VEGF expression [21].

A study in normal sheep pregnancies, published in 2008, showed an increased flow in the uterine arteries due to decreased vasoconstriction. This effect was noticed 4–7 days after injecting the vector, and the increased flow was sustained for up to 6 weeks (until the end of sheep pregnancies) probably because of neovascularization and the modification of vascular reactivity [38, 39]. In 2014, a study in sheep afflicted by FGR and treated using gene therapy with VEGF showed an increase in the growth rate and a decrease in the brain-sparing effect (assessed using the BPD/

AC or brain weight/liver weight ratio) in comparison with the group treated with placebo [40]. A 2016 study on Guinea pigs with induced FGR (the placental physiology of Guinea pigs is more similar to the human one than that of other animals) concluded that the treatment led to an increase in the growth rate and fewer fetuses were affected by severe FGR at birth [41]. Animal model studies have not shown evidence that the vector crosses the placental barrier or that VEGF is expressed in fetal tissues [38].

A multicenter clinical trial termed "Does vascular endothelial growth factor gene therapy safely improve outcome in severe early-onset fetal growth restriction?" (EVERREST) is being conducted since 2013 aiming to evaluate the safety and effectiveness of maternal gene therapy with VEGF in severe early-onset FGR [42]. At the moment, the group is conducting a prospective observational study in pregnancies with severe early-onset FGR to define the inclusion criteria, probably pregnant women with severe early-onset FGR with greater risks of fetal and neonatal death [43].

Although the method is invasive, no ethical or legal objections to the use of this therapy in clinical studies in pregnant women were found because the disease still lacks effective treatment and gene therapy with VEGF has the potential to cause vasodilation in maternal uteroplacental circulation [44].

Nanotechnology and Treatment Strategies Targeted at Uteroplacental Circulation

Numerous studies have focused on treatment strategies that may locally act on uteroplacental circulation or on trophoblastic tissue to improve placental function and increase uterine circulation [21].

Peptide sequences that selectively bind to the placenta and, therefore, do not interfere with the normal development can be used to carry proteins such as insulin-like growth factor type 2 specifically to the placental tissue. Insulin-like growth factors stimulate cell proliferation in the placenta and promote a greater placental supply of glucose and amino acids [45, 46]. Studies in mice have shown an increase in the placental and fetal weights [47]. Another treatment currently under study uses microRNA inhibitors, particularly miR145-3 and miR675, that have been identified as placental growth inhibitors. In rats, an increase in the placental and fetal weights was found when compared with controls. Tests with human trophoblastic tissue have also been conducted in the first trimester, decreasing miR145 expression and increasing cytotrophoblast proliferation [48]. Although these new treatment strategies seem promising, all of them require further studies to prove their safety and effectiveness.

Statins

Statins inhibit 3-hydroxy-3-methylglutaryl-coenzyme A reductase (HMG-CoA reductase), which is known for its cardioprotective effect by acting on lipids. However, statins also have anti-inflammatory and antioxidant effects, making them potentially beneficial for inadequate placentation [49]. Statins were classified into Food and Drug Administration (FDA) pregnancy category X in the 1980s. This happened mostly because, at that moment, there were no benefits justifying their use in pregnancy [50]. However, records of exposure to pravastatin in the United States (20 cases) and Canada (288 cases) show no association with fetal malformations [51, 52]. In addition, a prospective observational study conducted in Canada with 64 patients found no greater incidence of fetal malformations resulting from the exposure to pravastatin in the first trimester [53]. If studies with pravastatin show benefits during pregnancy, then this classification will probably be reviewed [54].

A study, published in 2013, on rats with reduced uteroplacental perfusion showed that rats treated with pravastatin improved maternal hypertension, decreased sFlt-1, and increased VEGF and fetal weight compared with controls [55]. In a study on 21 patients with antiphospholipid antibody syndrome treated with aspirin and low-molecular-weight heparin, 11 of these patients were also treated with pravastatin after developing preeclampsia or FGR. The results revealed an increase in the gestational age at delivery and an apparent improvement in the perinatal prognosis in patients who received pravastatin [56].

In England, a randomized double-blind clinical trial is being conducted in patients with early-onset preeclampsia between 24 weeks and 31 weeks and 6 days. The study will measure sFlt-1 levels 48 h after randomization and evaluate neonatal morbidity and mortality [49]. Another randomized double-blind clinical trial is being conducted in the United States with pregnant women between 12 weeks and 16 weeks and 6 days with a history of preeclampsia in prior pregnancies to evaluate the safety and pharmacokinetics of pravastatin in preeclampsia and FGR [57].

Conclusion

Since FGR is diagnosed, there are no proven effective therapies to reverse or at least interrupt the progressive course of placental insufficiency. Fetal surveillance and decision time to delivery are still the main strategies in the management of these fetuses. Some recommendations, like bed rest, despite widely prescribed, are not established to be benefic. Several studies with potential new possibilities of therapies are done, but we have to wait for the results before implementing these treatments in clinical practice.

References

1. Froen JF, Gardosi JO, Thurmann A, Francis A, Stray-Pedersen B. Restricted fetal growth in sudden intrauterine unexplained death. Acta Obstet Gynecol Scand. 2004;83:801–7.
2. Barker DJP, Gluckman PD, Godfrey KM. Fetal nutrition and cardiovascular disease in adult life. Lancet. 1993;341:938–41.
3. Mandruzzato GP, Bogatti P, Fisher L, Gigli C. The clinical significance of absent or reverse end diastolic flow in the fetal aorta and umbilical artery. Ultrasound Obstet Gynecol. 1991;1:192–6.
4. Nardozza LM, Caetano AC, Zamarian AC, Mazzola JB, Silva CP, Marçal VM, et al. Fetal growth restriction: current knowledge. Arch Gynecol Obstet. 2017;295:1061–77.

5. Waitzberg DL, Garla P. Contribution of omega-3 fatty acids for memory and cognitive function. Nutr Hosp. 2014;30:467–77.
6. Agostoni C, Marangoni F, Stival G, Gatelli I, Pinto F, Risé P, et al. Whole blood fatty acid composition differs in term versus mildly preterm infants: small versus matched appropriate for gestational age. Pediatr Res. 2008;64:298–302.
7. Brantsæter AL, Birgisdottir BE, Meltzer HM, Kvalem HE, Alexander J, Magnus P, et al. Maternal seafood consumption and infant birth weight, length and head circumference in the Norwegian Mother and Child Cohort Study. Br J Nutr. 2012;107:436–44.
8. Gaete MG, Atalah ES. Niveles de LC-PUFA n-3 en la leche maternal despues de incentivar el consumo de valimentosx marinos. Rev Chil Pediatr. 2003;74:158–65.
9. Olsen SF, Sørensen JD, Secher NJ, Hedegaard M, Henriksen TB, Hansen HS, et al. Randomised controlled trial of effect of fish-oil supplementation on pregnancy duration. Lancet. 1992;25:1003–7.
10. Saccone G, Berghella V, Maruotti GM, Sarno L, Martinelli P. Omega-3 supplementation during pregnancy to prevent recurrent intrauterine growth restriction: systematic review and meta-analysis of randomized controlled trials. Ultrasound Obstet Gynecol. 2015;46:659–64.
11. Saccone G, Saccone I, Berghella V. Omega-3 long-chain polyunsaturated fatty acids and fish oil supplementation during pregnancy: which evidence? J Matern Fetal Neonatal Med. 2016;29:2389–97.
12. Urrutia-Pereira M, Sole D. Vitamin D deficiency in pregnancy and its impact on the fetus, the newborn, and in childhood. Rev Paul Pediatr. 2015;33:104–13.
13. Bodnar LM, Catov JM, Zmuda JM, Cooper ME, Parrott MS, Roberts JM, et al. Maternal serum 25-hydroxyvitamin D concentrations are associated with small-for-gestational age births in white women. J Nutr. 2010;140:999–1006.
14. Robinson CJ, Wagner CL, Hollis BW, Baatz JE, Johnson DD. Maternal vitamin D and fetal growth in early-onset severe preeclampsia. Am J Obstet Gynecol. 2011;204:556.e1–4.
15. Gernand AD, Bodnar LM, Klebanoff MA, Parks WT, Simhan HN. Maternal serum 25-hydroxyvitamin D and placental vascular pathology in a multicenter US cohort. Am J Clin Nutr. 2013;98:383–8.
16. Gernand AD, Simhan HN, Caritis S, Bodnar LM. Maternal vitamin D status and small-for-gestational-age offspring in women at high risk for preeclampsia. Obstet Gynecol. 2014;123:40–8.
17. Khalessi N, Kalani M, Araghi M, Farahani Z. The relationship between maternal vitamin D deficiency and low birth weight neonates. J Family Reprod Health. 2015;9:113–7.
18. Miliku K, Vinkhuyzen A, Blanken LM, McGrath JJ, Eyles DW, Burne TH, et al. Maternal vitamin D concentrations during pregnancy, fetal growth patterns, and risks of adverse birth outcomes. Am J Clin Nutr. 2016;103:1514–22.
19. Wookey AF, Chollangi T, Yong HE, Kalionis B, Brennecke SP, Murthi P, et al. Placental vitamin D-binding protein expression in human idiopathic fetal growth restriction. J Pregnancy. 2017;2017:5120267.
20. El-Sayed MA, Saleh SA, Maher MA, Khidre AM. Utero-placental perfusion Doppler indices in growth restricted fetuses: effect of sildenafil citrate. J Mater Fetal Neonatal Med. 2018;31:1045–50.
21. Gromm KM, David AL. The role of aspirin, heparin, and other interventions in the prevention and treatment of fetal growth restriction. Am J Obstet Gynecol. 2018;218:S829–40.
22. Paauw ND, Terstappen F, Ganzevoort W, Joles JA, Gremmels H, Lely AT. Sildenafil during pregnancy a preclinical meta-analysis on fetal growth and maternal blood pressure. Hypertension. 2017;70:998–1006.
23. Pels A, Kenny LC, Alfirevic Z, Baker PN, von Dadelszen P, Gluud C, et al. STRIDER (Sildenafil The Rapy in dismal prognosis early onset fetal growth restriction): an international consortium of randomised placebo-controlled trials. BMC Pregnancy Childbirth. 2017;17:440.
24. Sladek SM, Magness RR, Conrad KP. Nitric oxide and pregnancy. Am J Phsyiol. 1997;272:441–63.
25. Gupta S, Chauhan M, Sen J, Nanda S. Effect of transdermal nitroglycerine on Doppler velocity waveforms of the uterine, umbilical and fetal middle cerebral arteries in patients with chronic placental insufficiency: a prospective RCT. J Clin Diagn Res. 2017;11:QC13–7.

26. Tiralongo GM, Pisani I, Vasapollo B, Khalil A, Thilaganathan B, Valensise H. Effect of a nitric oxide donor on maternal hemodynamics in fetal growth restriction. Ultrasound Obstet Gynecol. 2018;51:514–8.
27. Cureton N, Korotkova I, Baker B, Greenwood S, Wareing M, Kotamraju VR, et al. Selective targeting of a novel vasodilator to the uterine vasculature to treat impaired uteroplacental perfusion in pregnancy. Theranostics. 2017;7:3715–31.
28. Say L, Gülmezoglu AM, Hofmeyr GJ. Bed rest in hospital for suspected impaired fetal growth. Cochrane Database Syst Rev. 2000;2:CD000034.
29. Maloni JA, Alexander GR, Schluchter MD, Shah DM, Park S. Antepartum bed rest: maternal weight change and infant birth weight. Biol Res Nurs. 2004;5:177–86.
30. Figueroa R, Maulik D. Prenatal therapy for fetal growth restriction. Clin Obstet Gynecol. 2006;49:308–19.
31. Kovacevich GJ, Gaich SA, Lavin JP, Hopkins MP, Crane SS, Stewart J, et al. The prevalence of thromboembolic events among women with extended bed rest prescribed as part of the treatment for premature labor or preterm premature rupture of membranes. Am J Obstet Gynecol. 2000;182:1089–92.
32. Heaman M, Gupton A. Perceptions of bed rest by women with high-risk pregnancies: a comparison between home and hospital. Birth. 1998;25:252–8.
33. Laurin J, Persson PH. The effect of bed rest in hospital on fetal outcome in pregnancies complicated by intra-uterine growth retardation. Acta Obstet Gynecol Scand. 1987;66:407–11.
34. Brosens JJ, Pijnenborg R, Brosens IA. The myometrial junctional zone spiral arteries in normal and abnormal pregnancies: a review of the literature. Am J Obstet Gynecol. 2002;187:1416–23.
35. Brosens IA, Robertson WB, Dixon HG. The role of the spiral arteries in the pathogenesis of preeclampsia. Obstet Gynecol Annu. 1972;1:177–91.
36. Levine RJ, Lam C, Qian C, Yu KF, Maynard SE, Sachs BP, et al. Soluble endoglin and other circulating antiangiogenic factors in preeclampsia. N Engl J Med. 2006;355:992–1005.
37. Benton SJ, McCowan LM, Heazell AE, Grynspan D, Hutcheon JA, Senger C, et al. Placental growth factor as a marker of fetal growth restriction caused by placental dysfunction. Placenta. 2016;42:1–8.
38. David AL, Torondel B, Zachary I, Wigley V, Abi-Nader K, Mehta V, et al. Local delivery of VEGF adenovirus to the uterine artery increases vasorelaxation and uterine blood flow in the pregnant sheep. Gene Ther. 2008;15:1344–50.
39. Mehta V, Abi-Nader KN, Peebles DM, Benjamin E, Wigley V, Torondel B, et al. Long-term increase in uterine blood flow is achieved by local overexpression of VEGFA(165) in the uterine arteries of pregnant sheep. Gene Ther. 2012;19:925–35.
40. Carr DJ, Wallace JM, Aitken RP, Milne JS, Mehta V, Martin JF, et al. Uteroplacental adenovirus vascular endothelial growth factor gene therapy increases fetal growth velocity in growth-restricted sheep pregnancies. Hum Gene Ther. 2014;25:375–84.
41. Swanson AM, Rossi CA, Ofir K, Mehta V, Boyd M, Barker H, et al. Maternal therapy with Ad.VEGF-A165 increases fetal weight at term in a guinea-pig model of fetal growth restriction. Hum Gene Ther. 2016;27:997–1007.
42. Gancberg D, Hoeveler A, Draghia-Akli R. Introduction: gene therapy and gene transfer projects of the 7th Framework Programme for Research and Technological Development of the European Union (second part). Hum Gene Ther Clin Dev. 2015;26:77.
43. Spencer R, Ambler G, Brodszki J, Diemert A, Figueras F, Gratacós E, et al. EVERREST prospective study: a 6-year prospective study to define the clinical and biological characteristics of pregnancies affected by severe early onset fetal growth restriction. BMC Pregnancy Childbirth. 2017;17:43.
44. Sheppard M, Spencer RN, Ashcroft R, David AL, EVERREST Consortium. Ethics and social acceptability of a proposed clinical trial using maternal gene therapy to treat severe early-onset fetal growth restriction. Ultrasound Obstet Gynecol. 2016;47:484–91.
45. Harris LK. Could peptide-decorated nanoparticles provide an improved approach for treating pregnancy complications? Nanomedicine. 2016;11(17):2235–8.
46. Constancia M, Hemberger M, Hughes J, Dean W, Ferguson-Smith A, Fundele R, et al. Placental-specific IGF-II is a major modulator of placental and fetal growth. Nature. 2002;417:945–8.

47. King A, Ndifon C, Lui S, Widdows K, Kotamraju VR, Agemy L, et al. Tumor-homing peptides as tools for targeted delivery of payloads to the placenta. Sci Adv. 2016;2:e1600349.
48. Beards F, Jones LE, Charnock J, Forbes K, Harris LK. Placental homing peptide-microRNA inhibitor conjugates for targeted enhancement of intrinsic placental growth signaling. Theranostics. 2017;7:2940–55.
49. Spencer R, Carr D, David A. Treatment of poor placentation and the prevention of associated adverse outcomes – what does the future hold? Prenat Diagn. 2014;34:677–84.
50. U.S. Food and Drug Administration Drug bulletin. Fed Reg. 1980;44:37434–67.
51. Edison R, Muenke M. Mechanistic and epidemiologic considerations in the evaluation of adverse birth outcomes following gestational exposure to statins. Am J Med Genet. 2004;131A:287.
52. Ofori B, Rey E, Berard A. Risk of congenital anomalies in pregnant users of statin drugs. Br J Clin Pharmacol. 2007;64:496.
53. Taguchi N, Rubin ET, Hosokawa A. Prenatal exposure to HMG-CoA reductase inhibitor: effects on fetal and neonatal outcomes. Repro Tox. 2008;26:175.
54. Taguchi N, Rubin ET, Hosokawa A, Choi J, Ying AY, Moretti ME, Koren G, Ito S. Prenatal exposure to HMG-CoA reductase inhibitors: effects on fetal and neonatal outcomes. Reprod Toxicol. 2008;26:175–7.
55. Bauer AJ, Banek CT, Needham K, Gillham H, Capoccia S, Regal JF, et al. Pravastatin attenuates hypertension, oxidative stress and angiogenic imbalance in rat model of placental ischemia-induced hypertension. Hypertension. 2013;61:1103–10.
56. Lefkou E, Mamopoulos A, Dagklis T, Vosnakis C, Rousso D, Girardi G. Pravastatin improves pregnancy outcomes in obstetric antiphospholipid syndrome refractory to antithrombotic therapy. J Clin Invest. 2016;126:2933–40.
57. Costantine M, Cleary K, Eunice Kennedy Shriver National Institute of Child Health and Human Development Obstetric – Fetal Pharmacology Research Units Network. Pravastatin for the prevention of preeclampsia in high-risk pregnant women. Obstet Gynecol. 2013;121:349–53.

Obstetric Management

12

Ana Carolina Rabachini Caetano and Luciano Marcondes Machado Nardozza

Introduction

The biggest challenges in the management of fetal growth restriction (FGR) are the precise diagnosis of fetuses at risk of adverse perinatal outcomes, prevention of fetal death, and timing of delivery [1]. Because there is no effective treatment to reverse or stop the progression of placental insufficiency yet, fetal vitality assessment and the decision regarding timing of delivery are the main strategies in the management of these fetuses [2]. However, despite numerous studies, the literature lacks a consensus on how to monitor and when and how to delivery in FGR (expectant management, labor induction, or elective cesarean section) [1].

A clinical trial titled *The Growth Restriction Intervention Trial* randomly divided pregnant women with FGR between 24 and 36 weeks into two groups: immediate delivery ($n = 296$) and expectant management ($n = 292$); the patients were assigned when obstetricians were in doubt about when to recommend delivery. Of these patients, 40% had absent or reversed end-diastolic flow in the umbilical artery Doppler. The number of fetal deaths was lower in the immediate delivery group than in the expectant management group (two versus nine). There was no statistically significant difference in the combined rates of neonatal death and severe disability at the age of 2 years between the immediate delivery group and the expectant management group [19% versus 16%, odds ratio (OR) 1.1, confidence interval (CI) 95% (0.7–1.8)]; however, the percentage of pregnancies under 31 weeks was 13% in the immediate delivery group and 5% in the expectant management group [2]. The follow-up of children aged 6–13 years showed no difference between the groups in terms of cognition, language, and motor and behavioral development [3]. These

A. C. R. Caetano (✉) · L. M. M. Nardozza
Discipline of Fetal Medicine, Department of Obstetrics, Paulista School of Medicine, Federal University of São Paulo (EPM-UNIFESP), São Paulo, SP, Brazil

L. M. M. Nardozza et al. (eds.), *Fetal Growth Restriction*,
https://doi.org/10.1007/978-3-030-00051-6_12

data suggest that expectant management of very premature growth-restricted fetuses, when there is doubt about the timing of delivery, results in more fetal deaths, but immediate delivery resulted in a greater number of neonatal deaths and that neither of the two produced a better neurological prognosis [3, 4].

The study "TRUFFLE—Trial of Randomized Umbilical and Fetal Flow in Europe" assessed neurological development in infants aged 2 years with early FGR born before 32 weeks of pregnancy. The patients were divided into three groups of recommended timing of delivery according to different strategies of assessing fetal vitality, such as reduction in the computerized cardiotocography short-term variation, early changes in the ductus venosus (DV) Doppler (pulsatility index above 95th percentile), and late changes in the DV Doppler (absent A-wave). Most of the infants had their deliveries recommended for reasons other than those in the protocol for each group (maternal or other fetal conditions). Only 32% of the patients had their delivery recommended based on study criteria. The groups based on DV Doppler used cardiotocography as a safety criterion, whereas the reverse did not apply, i.e., DV Doppler was not a safety criterion for the cardiotocography group. Survival without impairment at the age of 2 years in the group based on the reduction in cardiotocography short-term variation was worse (77%) than that in the two groups that used DV Doppler (83%), without any statistically significant difference. However, on analyzing the surviving infants, the groups that used DV Doppler showed half the prevalence of neurological impairment in comparison to the cardiotocography group (7% versus 15%, $p = 0.049$). The hypothesis was that the slightly worse prognosis in the cardiotocography group is explained by the absence of information on the DV Doppler. Therefore, they concluded that, in order to optimize the decision on the timing of delivery in early FGR, fetuses should be monitored longitudinally with the DV Doppler and computerized cardiotocography [5].

A 2010 clinical trial with women with suspected FGR between 36 and 41 weeks showed no increased neonatal morbidity or incidence of cesarean section or operative vaginal delivery, when comparing groups of labor induction and expectant management. The authors concluded that expectant management could be conducted with strict control of fetal vitality, but it would be wise to induce labor at term in order to prevent neonatal morbidity and fetal death [6]. A 2017 study by Pilliod et al. concluded that at 38 weeks and later, the risk of fetal death in expectant management for another week exceeded the risk of immediate delivery, regardless of whether the estimated fetal weight was below the 10th, 5th, or 3rd percentile. However, the lower the percentile, the higher the risk [7]. A retrospective study published in 2018 assessed 2232 patients with FGR (characterized in the study as estimated fetal weight below the 10th percentile) and compared labor induction with expectant management between 34 and 38 + 6 weeks. The authors concluded that labor induction at 37 weeks decreases the prevalence of fetal death and, additionally, in late preterm, it is associated with lower rates of neonatal death and nonreassuring cardiotocography pattern [8].

Although many studies have been conducted, there is a lack of consistent evidence to safely recommend the timing of delivery in FGR. The aim of a FGR clinical management protocol is to combine the existing evidence on the various methods of evaluation of fetal vitality (cardiotocography, fetal biophysical profile, and Doppler), in order to achieve the best growth and lung maturity and thus minimize the risks of fetal and neonatal morbidity and mortality. This decision is often based on gestational age, etiology of growth restriction, and degree of fetal vitality impairment, in addition to the experience and technological resources available to assess the fetus and treat the neonate, who preferably should be delivered in a tertiary hospital. One type of management considered ideal by many authors and used in our service is longitudinal monitoring of fetal vitality, starting between 24 and 26 weeks (depending on the viability gestational age used by the service), with ultrasound, biophysical, and Doppler velocimetry methods. Combining multiple tests in the evaluation of fetal vitality improves the prediction of acidemia and fetal death in comparison to isolated tests [9]. The intervals for this evaluation depend on gestational age and signs of placental insufficiency.

In the management of these fetuses, the first important step is trying to distinguish actual FGR, associated with placental insufficiency and worse perinatal prognosis, from fetuses of small constitution, with practically normal perinatal prognosis [10]. Early and late FGRs are distinguishable when considered in groups. Early FGR usually starts with an abnormal umbilical artery Doppler, progressing to brain-sparing, abnormal venous Doppler, abnormal computerized cardiotocography, and finally abnormal fetal biophysical profile [9]. The primary change in late FGR is observed in the middle cerebral artery Doppler or the umbilical artery Doppler, without significant changes in the venous Doppler. Changes in the cerebroplacental ratio (CPR) might be the only existing sign of hypoxemia. Furthermore, fetal death is faster and more unexpected in late FGR; thus, fetal vitality control must be intensified from 34 weeks onward [9].

Despite pathophysiological differences in placental insufficiency, when dealing with individual fetuses, clinical features can overlap, especially at borderline gestational age. Therefore, the same management protocol can be used to monitor and decide the timing of delivery in both groups [10]. Grouping patients according to the stage of evolution, with similar monitoring, timing of delivery, and fetal risks is a type of management described in the literature [10]. Based on evidence available in the literature and the features of our service and of the population of patients and obstetricians in the Department of Obstetrics, Paulista School of Medicine – Federal University of São Paulo (EPM-UNIFESP), Brazil, we follow a management protocol based on the stages of evolution of FGR [11]. The protocol is summarized in Table 12.1.

Small for Gestational Age Fetuses

In fetuses with estimated weight between the 3rd and 10th percentiles, without changes in the Doppler, fetal vitality (Doppler and fetal biophysical profile) and fetal growth can be assessed every 2 weeks [10]. If the patient does not go into labor spontaneously, it can be induced at 40 weeks. Prostaglandins can be carefully used

Table 12.1 Management of fetal growth restriction according to the stages of evolution proposed in the Department of Obstetrics, Paulista School of Medicine – Federal University of São Paulo

Stage	Description	Viability monitoring	Birth
SGA fetus	3rd > EFW < 10th	Monitor vitality every 2 weeks	Birth at 40 weeks
Stage 1	EFW < 3rd EFW < 1st	Monitor vitality every 2 weeks until 34w and every week after 34w	Birth at 38 weeks Birth at 37 weeks
Stage 2	Abnormalities in UA, MCA, or CPR	Monitor vitality twice a week	Birth at 37 weeks
Stage 3	Absent-end diastole in UA	Hospitalization and daily monitoring	Birth at 34 weeks (elective cesarean)
Stage 4	UA with reversed-end diastole or DV PI >95th	Hospitalization and delivery	Delivery when viable (26–28 weeks) (elective cesarean)
Stage 5	Reversed wave DV/STV in cCTG <3 ms or FHR decelerations	Hospitalization and delivery	Delivery when viable 26–28 weeks (elective cesarean)

SGA small for gestational age, *EFW* estimated fetal weight, *UA* umbilical artery, *MCA* medial cerebral artery, *CPR* cerebroplacental ratio, *PI* pulsatility index, *DV* ductus venosus, *cCTG* computerized cardiotocography, *STV* short-term variation, *FHR* fetal heart rate

for labor induction, with strict control of intrapartum vitality, owing to the risk of hyperstimulation in fetuses that could present some degree of placental injury [11].

Stage 1: Fetal Growth Restriction with Normal Doppler (Mild Placental Insufficiency)

Stage 1 is characterized by an estimated fetal weight below the 3rd percentile, without changes in the Doppler. Fetal growth and vitality (Doppler and fetal biophysical profile) can be assessed every 2 weeks up to 34 weeks and weekly after that [11]. Delivery can be carefully induced at 38 weeks, avoiding, however, the use of prostaglandins [1]. If the estimated weight is below the 1st percentile, delivery is considered at 37 weeks [10, 11] (Fig. 12.1).

Stage 2: Fetal Growth Restriction with Moderate Placental Insufficiency (with Changes in the Doppler)

Stage 2 is characterized by the following changes in the Doppler: umbilical artery pulsatility index (PI) >95th percentile, middle cerebral artery PI <5th percentile, or CPR <5th percentile. Weekly assessment of fetal vitality (Doppler and fetal biophysical profile) is acceptable [10, 12]. In our service, we monitor fetal vitality twice a week and consider hospitalization of the patient after 34 weeks to optimize clinical control and check vitality daily [11]. Evidence suggests a low risk of fetal

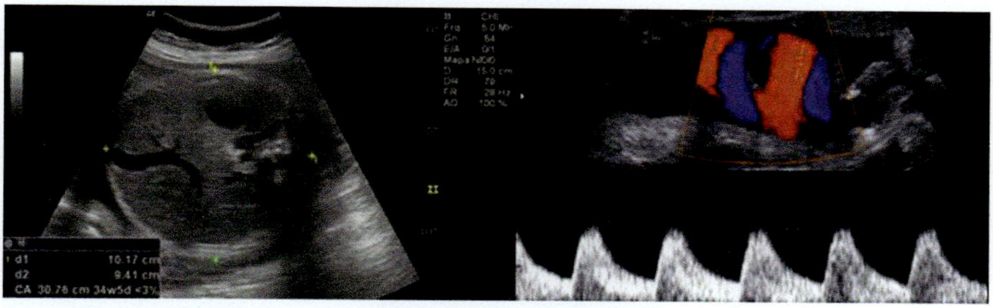

Fig. 12.1 Stage 1 – Fetal growth restriction (in the figure: abdominal circumference below the 3rd percentile), with normal Doppler velocimetry (in the figure: normal umbilical artery Doppler velocimetry)

deterioration before term, but it also shows no benefits in maintaining pregnancy after reaching term. Delivery induction at 37 weeks is acceptable, avoiding, however, the use of prostaglandins. There is a higher risk of intrapartum fetal distress [12]. Resolution by elective cesarean section is acceptable for patients with an unfavorable cervix and changes in the CPR [in our service, we consider it altered when it is less than 1] [13].

There are FGR management protocols in the literature that include mean uterine artery PI >95th percentile in the category above and recommend the resolution of delivery at 37 weeks [10]. A few studies showed that small fetuses with changes in the uterine artery Doppler have twice the risk of developing changes in the middle cerebral artery Doppler before delivery, which could be useful in planning fetal surveillance [14, 15]. However, longitudinal studies with serial assessment of uterine arteries failed to show any worsening of Doppler from diagnosis to delivery, so its use as a method to evaluate fetal vitality is questionable [15]. At our service, we use uterine artery Doppler as one of the FGR diagnostic criteria [according to the Delphi consensus [16]] but not as a management criterion (Fig. 12.2).

Stage 3: Fetal Growth Restriction with Severe Placental Insufficiency (Umbilical Artery Doppler with Absent End-Diastolic Flow)

Stage 3 is defined by the absence of end-diastolic flow in the umbilical artery Doppler or reversed end-diastolic flow in the aortic isthmus Doppler. Fetal monitoring every 2 days is acceptable [5]. To optimize the control of fetal vitality, in our service, patients are hospitalized after the limit of viability and evaluated on a daily basis (Doppler, fetal biophysical profile, and computerized cardiotocography) [11]. Delivery is recommended at 34 weeks by elective cesarean section, because the risk of fetal distress in labor induction exceeds 50% [10, 11] (Fig. 12.3).

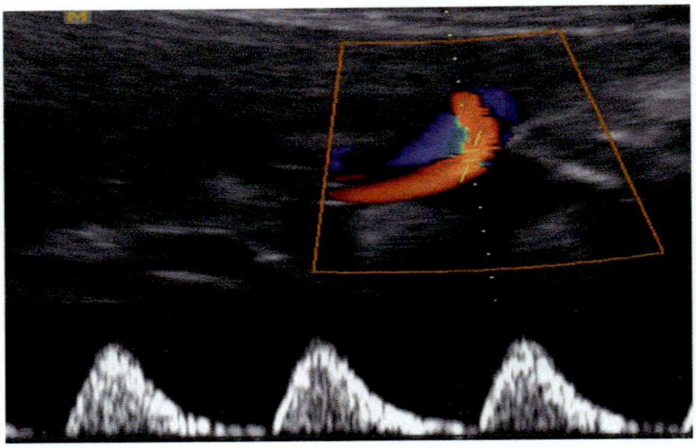

Fig. 12.2 Stage 2 – Umbilical artery Doppler velocimetry with increased resistance

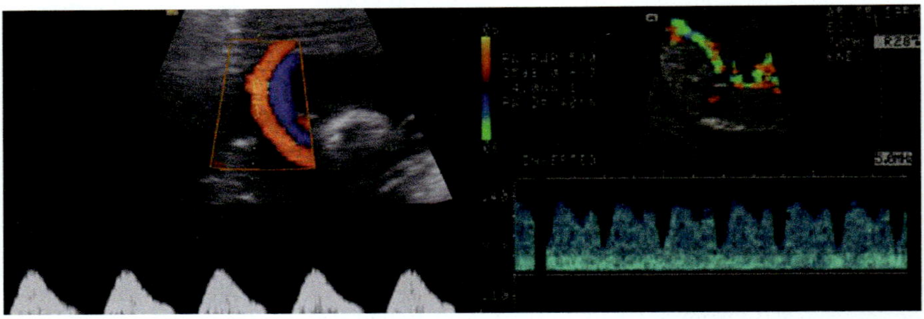

Fig. 12.3 Stage 3 – Absence of end-diastolic flow in the umbilical artery, with normal ductus venosus Doppler

Stage 4: Fetal Growth Restriction with Advanced Fetal Deterioration (Umbilical Artery Doppler with Reversed End-Diastolic Flow or Ductus Venosus with Pulsatility Index ˃95th Percentile)

Stage 4 is defined by reversed end-diastolic flow in the umbilical artery Doppler or a DV Doppler with PI ˃95th percentile. There is a high risk of fetal death and impairment of neurological development, and the following protocol should be followed: hospitalization and daily monitoring of fetal vitality with Doppler, fetal biophysical profile, and computerized cardiotocography. Some protocols in the literature recommend delivery from 30 weeks onward [10]; however, in our service, we have adopted delivery by elective cesarean section, after the neonatal intensive unit care (NIUC) limit of viability (26 weeks and estimated fetal weight ≥500 g or 28 weeks regardless of estimated fetal weight) [11]. In this stage, before 30 weeks, we can use the fetal biophysical profile to evaluate the possibility of expectant management at least for corticosteroid therapy and transfer to a tertiary service [9]. A fetal biophysical profile score of less than 6/10 is a recommendation for birth at the limit of viability due to its high association with acidemia [1]; nonetheless, we must emphasize that the fetal biophysical profile before 28 weeks changes on an average of 1 week after the changes in the venous Doppler [17], a period that could increase neonatal survival by 14% [1] (Fig. 12.4).

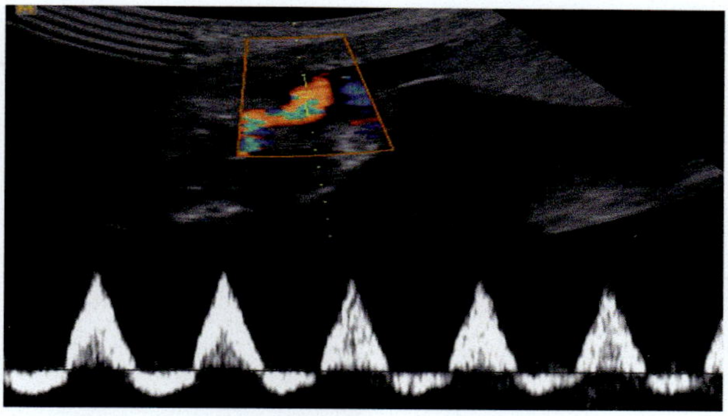

Fig. 12.4 Stage 4 – Umbilical artery Doppler with reversed end-diastolic flow

Stage 5: Fetal Growth Restriction with a High Probability of Fetal Acidosis and a High Risk of Fetal Death (Ductus Venosus Doppler with Reversed A-Wave, Computerized Cardiotocography <3 ms, or Fetal Heart Rate Decelerations)

Stage 5 is defined by ductus venosus Doppler with reversed A-wave, computerized cardiotocography short-term variation <3 ms, or fetal heart rate decelerations. Delivery is recommended by elective cesarean section at the moment of diagnosis, depending on the NIUC limit of viability [10, 11] (Fig. 12.5). In earlier gestational ages, parents should be advised according to the available data of viability without impairment, and their opinion should be taken into account in the decision on delivery [10]. We must emphasize that the survival rate described in the literature for newborns between 24 and 26 weeks with FGR is less than 50%, and the risk of severe morbidity is more than 80% [18]. Survival rates surpass 50% when fetuses reach 500 g or 26 weeks [1].

In any of these stages, whenever any change can indicate accelerated progression of the disease (e.g., the co-occurrence of preeclampsia) or any signs of fetal deterioration arise, the frequency of fetal vitality assessment must be increased until the gestational age for delivery is reached [1].

Amniotic Fluid Assessment

A systematic review conducted in 2008 with low- and high-risk pregnancies compared the amniotic fluid index with the deepest vertical pocket measurement, considered normal when greater or equal than 20 mm, as a method of amniotic fluid assessment. The authors concluded that the deepest vertical pocket measurement is more beneficial because assessing the amniotic fluid index increases oligohydramnios and labor induction rates without improving perinatal prognosis [19]. A meta-analysis including 18 clinical trials showed that an amniotic fluid index less than 50 mm is associated with a lower 5-min Apgar score and increased intrapartum fetal distress; however, it showed no association with fetal acidosis or perinatal death [20]. To date, the inclusion of oligohydramnios in FGR management protocols has found no consensus in the literature, and more studies are needed to validate its use [14].

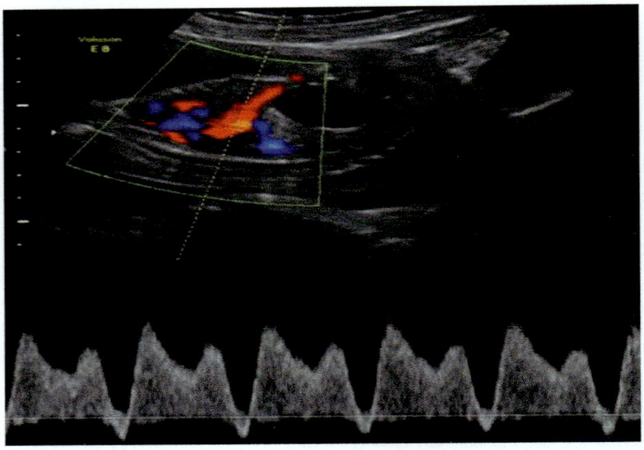

Fig. 12.5 Stage 5 – Reversed ductus venosus Doppler

Corticosteroids and Magnesium Sulfate

Antenatal corticosteroids should be used between 24 and 34 weeks and preferably in the week prior to the scheduled delivery (maximum 2 cycles) to accelerate fetal lung maturity and reduce the risk of intracranial bleeding [21]. A systematic review of the literature with a meta-analysis published in 2016 showed the benefits of using corticosteroids between 34 and 36 6/7 weeks in patients with immediate risk of late preterm birth [22]. It also concluded that, in cesarean sections planned between 37 and 38 + 6 weeks, parents can be advised about the benefits of a single dose of corticosteroids, such as decreased respiratory distress syndrome [22]. Nevertheless, soon after the use of corticosteroids, Doppler indices may show only a transitory improvement. For births before 32 weeks, the use of magnesium sulfate is recommended for neuroprotection [20]. Further studies on the use of corticosteroids and magnesium sulfate in specific groups of patients, such as those of restricted fetal growth, must be conducted [23].

Conclusion

As there is no effective treatment of FGR, the optimal clinical management is the main goal in these fetuses. There is no consensus in the literature on how to monitor and when and how to delivery in FGR. Besides that, a uniform management, based on protocol, improves perinatal outcome. A stage-based management protocol, as described in this chapter, can help the clinicians minimizing practice variations.

References

1. Seravalli V, Baschat AA. A uniform management approach to optimize outcome in fetal growth restriction. Obstet Gynecol Clin North Am. 2015;42:275–88.
2. Figueras F, Gardosi J. Intrauterine growth restriction: new concepts in antenatal surveillance, diagnosis, and management. Intrauterine growth restriction: new concepts in antenatal surveillance, diagnosis, and management. Am J Obstet Gynecol. 2011;204:288–300.

3. Thornton JG, Hornbuckle J, Vail A, Spiegelhalter DJ, Levene M. GRIT study group. Infant wellbeing at 2 years of age in the Growth Restriction Intervention Trial (GRIT): multicentred randomised controlled trial. Lancet. 2004;364:513–20.
4. Walker DM, Marlow N, Upstone L, Gross H, Hornbuckle J, Vail A, et al. The Growth Restriction Intervention Trial: long-term outcomes in a randomized trial of timing of delivery in fetal growth restriction. Am J Obstet Gynecol. 2011;204:34.e1–9.
5. Visser GHA, Bilardo CM, Derks JB, Ferrazzi E, Fratelli N, Frusca T, et al. Fetal monitoring indications for delivery and 2-year outcome in 310 infants with fetal growth restriction delivered before 32 weeks' gestation in the TRUFFLE study. Ultrasound Obstet Gynecol. 2017;50:347–52.
6. Boers KE, Vijgen SM, Bijilenga D, van der Post JA, Bekedam DJ, Kwee A, et al. Induction versus expectant monitoring for intrauterine growth restriction at term: randomised equivalence trial (DIGITAT). BMJ. 2010;341:c7087.
7. Pilliod RA, Page JM, Sparks TN, Caughey AB. The growth-restricted fetus: risk of mortality by each additional week of expectant management. J Matern Fetal Neonatal Med. 2017;3:1–6. https://doi.org/10.1080/14767058.2017.1381904.
8. Rabinovich A, Tsemach T, Novack L, Mazor M, Rafaeli-Yehudai T, Staretz-Chacham O, et al. Late preterm and early term: when to induce a growth restricted fetus? A population-based study. J Matern Fetal Neonatal Med. 2018;31:926–32.
9. Baschat AA. Integrated fetal testing in growth restriction: combining multivessel Doppler and biophysical parameters. Ultrasound Obstet Gynecol. 2003;21:1–8.
10. Figueras F, Gratacós E. Update on the diagnosis and classification of fetal growth restriction and proposal of a stage-based management protocol. Fetal Diagn Ther. 2014;36:86–98.
11. Nardozza LM, Caetano AC, Zamarian AC, Mazzola JB, Silva CP, Marçal VM, et al. Fetal growth restriction: current knowledge. Arch Gynecol Obstet. 2017;295:1061–77.
12. Figueras F, Gratacos E. Stage-based approach to the management of fetal growth restriction. Prenat Diagn. 2014;34:655–9.
13. Arias F. Accuracy of the middle-cerebral-to-umbilical-artery resistance index ratio in the prediction of neonatal outcome in patients at high risk for fetal and neonatal complications. Am J Obstet Gynecol. 1994;171:1541–5.
14. Cruz-Martinez R, Savchev S, Cruz-Lemini M, Mendez A, Gratacos E, Figueras F. Clinical utility of third-trimester uterine artery Doppler in the prediction of brain hemodynamic deterioration and adverse perinatal outcome in small-for-gestational-age fetuses. Ultrasound Obstet Gynecol. 2014;45:273–8.
15. Figueras F, Caradeux J, Crispi F, Eixarch E, Peguero A, Gratacos E. Diagnosis and surveillance of late-onset fetal growth restriction. Am J Obstet Gynecol. 2018;218:S790–S802.e1.
16. Gordijn SJ, Beune IM, Thilaganathan B, Papageorghiou A, Baschat AA, Baker PN, et al. Consensus definition of fetal growth restriction: a Delphi procedure. Ultrasound Obstet Gynecol. 2016;48:333–9.
17. Cosmi E, Ambrosini G, D'Antona D, Saccardi C, Mari G. Doppler, cardiotocography, and biophysical profile changes in growth-restricted fetuses. Obstet Gynecol. 2005;106:1240–5.
18. Baschat AA, Cosmi E, Bilardo CM, Wolf H, Berg C, Rigano S, et al. Predictors of neonatal outcome in early-onset placental dysfunction. Obstet Gynecol. 2007;109:253–61.
19. Nabhan AF, Abdelmoula YA. Amniotic fluid index versus single deepest vertical pocket as a screening test for preventing adverse pregnancy outcome. Cochrane Database Syst Rev. 2008;3:CD006593.
20. Chauhan SP, Sanderson M, Hendrix NW, Magann EF, Devoe LD. Perinatal outcome and amniotic fluid index in the antepartum and intrapartum periods: a meta-analysis. Am J Obstet Gynecol. 1999;181:1473–8.
21. Committee on Obstetric Practice. Antenatal corticosteroid therapy for fetal maturation. Committee opinion no. 713. Obstet Gynecol. 2017;130:e102–9.
22. Saccone G, Berghella V. Antenatal corticosteroids for maturity of term or near term fetuses: systematic review and meta-analysis of randomized controlled trials. BMJ. 2016;355:i5044.
23. Ting JY, Kingdom JC, Shah PS. Antenatal glucocorticoids, magnesium sulfate, and mode of birth in preterm fetal small for gestational age. Am J Obstet Gynecol. 2018;218:S818–28.

Postnatal Prognosis

13

Erich Cosmi, Matteo Andolfatto, Matteo Arata,
Marilia Calanducci, and Silvia Visentin

Fetal growth restriction (FGR) lacks a widely agreed upon definition in the literature. The most commonly used definition includes the presence of a fetus that does not reach its maximum growth potential owing to several pathological insults.

The causes of FGR may be related to the following conditions: (1) maternal problems: infections, chronic hypertension, diabetes mellitus, cardiovascular disease, or substance abuse (as smoke); (2) placental problems: inadequate vascular supply, chorioangioma, infarct, circumscribed placenta, confined placental mosaicism, or obliterative placental vasculopathy; (3) fetal problems: infections, chromosome disease, or genetic disease; (4) idiopathologies.

The etiology commonly understood to be the most frequent appears to be placental insufficiency [1–6]. There is, thus, vascular compromise, which inevitably leads to an increase in vascular resistance in the umbilical artery, limiting blood flow and, therefore, nourishment to the fetus [2, 4, 5]. The fetus implements compensation mechanisms that allow delivery of most nutrients to the major organs, i.e. adrenal glands, heart, and brain [7]. Cardiac output is also redistributed in favor of the left ventricle. This hemodynamic adaptation leads to a doubling of oxygen delivery from the umbilical vein to the myocardium and fetal brain [8]. A further mechanism of control and local compensation is activated at the cerebral level. In fact, by dilating the vessels that supply the nuclei of the brain base with blood, there is preferential flow toward these structures and away from the cerebral cortex. The

E. Cosmi (✉)
University of Padua School of Medicine, Deparment of Woman and Child Health, Padua, Italy

Department of Woman and Child Health, Maternal Fetal Medicine Unit, University of Padua, Padua, Italy

M. Andolfatto · M. Arata · M. Calanducci · S. Visentin
Department of Woman and Child Health, Maternal Fetal Medicine Unit, University of Padua, Padua, Italy

L. M. M. Nardozza et al. (eds.), *Fetal Growth Restriction*,
https://doi.org/10.1007/978-3-030-00051-6_13

reduction of cardiac flow to certain organs places them in a suboptimal condition. When the liver, the main producer of fetal proteins, receives 30% less blood than usual it becomes limited in its operation, which results in a low fetal body weight from FGR. From an ultrasound point of view, the evaluation of maternal vessels (uterine arteries) plays a predominantly diagnostic role and has a high negative predictive value [9, 10]. These vessels are generally assessed during the first and second trimesters of pregnancy. Normal pulsatility index values preclude, with high probability, the emergence of pre-eclampsia or FGR [9, 10]. With regard to fetal vessels, the first Doppler abnormality corresponds to an increase in the pulsatility index in the umbilical artery (PIUA).

In normal fetuses, in fact, a large percentage of cardiac output supply the vascular bed, one third during II trimester and one fifth near term [11]. In FGR fetuses, a lower quantity of blood is directed to the placenta while normal cardiac output is maintained. The purpose of this is so that umbilical blood can recirculate widely in the fetal body to obtain a more efficient extraction of oxygen and nutrients. A reactive polycythemia is often present as a further compensation method [8, 11]. At this stage the fetus enters a phase of compensation. Specifically, the compensation state allows a satisfactory fetal condition that could continue for a long time. As long the fetus in in this condition, there are only Doppler changes. With the progression of the pathology, and therefore of the obstruction of vascular flow, absent end diastolic flow (AEDF) and reverse end diastolic flow (REDF) develop [12]. The cerebral compensation is manifested itself by changes in the Doppler reading, such as a vasodilatation of the middle cerebral artery [12]. When the metabolic stress becomes more intensive, the fetus is no longer able to meets the demands of single organs, which leads to a state of decompensation and fetal suffering. Absolutely late sign and acute cardiac compromise index is represented by the absent or the reverse at the level of the venous duct, which leads to a state of hypercarbia and cardiac compromize resembled by absent or reverse A wave in Doctus venosus [13].

Following a morphofunctional alteration of the placental bed, in fact, the fetus is not allowed to reach its (genetically predetermined) maximum development and lacks in fact the environmental and metabolic requirements for such development.

The gestational age in which the pathology develops is also fundamental in the diagnostic, therapeutic, and prognostic framework. The development of the disease below 32 weeks (early FGR) greatly increases the risk of rapid progression of the disease itself, thus having a more precocious and more severe prognosis than late FGR [6]. The fetal response to placental dysfunction evolves from early compensatory reactions to late multiple organ failure disorders. This response contributes to fetal intrauterine programming and, as a result, short- and long-term morbidity [6]. The consequence is a smaller fetus than expected. Fundamental, however, both in terms of management and prognosis, is the correct classification of a small fetus, specifically a correct differentiation between the small for gestational age (SGA) and a true FGR.

Recently the Delphi definition, formulated by expert consensus, both for early and late FGR [14], has emerged as the most widely used classification. It divides early and late FGR as follows:

- Early FGR (< 32 weeks)
  - Solitary parameters
    1. Abdominal circumference (AC) < 3(rd) centile
    2. Estimated fetal weight (EFW) < 3(rd) centile
    3. AEDF in the umbilical artery (UA)
  - Contributory parameters: AC or EFW < 10(th) centile combined with a pulsatility index (PI) > 95(th) centile in either the UA or uterine artert
- Late FGR (≥ 32 weeks)
  - Solitary parameters
    1. AC < 3(rd) centile or
    2. EFW < 3(rd) centile
  - Contributory parameters:
    1. EFW or AC < 10(th) centile
    2. AC or EFW crossing centiles by > two quartiles on growth charts
    3. Cerebroplacental ratio < 5(th) centile or UA-PI >95(th) centile

Furthermore, a series of functional morphological modifications is made. From a hemodynamic point of view, there is a tendency to increase pressure. The main determinants of this condition are vascular and renal factors. The whole vascular bed is in fact characterized by the presence of forces that constantly act on the endothelium in a varied and turbulent manner, changing in intensity, direction, and frequency. Thus we have both forces acting perpendicular to the vessel and forces acting tangentially [15]. Thus, an increase in the average arterial pressure causes greater trauma to the vessel, leading to unavoidable cellular modifications, including cell proliferation, apoptosis, and matrix modification, with its destruction and new synthesis [15].

A condition of chronic hypoxemia, when decompensated, can negatively involve different organs. At the heart level, hypoxemia can result in hypoxia. Fibrocells furthest from the vessel are the first to undergo cell death. This results in the formation of scars that further limit the contractile capacity of the heart. The remaining myocytes undergo compensatory hypertrophy in an attempt to meet the increased peripheral and cardiac muscle demands. This situation puts the heart in a suboptimal condition already in the fetal phase of life.

Thus, as an adult, a person who experienced FGR is more likely to have difficulties meeting increased cardiac and peripheral muscle demands in the course of physical exertion, making the heart more fragile and, therefore, prone to damage or acute myocardial infarction [16, 17].

Developments in molecular biology have allowed for the creation of microarrays that facilitate the evaluation of gene expression during stressful fetal conditions [18]. They might also lead to a deepening of the molecular mechanisms of this phenomenon from a therapeutic point of view, making it possible to regressively remodel cardiac muscle (and therefore help to develop a more normal heart) already in utero.

Another very important organ in the context of FGR is the kidney. In fact, fetuses suffering from FGR, which typically shows up as a vitamin A deficiency [19], see a reduction in the number of glomeruli and nephrons, followed by renal hyperfiltration with the result of glomerulosclerosis and an increased risk of developing hypertension in adulthood [20]. However, this is a risk factor for renal damage too, so it can trigger a self-perpetuating cycle of renal and hemodynamic damage. Some studies in the literature have shown that these fetuses undergo genetic reprogramming with an increase in apical sodium transporters in the nephrons [21, 22]. This could increase the risk of salt-dependent hypertension in adulthood.

In fact, it seems that already during intrauterine life there is a genetic programming of the fetus to help it cope with the difficulties of living in its environment. But this also changes fetal hemodynamics, unavoidably affecting adult life. This consideration was already hypothesized in 1997 in a very large cohort study of nearly 150,000 adolescents in Sweden that demonstrated that systolic blood pressure was significantly higher in young men with the lowest birth weight [23].

Endothelial dysfunction is thought to be an innate trait in individuals with FGR and that this innate predisposition inevitably also affects neonatal and adult life. Useful methods for assessing endothelial dysfunction may be aorta intima-media thickness (aIMT), carotid intima-media thickness (cIMT), carotid stiffness, central pulse wave velocity, brachial artery flow-mediated dilation, endothelium-dependent microvascular vasodilatation, and echocardiographic evaluation [24–30]. Recent studies have shown that prenatal programming leads to an increase in apical sodium transporters in multiple nephron segments that could lead to salt-sensitive hypertension, as described in models of developmental hypertension and glucocorticoids and placental dysfunction [21].

Barker theory considers what may happen to a fetus in a condition of maternal malnutrition. In the case of nutritional deprivation, endocrine-metabolic changes occur in the unborn child. The ultimate aim is to strengthen the fetus, make it less needy in terms of nutrients for development, which represents a prophylactic mechanism in case of subsequent food shortages. This may certainly be very useful in acute conditions, and perhaps also from an evolutionary point of view if the conditions and the environment in which the newborn and then the adult will live are difficult to sustain. In the case of subsequent abundance of food, in contrast, typically this intrauterine imprint inevitably predisposes the fetus to developing diseases such as metabolic syndrome or diabetes. And this is generally what happens later in life. The lack of nourishment is not due to an actual lack of food but to a placental dysfunction.

Unfortunately, the fetus cannot understand the difference, so it is "forged" in a counterproductive way. In fact FGR will occur, but the child will be predisposed to rapid weight gain in the first years of life, as well as to adolescent obesity and increased risk of cardiovascular disease (CVD), stroke, glucose intolerance, and type II diabetes in adulthood [31–33]. Thus, FGR leads to intrinsic vascular damage, which contributes to hemodynamic alterations. However, additional factors damage a vessel that has already been structurally altered. In fact, we have seen that in this type of fetus suffers from an increase in sympathetic tone and an alteration of the lipid condition, leading to dyslipidemia [22, 34]. Thus, multiple actors and conditions arise, including nutritional and metabolic ones, that contribute to the formation of atherosclerotic plaques. Endothelial cells, smooth muscle cells, and cells of the immune system are definitely involved, and later, calcium crystals are also deposited [35, 36].

In fact, first of all, various types of cells migrate and move in the intimal space, contributing to its thickening. The cells present are leukocytes, monocytes, macrophages (identified by the specific marker CD68), smooth muscle cells, and quiescent (identified by the specific marker CD31) or activated (identified by the specific E-selectin marker) endothelial cells , the latter two typical of preinjury atherosclerosis [37]. The condition is further exacerbated by the deposition of interstitial glycosaminoglycans, always at the level of this layer [38].

Some authors [24–26] have confirmed that ultrasound-based measurement of aIMT was inversely proportional, both in fetuses and in newborns, to EFW, hypothesizing how various Doppler anomalies of UA and low birth weight (LBW) could be correlated with an abnormal vascular structure and endothelial damage. It is hypothesized that such histological changes cause greater arterial stiffness and that this correlates with an increase in the aortic PI [25]. This fact is not to be underestimated, because it represents, from a cardiovascular point of view, a higher risk factor, similar to hypertension [39]. This applies to both single pregnancies and twin pregnancies [40]. When twins have both biometric and flowmeter alterations (thus falling within the definition of FGR placenta dependent), it has been shown that they also have a greater thickness of the aorta in the studied ultrasound, leading to hemodynamic changes in the vascular tree. This happens regardless of gender or chorionicity.

Unfortunately these lesions do not have only a histological significance, but they manifest themselves clinically and, depending on the degree of development of atherosclerotic plaques, can also lead to massive compromise, with the final result being death. Some studies report autopsies on children (aged between 2 and 15 years) in which a possible cardiovascular cause has been excluded, showing the presence of lipid striae and fibro-atherosclerotic lesions on the wall of the aorta [41]. Specifically, anatomical pathological analysis of these lesions showed that they actually generated a thickening of the intima, thus confirming the ultrasound data. Immunohistochemical investigations have revealed the presence of condensed elastic fibers to form a strongly defined and marked internal elastic membrane [37]. Therefore, in conclusion, the plaques that involve marked functional morphological alterations of the vessels develop progressively over time, starting from an intrinsically pathological vascular structure, eventually leading to very unfavorable prognosis.

The importance of differentiating between an adequate gestational age (AGA) fetus and an FGR one was mentioned previously. In addition to the biometric and flowmetry parameters, a valid aid may also be provided by metabolomics, based on a different distribution of the essential amino acids [42–44]. Specifically, we have seen how sphingosine 1-phosphate, a molecule expressed in the cardiovascular system, is involved in the pathophysiology of diseases associated with endothelial dysfunction [45]. This molecule has as its precursor the ceramide, which, if increased, can induce an endothelium-dependent release of thromboxane A2, involved in hypertension and inflammation and has a vasoactive effect [45].

Therefore, during intrauterine life, these changes must also be considered in the large pathophysiological picture that determines the vascular bed in a pathological way, predisposing such fetuses to pathologies such as hypertension and nephropathy, especially glomerulonephritis, with a decrease in the number of nephrons in proportion to body weight at birth [24, 34, 46]. Even the heart muscle suffers from this systemic remodeling. A prospective cohort study (FGR children aged 3–6 years) showed that the prevalence of globular hearts and impaired myocardial relaxation increased. This leads to an inevitable increase in postload and compromise of cardiac compliance [21].

Numerous studies show an increase in aIMT and microalbuminuria in FGR fetuses compared to AGA fetuses, both in single and twin pregnancies, probably contributing also to an early and pathological stiffening of the arterial vascular tree. It is important to underline that intrauterine fetal remodeling does not occur only in severe FGR, typically early FGR, but can also occur in late FGR. Some studies on SGA infants have shown a correlation between weight recovery after birth (therefore substantial fat accumulation) and increase in blood pressure in subsequent ages, regardless of birth weight [34, 47–49]. Not all studies agree on this, but very likely the diversity of results also depends on the different statistical methods of analysis used and the different sample groups considered [50].

Other studies showed that infants with the lowest birth weight and who had a strong nutritional reward in the postbirth period developed a higher cIMT in adulthood compared to those adults who had been normal size fetuses and with normal postnatal growth [47, 51]. It is clear that the rapid accumulation of fat in the postnatal period should be avoided in order to limit the risk of developing increased blood pressure in adulthood. Further research is needed to understand more thoroughly whether FGR with postnatal weight recovery also carries a greater risk of developing cardiovascular adverse events and obesity in adulthood [52].

Prospective Studies

Baker's hypothesis was corroborated by numerous in vivo prospective studies, which related FGR patients with the development of cardiovascular, metabolic, and blood diseases in adulthood [53, 54]. Until recently, most studies focused on the phenotype resulting from changes in maternal nutrition. Today there is a greater interest in the study of the mechanisms through which this phenotype is created. In this context it is fundamental to investigate the role of overnutrition and undernutrition at the prenatal age with experimental and epidemiological methods, thereby allowing for a balancing of the link between genotype and saver phenotype.

The deepening of the molecular and epigenetic pathways involved in this field might make it possible to reveal the mechanisms underlying CVD and renal diseases in adulthood. In this sense, in vitro research is fundamental, mainly through animal models. The fundamentals of research for the future will be represented by the medicine of reproduction, nutrition, and the study of the vascular system, as well as metabolomics. Evaluation of these aspects will allow researchers to reach new therapeutic targets with important implications for the wellbeing of the general population [55].

In this context it is important to note the role of FGR diagnosis and in particular follow-up during adulthood. To date, pediatric guidelines do not include FGR as a risk factor for childhood diseases, but it would be desirable for it to be considered. This would make it possible to monitor on a large scale the cardiovascular, hypertensive, and metabolic problems in these children and to intervene with primary and secondary prevention. It has been shown that lifestyle interventions, such as physical activity promotion, passive smoking protection, and weight control, greatly improve cardiovascular wellbeing of these children [56]. It is interesting to note, then, recent evidence showing that high doses of omega-3 fatty acids help to reduce cases of hypertension and can slow down the progression of atherosclerosis in FGR children [57, 58] and play a preventive role in the thickening of the arterial part that occurs in these children after birth [59].

In conclusion, such evidence suggests the desirability for postnatal monitoring of FGR fetuses to become routine, allowing for important interventions to improve the quality of life of patient using strategies that include lifestyle changes and possibly pharmacological or nutraceutical interventions.

References

1. American College of Obstetricians and Gynecologists. ACOG Practice bulletin no. 134: fetal growth restriction. Obstet Gynecol. 2013;121:1122–33.
2. Unterscheider J, Daly S, Geary MP, Kennelly MM, McAuliffe FM, O'Donoghue K, et al. Optimizing the definition of intrauterine growth restriction: the multicenter prospective PORTO Study. Am J Obstet Gynecol. 2013;208:290.e1–6.
3. Gardosi J, Mongelli M, Wilcox M, Chang A. An adjustable fetal weight standard. Ultrasound Obstet Gynecol. 1995;6:168–74.
4. Royal College of Obstetricians and Gynecologists. The investigation and management of the small-for-gestational-age fetus (guideline no. 31). London: Royal College of Obstetricians and Gynecologists; 2002.
5. Society for Maternal-Fetal Medicine Publications Committee, Berkley E, Chauhan SP, Abuhamad A. Doppler assessment of the fetus with intrauterine growth restriction. Am J Obstet Gynecol. 2012;206:300–8.
6. Baschat AA, Cosmi E, Bilardo CM, Wolf H, Berg C, Rigano S, et al. Predictors of neonatal outcome in early-onset placental dysfunction. Obstet Gynecol. 2007;109:253–61.
7. Garg M, Thamotharan M, Dai Y, Lagishetty V, Matveyenko AV, Lee WN, et al. Glucose intolerance and lipid metabolic adaptations in response to intrauterine and postnatal calorie restriction in male adult rats. Endocrinology. 2013;154:102–13.
8. Al-Ghazali W, Chita SK, Chapman MG, Allan LD. Evidence of redistribution of cardiac output in asymmetrical growth retardation. Br J Obstet Gynaecol. 1989;96:697–704.
9. Słowakiewicz K, Perenc M, Sieroszewski P. Biochemical prenatal tests and uterine artery Doppler examination in prediction of PIH and IUGR in the third trimester of pregnancy. Ginekol Pol. 2010;81:352–7.
10. Valensise H, Romanini C. Uterine Doppler in the identification of patients at risk for hypertension and IUGR. J Perinat Med. 1994;22(Suppl 1):69–72.

11. Rizzo G, Capponi A, Cavicchioni O, Vendola M, Arduini D. Low cardiac output to the placenta: an early hemodynamic adaptive mechanism in intrauterine growth restriction. Ultrasound Obstet Gynecol. 2008;32:155–9.
12. Jang DG, Jo YS, Lee SJ, Kim N, Lee GS. Perinatal outcomes and maternal clinical characteristics in IUGR with absent or reversed end-diastolic flow velocity in the umbilical artery. Arch Gynecol Obstet. 2011;284:73–8.
13. Picconi JL, Hanif F, Drennan K, Mari G. The transitional phase of ductus venosus reversed flow in severely premature IUGR fetuses. Am J Perinatol. 2008;25:199–203.
14. Gordijn SJ, Beune IM, Thilaganathan B, Papageorghiou A, Baschat AA, Baker PN, et al. Consensus definition of fetal growth restriction: a Delphi procedure. Ultrasound Obstet Gynecol. 2016;48:333–9.
15. White CR, Haidekker M, Bao X, Frangos JA. Temporal gradients in shear, but not spatial gradients, stimulate endothelial cell proliferation. Circulation. 2001;103:2508–13.
16. McMillen IC, Robinson JS. Developmental origins of the metabolic syndrome: prediction, plasticity, and programming. Physiol Rev. 2005;85:571–633.
17. Li G, Xiao Y, Estrella JL, Ducsay CA, Gilbert RD, Zhang L. Effect of fetal hypoxia on heart susceptibility to ischemia and reperfusion injury in the adult rat. J Soc Gynecol Investig. 2003;10:265–74.
18. Resnick N, Yahav H, Shay-Salit A, Shushy M, Schubert S, Zilberman LC, et al. Fluid shear stress and the vascular endothelium: for better and for worse. Prog Biophys Mol Biol. 2003;81:177–99.
19. Lelievre-Pegorier M, Vilar J, Ferrier ML, Moreau E, Freund N, Gilbert T, et al. Mild vitamin A deficiency leads to inborn nephron deficit in the rat. Kidney Int. 1998;54:1455–62.
20. Brenner BM, Garcia DL, Anderson S. Glomeruli and blood pressure. Less of one, more the other? Am J Hypertens. 1988;1:335–47.
21. Baum M. Role of the kidney in the prenatal and early postnatal programming of hypertension. Am J Physiol Renal Physiol. 2010;298:F235–47.
22. Mizuno M, Siddique K, Baum M, Smith S. Prenatal programming of hypertension induces sympathetic over activity in response to physical stress. Hypertension. 2013;61:180–6.
23. Nilsson PM, Ostergren PO, Nyberg P, Söderström M, Allebeck P. Low birth weight is associated with elevated systolic blood pressure in adolescence: a prospective study of a birth cohort of 149,378 Swedish boys. J Hypertens. 1997;15:1627–31.
24. Skilton MR, Evans N, Griffiths KA, Harmer JA, Celermajer DS. Aortic wall thickness in newborns with intrauterine growth restriction. Lancet. 2005;365:1484–6.
25. Cosmi E, Visentin S, Fanelli T, Mautone AJ, Zanardo V. Aortic intima media thickness in fetuses and children with intrauterine growth restriction. Obstet Gynecol. 2009;114:1109–14.
26. Järvisalo MJ, Jartti L, Näntö-Salonen K, Irjala K, Rönnemaa T, Hartiala JJ, et al. Increased aortic intima-media thickness: a marker of preclinical atherosclerosis in high-risk children. Circulation. 2001;104:2943–7.
27. Comas M, Crispi F, Cruz-Martinez R, Figueras F, Gratacos E. Tissue Doppler echocardiographic markers of cardiac dysfunction in small-for-gestational age fetuses. Am J Obstet Gynecol. 2011;205:57.e1–6.
28. Ley D, Stale H, Marsal K. Aortic vessel wall characteristics and blood pressure in children with intrauterine growth retardation and abnormal fetal aortic blood flow. Acta Paediatr. 1997;86:299–305.
29. Norman M, Martin H. Preterm birth attenuates association between low birth weight and endothelial dysfunction. Circulation. 2003;108:996–1001.
30. Leeson CP, Whincup PH, Cook DG, Donald AE, Papacosta O, Lucas A, et al. Flow-mediated dilation in 9- to 11-year-old children: the influence of intrauterine and childhood factors. Circulation. 1997;96:2233–8.
31. Barker DJ. The developmental origins of well-being. Philos Trans R Soc Lond Ser B Biol Sci. 2004;359:1359–66.
32. Rich-Edwards JW, Kleinman K, Michels KB, Stampfer MJ, Manson JE, Rexrode KM, et al. Longitudinal study of birth weight and adult body mass index in predicting risk of coronary heart disease and stroke in women. BMJ. 2005;330:1115.

33. Liao D, Arnett DK, Tyroler HA, Riley WA, Chambless LE, Szklo M, et al. Arterial stiffness and the development of hypertension: the ARIC study. Hypertension. 1999;34:201–6.
34. Koklu E, Kurtoglu S, Akcakus M, Koklu S, Buyukkayhan D, Gumus H, et al. Increased aortic intima-media thickness is related to lipid profile in newborns with intrauterine growth restriction. Horm Res. 2006;65:269–75.
35. Minshall RD, Tiruppathi C, Vogel SM, Malik AB. Vesicle formation and trafficking in endothelial cells and regulation of endothelial barrier function. Histochem Cell Biol. 2002;117:105–12.
36. Furchgott RF, Zawadzki JV. The obligatory role of the endothelial cells in the relaxation of arterial smooth muscle by acetylcholine. Nature. 1980;288:373–6.
37. Lo Vasco VR, Salmaso R, Zanardo V, Businaro R, Visentin S, Trevisanuto D, et al. Fetal aorta wall inflammation in ultrasound detected aortic intima/media thickness and growth retardation. J Reprod Immunol. 2011;91:103–7.
38. Meyer WW, Lind J, Yao AC, Kauffman SL. Early arterial lesions in infancy and childhood and ways of prevention. Paediatrician. 1982;11:136–56.
39. Zanardo V, Fanelli T, Weiner G, Fanos V, Zaninotto M, Visentin S, et al. Intrauterine growth restriction is associated with persistent aortic wall thickening and glomerular proteinuria during infancy. Kidney Int. 2011;80:119–23.
40. Visentin S, Grisan E, Zanardo V, Bertin M, Veronese E, Cavallin F, et al. Developmental programming of cardiovascular risk in intrauterine growth-restricted twin fetuses according to aortic intima thickness. J Ultrasound Med. 2013;32:279–84.
41. McGill HC Jr, McMahan CA, Herderick EE, Malcom GT, Tracy RE, Strong JP. Origin of atherosclerosis in childhood and adolescence. Am J Clin Nutr. 2000;72:1307S–15S.
42. Cecconi D, Lonardoni F, Favretto D, Cosmi E, Tucci M, Visentin S, et al. Changes in amniotic fluid and umbilical cord serum proteomic profiles of fetuses with intrauterine growth retardation. Electrophoresis. 2011;32:3630–7.
43. Favretto D, Cosmi E, Ragazzi E, Visentin S, Tucci M, Fais P, et al. Cord blood metabolomic profiling in intrauterine growth restriction. Anal Bioanal Chem. 2012;402:1109–21.
44. Cosmi E, Visentin S, Favretto D, Tucci M, Ragazzi E, Viel G, et al. Selective intrauterine growth restriction in monochorionic twin pregnancies: markers of endothelial damage and metabolomic profile. Twin Res Hum Genet. 2013;16:816–26.
45. Spijkers LJ, van den Akker RF, Janssen BJ, Debets JJ, De Mey JG, Stroes ES, et al. Hypertension is associated with marked alterations in sphingolipid biology: a potential role for ceramide. PLoS One. 2011;6:e21817.
46. Brenner BM, Lawler EV, Mackenzie HS. The hyperfiltration theory: a paradigm shift in nephrology. Kidney Int. 1996;49:1774–7.
47. Leunissen RW, Kerkhof GF, Stijnen T, Hokken-Koelega AC. Effect of birth size and catch-up growth on adult blood pressure and carotid intima-media thickness. Horm Res Paediatr. 2012;77:394–401.
48. Uiterwaal CS, Anthony S, Launer LJ, Witteman JC, Trouwborst AM, Hofman A, et al. Birth weight, growth, and blood pressure: an annual follow-up study of children aged 5 through 21 years. Hypertension. 1997;30:267–71.
49. Adair LS, Cole TJ. Rapid child growth raises blood pressure in adolescent boys who were thin at birth. Hypertension. 2003;41:451–6.
50. Huxley R, Neil A, Collins R. Unravelling the fetal origins hypothesis: is there really an inverse association between birth weight and subsequent blood pressure? Lancet. 2002;360:659–65.
51. Oren A, Vos LE, Uiterwaal CS, Gorissen WH, Grobbee DE, Bots ML. Birth weight and carotid intima-media thickness: new perspectives from the atherosclerosis risk in young adults (ARYA) study. Ann Epidemiol. 2004;14:8–16.
52. Santos MS, Joles JA. Early determinants of cardiovascular disease. Best Pract Res Clin Endocrinol Metab. 2012;26:581–97.
53. Barker DJ. Fetal origins of coronary heart disease. BMJ. 1995;311:171–4.
54. Tintu A, Rouwet E, Verlohren S, Brinkmann J, Ahmad S, Crispi F, et al. Hypoxia induces dilated ardiomyopathy in the chick embryo: mechanism, intervention, and long-term consequences. PLoS One. 2009;4:e5155.

55. Skilton MR, Mikkila V, Wurtz P, Ala-Korpela M, Sim KA, Soininen P, et al. Fetal growth, omega-3 (ω-3) fatty acids, and progression of subclinical atherosclerosis: preventing fetal origins of disease? The Cardiovascular Risk in Young Finns Study. Am J Clin Nutr. 2013;97:58–65.
56. Williams CL, Hayman LL, Daniels SR, Robinson TN, Steinberger J, Paridon S, et al. Cardiovascular health in childhood: a statement for health professionals from the Committee on Atherosclerosis, Hypertension, and Obesity in the Young (AHOY) of the Council on Cardiovascular Disease in the Young, American Heart Association. Circulation. 2002;106:143–60.
57. Skilton MR, Raitakari OT, Celermajer DS. High intake of dietary long-chain ω-3 fatty acids is associated with lower blood pressure in children born with low birth weight: NHANES 2003–2008. Hypertension. 2013;61:972–6.
58. Skilton MR, Mikkila V, Wurtz P, Ala-Korpela M, Sim KA, Soininen P, et al. Fetal growth, omega-3 (ω-3) fatty acids, and progression of subclinicalatherosclerosis: preventing fetal origins of disease? The Cardiovascular Risk in Young Finns Study. Am J Clin Nutr. 2013;97:58–65.
59. Skilton MR, Ayer JG, Harmer JA, Webb K, Leeder SR, Marks GB, et al. Impaired fetal growth and arterial wall thickening: a randomized trial of ω-3 supplementation. Pediatrics. 2012;129:e698–703.

Neurological Complications

14

Danilo Buca, Marco Liberati, and Francesco D'Antonio

Introduction

Fetal growth restriction (FGR) encompasses a heterogeneous group of anomalies characterized by the inability of the fetus to achieve its growth potential in utero. Placental insufficiency is the most common cause of FGR, affecting about 5–10% of all pregnancies, and is characterized by progressive placental dysfunction commonly leading to altered fetal metabolism, blood redistribution, and impaired fetal growth [1].

FGR represents one of the most common causes of perinatal mortality and morbidity and has also been shown to be associated with a large variety of adverse long-term outcomes, including impaired cardiac function, metabolic and hematological disorders, cognitive dysfunction, and cerebral palsy [2–5].

Assessing the neurodevelopmental status of children affected by early FGR may be challenging; gestational age at birth remains the main determinant of perinatal outcome in singleton pregnancies, and the higher prevalence of neurologic and developmental complications reported in fetuses affected by FGR may be the

D. Buca
Department of Obstetrics and Gynaecology, University of Chieti, Chieti, Italy

M. Liberati
Women's Health and Perinatology Research Group, Department of Clinical Medicine, Faculty of Health Sciences, UiT – The Arctic University of Norway, Tromsø, Norway

Department of Obstetrics and Gynaecology, University Hospital of Northern Norway, Tromsø, Norway

F. D'Antonio (✉)
Department of Clinical Medicine, Faculty of Health Sciences,
UiT – The Arctic University of Norway, Tromsø, Norway
e-mail: francesco.dantonio@uit.no

L. M. M. Nardozza et al. (eds.), *Fetal Growth Restriction*,
https://doi.org/10.1007/978-3-030-00051-6_14

consequence of severe prematurity rather than growth restriction per se, with only few studies reporting stratified analyses for early and late FGR. Furthermore, the large majority of published studies do not try to correlate the neurodevelopmental outcome of FGR infants with the different parameters of fetal well-being used in clinical practice, such as umbilical artery (UA), middle cerebral artery (MCA), ductus venosus (DV), and cardiotocography (CTG). This is fundamental because early FGR may present with different phenotypes characterized by several degrees of hemodynamic and metabolic compromise which may be quantified on ultrasound [1]. In this scenario, labeling a FGR fetus exclusively according to the time at delivery and magnitude of fetal smallness may not account for the large variety of clinical phenotypes a FGR fetus can present with. Lack of outcome stratification according to the Doppler findings represents the main weakness of postnatal imaging studies on early FGR. Prenatal management and counseling of early FGR is based upon the magnitude of Doppler anomalies, and lack of information on such parameters makes prenatal counseling inaccurate.

Objective quantification of the actual burden of neurologic and developmental disabilities in fetuses affected by FGR is also affected by the large heterogeneity in the definition of FGR reported in the published literature. Fetal smallness is commonly used as a surrogate for FGR and an estimated fetal weight (EFW) or abdominal circumference (AC) less than the 10th centile the most commonly adopted cutoffs to define a fetus as growth restricted. The term "small for gestational age" (SGA) has also interchangeably used with FGR. By arbitrary convention, placental-related cases are usually defined as (true) FGR, while "nonplacental" cases are referred as SGA. FGR is commonly defined as SGA with abnormal Doppler indices such as UA pulsatility index (PI) above the 95th centile or mean uterine artery (UtA) PI above the 95th centile [6].

Despite this, it is important to understand that a fetus does not need to be small to be growth restricted and that FGR and SGA are not synonymous. The majority of FGR are SGA, while 50–70% of SGA are constitutionally small and have grown appropriately [7].

The term neurodevelopmental outcome is also misleading and inappropriate when dealing with neurodevelopmental anomalies, because it includes a wide spectrum of signs that are not always easily measured and that represent a continuous interaction between pathological, environmental, and adaptive factors. Time at assessment represents another peculiar issue; early neuropsychological examination may not accurately predict neurodevelopmental outcomes during later life, while late assessment may be biased by the influence of socioeconomic, parenting, environmental, and educational factors, which may significantly affect developmental measures, especially when looking for subtle difference. Finally, assessment of a control population may represent another considerable source of bias when assessing the diagnostic performance of children affected by brain anomalies. The risk for a given abnormal neurodevelopmental measure is commonly computed upon a control population which should theoretically include "health" individuals, free from the anomaly, and implies the knowledge of how this measure is abnormal in the cohort not affected by the anomaly.

Severity of growth disturbance, magnitude of Doppler anomalies, and gestational age at birth are the main determinants of perinatal outcome in fetuses affected by FGR [1]. In clinical practice, FGR is commonly classified according to the time at occurrence in early and late FGR which reflects two conditions with different pathophysiology, clinical phenotype, and prognosis.

Therefore, in the present chapter, we will report the neurological outcome of fetuses and infants affected by early and late FGR, respectively.

Early Fetal Growth Restriction

Early FGR is defined as growth restriction occurring before 32 weeks of gestation and presenting with a AC/EFW <3rd centile and abnormal UA flow pattern (absent end-diastolic flow) or with AC/EFW <10th centile combined with uterine artery or UA pulsatility index >95th centile [8].

Early FGR is characterized by a progressive reduction of placental perfusion due to a decrease in villous cross-sectional vascular area, leading to reduced substrate availability in the liver. Progressive fetal hypoxemia induces proportional elevation in the umbilical artery (UA) Doppler PI and a peculiar redistribution of cardiac output especially toward the frontal and median regions of fetal brain, aiming at preserving normal cell processes when oxygen availability is low [9, 10]. On ultrasound, such redistribution translates into a reduced PI of the anterior and especially middle cerebral artery (MCA). With advancing stages of placental deterioration, absent and reverse diastolic flow in the UA occurs, and there is a loss of the compensatory cerebral vasodilatation with normalization or increase in MCA PI. Cardiac performance deteriorates due to chronic hypoxemia and nutritional deprivation leading to increase atrial pressure and progressive reduction of the diastolic flow in the DV. Preterminal stages of early FGR are characterized by the presence of reverse atrial flow in the DV and pulsatile umbilical venous flow which usually anticipate death.

Early FGR has been shown to be associated with an increased risk of abnormal neurodevelopmental measures, such as cognitive function, attention capacity, and school performance [9, 10]. Although the pathophysiology of the brain-related damage in early FGR has not been completely elucidated yet, recent evidences suggest abnormal cerebral perfusion as one of the main determinants in inducing abnormal brain development and function. Fetal cardiovascular adaptation to impaired placental function and chronic hypoxemia induces a peculiar redistribution of cardiac output to the brain, especially to those areas perfused by ACA and MCA. Classically considered a protective mechanism to preserve cerebral functions when oxygen availability is low, brain sparing does not entirely seem to protect brain development [1].

Infants affected by early FGR have been shown to have smaller head circumference, brain, and cortical gray matter volumes compared to age-matched appropriately grown infants [2, 11, 12] on magnetic resonance imaging (MRI) and that such findings correlate with neurodevelopmental outcome. Fetal size is one of the main determinants of neurological outcome in infants, and reduced fetal head volume has been associated with cerebral palsy and psychomotor and cognitive development [11, 13]. Furthermore, decreased white matter in the hippocampus and cerebellum has been also reported in fetuses affected by early FGR compared to controls [14–16]. Preterm FGR infants with brain sparing and who underwent MRI at term-equivalent age further demonstrate a slowdown in myelination and reduced posterior white matter volume in the absence of white matter lesions [17]. These differences could be related to some results of epigenetic mechanisms derived from the adaptation of the developing brain to a hypoxic environment, which can lead to fetal reprogramming in brain organization, rather than true brain damage [2, 14, 18].

Recent evidences on the suboptimal brain development come also from studies using new imaging technique such as diffusion tensor imaging and connectome analysis which showed altered white matter organization in the prefrontal and limbic networks in preterm children born with FGR, compared with preterm children with appropriate birth weight [19]. These structural brain network measures also correlate with neurobehavioral impairments such as hyperactivity or cognitive deficits, in the executive function domain at school age [20]. However, it is important to underline the fact that some of the neurological complications observed in postnatal studies on early FGR may be the consequence of prematurity rather than placental insufficiency.

Two randomized controlled trials have tried to assess the neurodevelopmental status of fetuses affected by early FGR. In the Growth Restriction Intervention (GRIT) trial, 587 small babies at 24–36 weeks of gestation were randomized to immediate delivery or expectant management. Mode of delivery and monitoring strategies for the delayed delivery group was left up to the attending obstetrician. The risk of intrauterine death was higher in the delayed delivery group, while at 2 years of age, the prevalence of disability tended to be higher in the immediate delivery group. However, no major differences between the two management options were observed with comparable Griffiths developmental scores between the two groups. More importantly, a reevaluation of the study population at 6–13 years of age showed no differences in motor or intellectual disabilities between the two groups [21]. The major weaknesses of the study were the inclusion of cases likely to be affected by late FGR, lack of standardized protocol for antenatal monitoring, and thresholds for delivery based exclusively upon clinician's uncertainty on whether to deliver or continue the pregnancy. The TRUFFLE trial has evaluated the 2-year neurodevelopmental and intermediate perinatal outcomes in infants with very preterm fetal growth restriction, randomizing singleton pregnancies affected by early FGR (at 26–32 weeks of gestation), defined as AC <10th percentile and UA-PI >95th percentile, to three timing of delivery plans, which differed according to antenatal monitoring strategies: reduced short-term variation (STV) at CTG, early DV changes (pulsatility index >95th percentile), or late DV changes (A wave at or below baseline). Primary outcome of the study was survival without cerebral palsy or neurosensory impairment or with a Bayley III developmental score 33 of >85, at 2 years of age [22]. Intrauterine demise occurred in 2.5% of the study population, while 5% experienced neonatal death; 24% of children had severe morbidity.

There was no difference in the proportion of infants surviving without neuroimpairment between the three different monitoring strategies. However, among survivors, delivery based upon late DV changes was associated with a higher prevalence of infants free from neurodevelopmental disabilities compared with that based upon CTG (95%, 95%, 95% CI 90–98 vs 85%, 95% CI 78–90). These findings suggest that optimal time at delivery may preserve cerebral function in infants affected by early FGR in utero, thus highlighting the need for an appropriate antenatal monitoring once prenatal diagnosis of early FGR is achieved.

Ultrasound is the primary imaging tool to diagnose and follow up fetuses affected by early FGR, and several studies have tried to correlate individual ultrasound parameters with different neurodevelopmental measures. UA Doppler anomalies, such as AREDF, have been linked with mental retardation, lower psychomotor development, and Bayley and Kaufman score at 2 years of age in infants affected by FGR delivered preterm compared to controls [12, 23–25]) although such association was not consistently reported in the published literature. In the study by Brodszki et al., the risk of cerebral palsy was not different in FGR fetuses with UA-AREDV compared with AGA controls [26]. Shand et al. reported no correlation between UA Doppler anomalies and neurodevelopmental outcome at 2 years of age once the analysis was corrected for gestational age at birth; however, fetuses with UA-AERDF had a higher prevalence of major and minor neurological sequelae at 6 years of age compared to controls, although the QI was similar between the two groups [27]. Interestingly, in children delivered at later gestation, UA findings seem to strongly correlate with neurodevelopmental outcome. Wienerroither et al. reported that children delivered at around 34 weeks of gestation, FGR infants with previous UA-ARED, had lower score in fine motor and Kaufman tests compared to controls at 6 years of age, while in the study by Schreuder et al., cognitive delay and visual impairment were more commonly observed in infants presenting in utero with UA Doppler anomalies even after correction for gestational age [28].

Classically considered a protective mechanism to preserve cerebral performance, brain sparing does not entirely seem to protect brain development, and several studies have tried to correlate Doppler findings in the MCA with neurodevelopmental outcome. Scherjon et al. explored the association between umbilico-cerebral ratio (UCR), maturation of visual evoked potentials (VEP), and cognitive outcome in infants delivered at 25 and 33 weeks' gestation over an 11-year period. At 6 months, infants with a raised UCR had shorter visual evoked potential latencies compared to controls, suggesting a potential beneficial and protective mechanism of brain sparing on cerebral development. These findings were confirmed at 3 years of age, when, after adjustment for obstetric variables, adverse outcome was related to neonatal cranial ultrasound abnormality and low head circumference but not U/C ratio [29]. At 5 years of follow-up, mean IQ score was significantly lower for children born with a raised U/C ratio compared with children with a normal U/C ratio, while VEP latencies decreased significantly in infants with a normal U/C ratio, suggesting that brain sparing may be associated with a poor cognitive outcome later in childhood [30]. Finally, at the final follow-up (11 years), the authors reported no association between brain sparing itself and behavioral problems. When interpreting the results of this study, it is important to highlight the fact that steroids were administered exclusively to small fetuses presenting with abnormal UCR values; in this scenario, it is entirely plausible that the reported failed association between brain sparing and neurodevelopmental outcome might have been the result of the lack of steroid administration.

More recently, in a sub-analysis of the TRUFFLE trial, Stampalija et al. reported that higher MCA PI at inclusion but not within 1 week before delivery was associated with neonatal survival without severe morbidity, while MCA PI index and umbilico-cerebral ratio Z-score at inclusion were associated with 2-year survival with normal neurodevelopmental outcome as were gestation at delivery and birth weight/p50 ratio. Despite this, the authors concluded that the impact of MCA and its ratios in determining survival free from neurological impairment was less relevant than gestational age at delivery and birth weight and unlikely to be informative in optimizing the timing of delivery in early FGR [31].

Late stages of placental insufficiency are characterized by progressive cardiac performance deterioration leading to increase atrial pressure and progressive reduction of the diastolic flow in the DV, commonly associated with fetal academia. Only few studies look at the association between DV Doppler findings and abnormal neurodevelopmental outcome; such studies are affected by the small sample size, heterogeneity in inclusion criteria, and management option. Baschat et al. prospectively followed 72 survivors affected by early FGR at 2 years of age. The authors reported that gestational age at delivery was associated with cerebral palsy, UA-AREDV with global developmental delay, and birth weight with neurodevelopmental delay, while no association was found between abnormal venous Doppler findings and outcome (Baschat 2009). The findings from the TRUFFLE trial are discussed above. Likewise, in the study by Leppanen et al., abnormal UA-PI and UA-PI/MCA PI ratio but not DV were associated with adverse cognitive outcome at 2 years of age, while Torrance et al. reported that abnormal neurodevelopmental outcome at 2 years was exclusively predicted by low birth weight, fetal acidosis, and placental villitis [32, 33].

Late Fetal Growth Restriction

Early FGR is defined as growth restriction occurring before 34 weeks of gestation and presenting with a AC/EFW <3rd centile or at least two out of the following criteria: AC/EFW <10th centile, AC/EFW crossing centiles >2 quartiles on growth centiles, or cerebroplacental ratio (CPR) <5th centile or UA-PI >95th [8].

Identification of fetuses affected by late FGR is more challenging; in the general population, fetal smallness presents with a large variety of different clinical phenotypes: those reflecting the presence of placental insufficiency, defined as "true FGR," and those not presenting signs of impaired placental function, commonly labeled as "constitutional" small (for gestational age (SGA) fetuses. Distinction between late FGR and SGA is fundamental as they represent two peculiar clinical conditions with different natural histories, pathophysiologies, and prognoses. FGR is affected by a high burden of short- and long-term adverse outcomes, while SGA fetuses are associated with virtually normal perinatal outcome. Despite this, prenatal identification of true FGR in late pregnancy may be difficult; UA Doppler does not predict adverse outcome and may be normal in such cases, while assessment of MCA Doppler is not routinely performed in fetuses at term [1].

Such difficulties in prenatal identification of true FGR are responsible for the large heterogeneity in the reported incidence of abnormal neurodevelopmental outcome in small babies at term with the large majority of the previously published literature differing as regards definition of fetal smallness, neurodevelopmental tool used, and stratification according to Doppler findings.

In the systematic review by Arcangeli et al., the authors reported that standardized neurodevelopmental scores in SGA babies were 0.32 SD (95% CI, 0.25–0.38) below those for normal controls, while insufficient data were available for FGR babies [34]. However, there was large heterogeneity in the clinical definition of SGA, with most studies not reporting data on Doppler; furthermore, neurodevelopmental assessment varies among the included studies.

Decreased PI in the MCA has been recently reported to represent an additional risk factor for abnormal neurodevelopmental performance in small babies at term. Eixarch et al. reported that small fetuses with MCA PI <5th centile had a higher incidence of suboptimal neurodevelopmental outcome, especially in communication and problem-solving areas, compared with those with normal MCA PI, while there was no difference in the short-term perinatal outcomes between the two groups [35]. Furthermore, a recent systematic review exploring the role of brain redistribution in determining the outcome of small fetuses at term reported that cerebral redistribution was associated with increased risk of motor, state organizational problems, and lower mean percentile scores in communication and problem-solving at 2 years of age [3].

In this scenario, reduced MCA pulsatility index may represent a status of suboptimal brain perfusion and worsening chronic hypoxemia due to impaired placental function. The role of abnormal Doppler findings in the MCA on brain structure and function has been recently explored by studies using new imaging techniques to assess fetal brain, such as MRI spectroscopy and connectomics, which showed that SGA fetuses with signs of cerebral blood flow redistribution have peculiar abnormalities in brain structure and metabolism compared to AGA fetuses [4, 12, 19, 36]. More importantly, these studies showed that even SGA fetuses not presenting with abnormal Doppler findings may show signs of impaired brain structure and metabolism, although the magnitude of such changes was generally lower than in FGR fetuses.

Despite this growing body of evidence suggesting that small fetuses at term presenting with abnormal Doppler findings in the MCA are at higher risk of abnormal neurodevelopmental outcome, further studies are needed in order to clarify whether elective delivery may prevent adverse outcome or preserve the neurodevelopmental performance of these children.

Conclusions

FGR is associated with a high burden of neurologic and neurodevelopmental complications compared to appropriately grown fetuses. The magnitude of such complications is primarily determined by gestational age at birth in early FGR, while abnormal cerebral Doppler increases the risk of neurodevelopmental delay in late FGR. Despite this, in view of the large heterogeneity in inclusion criteria, outcome measures, and times at follow-up, further studies sharing objective protocols of prenatal management and postnatal assessment are needed in order to elucidate the actual incidence of abnormal developmental outcome in fetuses affected by growth restriction, identify optimal cutoff to predict compromise, and explore whether elective delivery may improve the neuropsychological performance of these children.

Appendix

Summary of the main abnormal neurodevelopmental measures observed in infants affected by early fetal growth restriction in utero.

- Lower scores on cognitive testing
- Difficulties in schools or require special education
- Gross motor and minor neurologic dysfunction
- Behavioral problems (attention deficit hyperactivity syndrome)
- Growth failure
- Lower strength and work capacity
- Cerebral palsy
- Low social competence
- Poor academic performance
- Lower levels of intelligence
- Hyperactive behavior
- Poor perceptual performance
- Poor visuomotor perception, motor incompetence, reading, and mathematics learning

Structural Anomalies

- Reduced head circumference
- Reduced total and gray matter volume
- Reduced hippocampal and cerebellar volume
- Reduced total number of cells
- Reduced myelin content
- Thinning cortex
- Delayed myelination
- Reduced connectivity

Motor Anomalies

- Reduced gross and fine motor skills
- Reduced visuomotor skills
- Clumsiness
- Cerebral palsy

Cognitive and Learning Anomalies

- Reduced IQ/executive function
- Reduced verbal IQ
- Poor memory
- Reduced IQ/executive function
- Reduced verbal IQ
- Poor memory

Behavioral Anomalies

- Attention and interaction
- Hyperactivity
- Mood and irritability
- Anxiety

References

1. Figueras F, Gratacos E. An integrated approach to fetal growth restriction. Best Pract Res Clin Obstet Gynaecol. 2017;38:48–48.
2. Tolsa CB, Zimine S, Warfield SK, Freschi M, Sancho Rossignol A, Lazeyras F, et al. Early alteration of structural and functional brain development in premature infants born with intrauterine growth restriction. Pediatr Res. 2004;56:132–8.
3. Meher S, Hernandez-Andrade E, Basheer SN, Lees C. Impact of cerebral redistribution on neurodevelopmental outcome in small-for-gestational-age or growth-restricted babies: a systematic review. Ultrasound Obstet Gynecol. 2015;46:398–404.
4. Sanz-Cortes M, Simoes RV, Bargallo N, Masoller N, Figueras F, Gratacos E. Proton magnetic resonance spectroscopy assessment of fetal brain metabolism in late-onset 'small for gestational age' versus 'intrauterine growth restriction' fetuses. Fetal Diagn Ther. 2015;37:108–16.
5. Crispi F, Miranda J, Gratacós E. Long-term cardiovascular consequences of fetal growth restriction: biology, clinical implications, and opportunities for prevention of adult disease. Am J Obstet Gynecol. 2018;218:S869–79.
6. Gómez O, Figueras F, Martínez JM, del Río M, Palacio M, Eixarch E, et al. Sequential changes in uterine artery blood flow pattern between the first and second trimesters of gestation in relation to pregnancy outcome. Ultrasound Obstet Gynecol. 2006;28:802–8.
7. Alberry M, Soothill P. Management of fetal growth restriction. Arch Dis Child Fetal Neonatal Ed. 2007;92:F62–7.

8. Gordijn SJ, Beune IM, Thilaganathan B, Papageorghiou A, Baschat AA, Baker PN, et al. Consensus definition of fetal growth restriction: a Delphi procedure. Ultrasound Obstet Gynecol. 2016;48:333–9.
9. Baschat AA. Neurodevelopment following fetal growth restriction and its relationship with antepartum parameters of placental dysfunction. Ultrasound Obstet Gynecol. 2011;37:501–14.
10. Baschat AA. Neurodevelopment after fetal growth restriction. Fetal Diagn Ther. 2014;36:136–42.
11. Harel S, Tomer A, Barak Y, Binderman I, Yavin E. The cephalization index: a screening device for brain maturity and vulnerability in normal and intrauterine growth retarded newborns. Brain and Development. 1985;7:580–4.
12. Padilla N, Perapoch J, Carrascosa A, Acosta-Rojas R, Botet F, Gratacós E. Twelve-month neurodevelopmental outcome in preterm infants with and without intrauterine growth restriction. Acta Paediatr. 2010;99:1498–503.
13. Harvey D, Prince J, Bunton J, Parkinson C, Campbell S. Abilities of children who were small-for-gestational-age babies. Pediatrics. 1982;69:296–300.
14. Lodygensky GA, Seghier ML, Warfield SK, Tolsa CB, Sizonenko S, Lazeyras F, et al. Intrauterine growth restriction affects the preterm infant's hippocampus. Pediatr Res. 2008;63:438–43.
15. Padilla N, Falcón C, Sanz-Cortés M, Figueras F, Bargallo N, Crispi F, et al. Differential effects of intrauterine growth restriction on brain structure and development in preterm infants: a magnetic resonance imaging study. Brain Res. 2011;1382:98–108.
16. Padilla N, Junqué C, Figueras F, Sanz-Cortes M, Bargalló N, Arranz A, et al. Differential vulnerability of gray matter and white matter to intrauterine growth restriction in preterm infants at 12 months corrected age. Brain Res. 2014;1545:1–11.
17. Ramenghi LA, Martinelli A, De Carli A, Brusati V, Mandia L, Fumagalli M, et al. Cerebral maturation in IUGR and appropriate for gestational age preterm babies. Reprod Sci. 2011;18:469–75.
18. Hernandez-Andrade E, Figueroa-Diesel H, Jansson T, Rangel-Nava H, Gratacos E. Changes in regional fetal cerebral blood flow perfusion in relation to hemodynamic deterioration in severely growth-restricted fetuses. Ultrasound Obstet Gynecol. 2008;32:71–6.
19. Batalle D, Eixarch E, Figueras F, Muñoz-Moreno E, Bargallo N, Illa M, et al. Altered small-world topology of structural brain networks in infants with intrauterine growth restriction and its association with later neurodevelopmental outcome. NeuroImage. 2012;60:1352–66.
20. Fischi-Gómez E, Vasung L, Meskaldji DE, Lazeyras F, Borradori-Tolsa C, Hagmann P, et al. Structural brain connectivity in school-age preterm infants provides evidence for impaired networks relevant for higher order cognitive skills and social cognition. Cereb Cortex. 2015;25:2793–805.
21. GRIT Study Group. A randomised trial of timed delivery for the compromised preterm fetus: short term outcomes and Bayesian interpretation. BJOG. 2003;110:27–32.
22. Lees CC, Marlow N, van Wassenaer-Leemhuis A, Arabin B, Bilardo CM, Brezinka C, et al. 2 year neurodevelopmental and intermediate perinatal outcomes in infants with very preterm fetal growth restriction (TRUFFLE): a randomised trial. Lancet. 2015;385:2162–72.
23. Vossbeck S, de Camargo OK, Grab D, Bode H, Pohlandt F. Neonatal and neurodevelopmental outcome in infants born before 30 weeks of gestation with absent or reversed end-diastolic flow velocities in the umbilical artery. Eur J Pediatr. 2001;160:128–34.
24. Baschat AA, Viscardi RM, Hussey-Gardner B, Hashmi N, Harman C. Infant neurodevelopment following fetal growth restriction: relationship with antepartum surveillance parameters. Ultrasound Obstet Gynecol. 2009;33:44–50.
25. Valcamonico A, Accorsi P, Battaglia S, Soregaroli M, Beretta D, Frusca T. Absent or reverse end-diastolic flow in the umbilical artery: intellectual development at school age. Eur J Obstet Gynecol Reprod Biol. 2004;114:23–8.
26. Brodszki J, Morsing E, Malcus P, Thuring A, Ley D, Marsál K. Early intervention in management of very preterm growth-restricted fetuses: 2-year outcome of infants delivered on fetal indication before 30 gestational weeks. Ultrasound Obstet Gynecol. 2009;34:288–96.

27. Shand AW, Hornbuckle J, Nathan E, Dickinson JE, French NP. Small for gestational age preterm infants and relationship of abnormal umbilical artery Doppler blood flow to perinatal mortality and neurodevelopmental outcomes. Aust N Z J Obstet Gynaecol. 2009;49:52–8.
28. Schreuder AM, McDonnell M, Gaffney G, Johnson A, Hope PL. Outcome at school age following antenatal detection of absent or reversed end diastolic flow velocity in the umbilical artery. Arch Dis Child Fetal Neonatal Ed. 2002;86:F108–14.
29. Scherjon SA, Oosting H, Smolders-DeHaas H, Zondervan HA, Kok JH. Neurodevelopmental outcome at three years of age after fetal 'brain-sparing'. Early Hum Dev. 1998;52:67–79.
30. Scherjon S, Briet J, Oosting H, Kok J. The discrepancy between maturation of visual-evoked potentials and cognitive outcome at five years in very preterm infants with and without hemodynamic signs of fetal brain-sparing. Pediatrics. 2000;105:385–91.
31. Stampalija T, Arabin B, Wolf H, Bilardo CM, Lees C. TRUFFLE investigators. Is middle cerebral artery Doppler related to neonatal and 2-year infant outcome in early fetal growth restriction? Am J Obstet Gynecol. 2017;216:521.e1–521.e13.
32. Leppanen M, Ekholm E, Palo P, Maunu J, Munck P, Parkkola R, et al. Abnormal antenatal Doppler velocimetry and cognitive outcome in very-low birth weight infants at 2 years of age. Ultrasound Obstet Gynecol. 2010;36:178–85.
33. Torrance HL, Bloemen MC, Mulder EJ, Nikkels PG, Derks JB, de Vries LS, et al. Predictors of outcome at 2 years of age after early intrauterine growth restriction. Ultrasound Obstet Gynecol. 2010;36:171–7.
34. Arcangeli T, Thilaganathan B, Hooper R, Khan KS, Bhide A. Neurodevelopmental delay in small babies at term: a systematic review. Ultrasound Obstet Gynecol. 2012;40:267–75.
35. Eixarch E, Meler E, Iraola A, Illa M, Crispi F, Hernandez-Andrade E, et al. Neurodevelopmental outcome in 2-year-old infants who were small-for-gestational age term fetuses with cerebral blood flow redistribution. Ultrasound Obstet Gynecol. 2008;32:894–9.
36. Wienerroither H, Steiner H, Tomaselli J, Lobendanz M, Thun-Hohenstein L. Intrauterine blood flow and long-term intellectual, neurologic, and social development. Obstet Gynecol. 2001;97:449–53.

Maternal Cardiovascular Involvement

15

Maya Reddy, Annie Kroushev, Kirsten Palmer,
Daniel Rolnik, and Fabricio Da Silva Costa

Measurement of Cardiac Function

The measurement of cardiac indices is important in understanding the maternal haemodynamic changes that occur in both physiological and pathological states of pregnancy. Traditionally, the invasive Swanz Ganz pulmonary artery catheter was the gold standard for measuring cardiac function. However, non-invasive transthoracic echocardiography has shown excellent correlation with these invasive techniques and as a result has become an equivalent gold standard [1].

More recently, there has been increasing interest in the use of other non-invasive cardiac monitors such as Ultrasound Cardiac Output Monitor (USCOM®), Non-invasive Cardiac Output Monitor (NICOM®) and an inert gas rebreathing method (INNOCOR®). The main advantage of these monitors is that healthcare professionals with different levels of experience can use them as point-of-care systems to assess cardiac function. Various studies have validated these cardiac monitors in non-pregnant individuals and have shown good reproducibility and correlation with echocardiograms and pulmonary artery catheterisation [2, 3]. Furthermore, studies in pregnancy have also demonstrated a reasonable correlation between the USCOM and NICOM cardiac output monitors when compared with echocardiography [4, 5].

M. Reddy · A. Kroushev · K. Palmer · D. Rolnik · F. Da Silva Costa (✉)
Department of Obstetrics and Gynaecology, Monash University and Perinatal Services, Monash Medical Centre, Melbourne, VIC, Australia

L. M. M. Nardozza et al. (eds.), *Fetal Growth Restriction*,
https://doi.org/10.1007/978-3-030-00051-6_15

Echocardiograms Explained: What Information Can You Obtain?

Heart rate and rhythm, cardiac output, and stroke volume

Valvular morphology and function

Cardiac morphology

This is valuable in assessing atrial and ventricular dilation, and concentric and eccentric ventricular hypertrophy. Left ventricular hypertrophy is measured through the thickness of the inter-ventricular septum and posterior left ventricular wall.

Systolic function

This can be evaluated through assessing stroke volume, cardiac output and left ventricular ejection fraction. Measurement of myocardial contractility is also valuable in assessing systolic function.

Diastolic function

This is evaluated through measuring the flow across the mitral valve during diastole as well as through assessment of left atrial size and volume. Diastolic dysfunction is an important factor in cardiovascular disease and often precedes systolic dysfunction. It is characterized by:

1. Increased left atrial size
2. Increased isovolumetric relaxation time (IVRT): this is the time between closure of the aortic valve at the end of systole and the opening of the mitral valve at the beginning of diastole, i.e. the time taken to build an adequate pressure gradient between the left atrium and ventricle.
3. Abnormal E/A ratio: the E/A ratio is a measurement of flow through early and late diastole. Due to the large pressure gradient, early diastole is characterized by rapid flow across the mitral valve resulting in a peak in flow called the E wave. The "a wave" is a reflection of increased filling velocities in late diastole due to an atrial contraction.
4. Prolonged Deceleration time: the deceleration time refers to the interval between the peak of the E wave and the beginning of diastasis. Diastasis refers to the period where flow across the mitral valve decreases as a result of rising ventricular pressures.
5. Increased E/e' ratio: this refers to the ratio of flow across the mitral valve through early diastole (the E wave) and the mitral annular early diastolic velocity (e' wave). This is reflective of increased atrial pressures.

Measurement of Vascular Function

Peripheral arterial measurements are also valuable in assessing physiological and pathological changes of pregnancy. Pregnancy is characterized by vascular remodelling across the entire arterial tree. In general, the physiological changes within this vasculature are designed to increase flow so as to allow for greater perfusion of the uteroplacental unit. Vascular function is predominantly assessed through measurement of arterial stiffness across the aortic, brachial, carotid, ophthalmic and uterine arteries. The main measures of arterial stiffness include:

1. Central and brachial blood pressure—traditional measurements of blood pressure are performed at the brachial artery. Systolic pressures, however, vary through the arterial tree, and more recent studies have shown that arterial pressures measured at the level of the aorta (central BP) are better correlated with cardiovascular events [6]. In pregnancy, while both brachial and central blood pressures decrease with gestation, central BP appears to have a more pronounced decline [7].
2. Augmentation index (AIx)—the augmentation index is a measure of systemic arterial stiffness and can indicate left ventricular workload and endothelial function [8]. This index is a reflection of the components of blood pressure and is made up of two discrete parts. The first component is forward flow and encompasses the blood that is pumped out from the heart into the bloodstream at the point of measurement. The second component is the backward flow that occurs due to the reflected wave of blood. As a result of changes in arterial calibre, arterial pathway and vessel plaques through the arterial tree, some proportion of blood flow is reflected back up the arterial tree and forms this reflected wave [9]. The augmentation index is the percentage of pulse pressure due to the reflected wave. Through the use of non-invasive blood pressure equipment, the arterial waveform, central blood pressure and central augmentation pressure can be detected [9]. These non-invasive techniques have been well validated in catheterization laboratories [9]. While the AIx remains within the normal range throughout pregnancy, it does show a slight decrease over the first two trimesters before increasing towards term [8].
3. Pulse wave velocity (PWV)—"PWV is defined as the velocity at which the pressure waves, generated by the systolic contraction of the heart, propagate along the arterial tree" [10]. Practically, it is measured over the carotid and femoral arteries through the use of non-invasive pressure sensors to measure arterial tonometry [11]. Measurement of PWV is considered the gold standard for assessing arterial stiffness and is inversely proportional to arterial elasticity and compliance [11]. PWV follows a similar course to AIx through pregnancy [8].

Normal Cardiovascular Adaptation to Pregnancy

Cardiac Output, Stroke Volume and Heart Rate

Cardiac output rises steadily through pregnancy, increasing to a maximum of 30–50% above non-pregnant values near term (Fig. 15.1) [13]. The sharpest rise incardiac output occurs in the first 8 weeks of gestation with a continued increase throughout the second trimester [13]. The rise in cardiac output is a result of an interplay between factors affecting preload and afterload including:

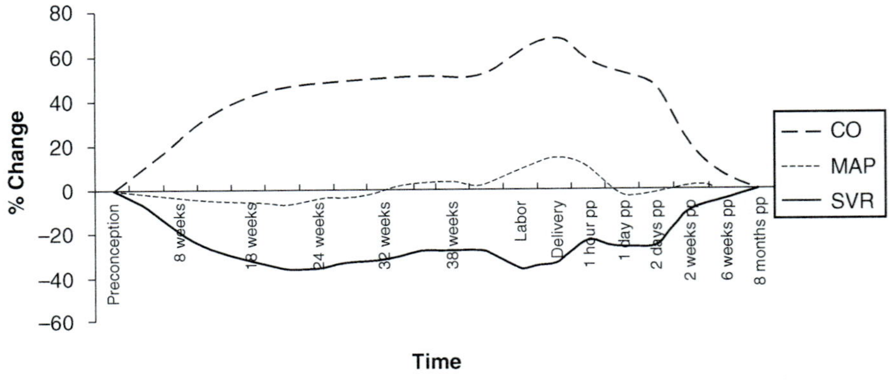

Fig. 15.1 Haemodynamic changes in pregnancy, labour and postpartum. Time on the x-axis changes scale. (Adapted from the Cornette and Roos-Hesselink [12], with permission from Springer). CO cardiac output, MAP mean arterial pressure, PP postpartum, SVR systemic vascular resistance

(a) Increased blood volume—this results in a rise in left ventricular preload, which can be assessed through measuring left atrial diameter and left ventricular end-diastolic dimensions [14].
(b) Drop in systemic vascular resistance—this is largely a reflection of vasodilation and results in a decrease in afterload [14].
(c) Increased maternal heart rate—resting heart rate increases by 10–30 beats per minute, reaching a peak in the third trimester. While in early pregnancy the rise in cardiac output is mainly related to a rise in stroke volume, in later pregnancy, this rise in heart rate plays a larger role [14].

Contractility, Ejection Fraction and Cardiac Remodelling

The haemodynamic changes in pregnancy create a state of volume overload, which results in *temporary* eccentric cardiac remodelling and left ventricular hypertrophy [15]. Studies have shown that the left ventricular wall thickness and mass increase by 28% and 52%, respectively [16]. Despite these changes, cardiac contractility, and right and left ventricular ejection fraction are preserved in pregnancy [15].

Blood Pressure and Systemic Vascular Resistance

During pregnancy, systemic vascular resistance (SVR/TVR) drops to 30% below non-pregnant values. SVR declines throughout pregnancy, reaching a trough in the early third trimester (Fig. 15.1) [15]. The drop in SVR contributes to a decrease in arterial pressures, which reach a nadir in the second trimester (a drop of 5–10 mmHg)

[17]. Mean arterial pressure (MAP) begins to rise in the third trimester and returns to non-pregnant levels in the puerperium [17].

These changes to blood pressure and SVR are mediated by a rise in oestrogen, progesterone, nitric oxide and relaxin [16]. Furthermore, the decrease in SVR can also be attributed to trophoblast invasion of the spiral arteries and the subsequent drop in uteroplacental resistance. In fact, some studies have suggested that this contributes to 20–26% of the reduction in SVR in the second trimester [18].

Changes in Blood Volume

The vasodilation and drop in SVR in pregnancy cause activation of the renin-angiotensin-aldosterone system, which in turn increases circulatory volume [16]. As a result, plasma volume increases by 40–45%, reaching a peak at 30–34 weeks' gestation [16]. This rise in plasma volume has an important role in maternal haemodynamics as it (1) contributes to the rise in preload, which plays an important role in increasing cardiac output, (2) facilitates the delivery of nutrients and removal of waste products from the uteroplacental unit, and (3) provides a reserve for blood loss during delivery. Due to an increase in plasma erythropoietin levels, red blood cell mass also rises in pregnancy to 15–20% above non-pregnant levels [19]. This helps support the higher oxygen requirement of pregnancy. As the increase in red blood cell mass is lower than the rise in plasma volume, a dilutional anaemia ensues [16].

The Role of Maternal Haemodynamics in the "Placental Syndromes" of Pre-eclampsia and Fetal Growth Restriction

PE and FGR are conditions that are thought to arise from the common pathological pathway of placental dysfunction. The underlying mechanisms leading to placental dysfunction and contributing to these "placental syndromes" are likely multifactorial and the focus of much debate. Traditionally, it has been hypothesized that impaired fetal growth and placental insufficiency are a product of inadequate trophoblast invasion, causing incomplete remodelling of the spiral arteries and the persistence of a high resistance placental vascular bed. This results in placental ischaemia-reperfusion injuries and poor fetal perfusion, which thereby impairs fetal growth. Placental ischaemia also triggers the release of anti-angiogenic factors into the maternal circulation. This causes an imbalance of pro-angiogenic and anti-angiogenic factors, resulting in endothelial dysfunction and the subsequent clinical manifestations of PE (Fig. 15.2) [20, 21]. Predictive models for PE and FGR use markers of placental function such as uterine artery Dopplers, PAPP-A and PlGF. While these markers have shown promise in predicting early-onset disease, their value in late-onset FGR and PE is somewhat limited. Thus, while the placental hypothesis is likely central to the pathogenesis of FGR and PE, it does not explain

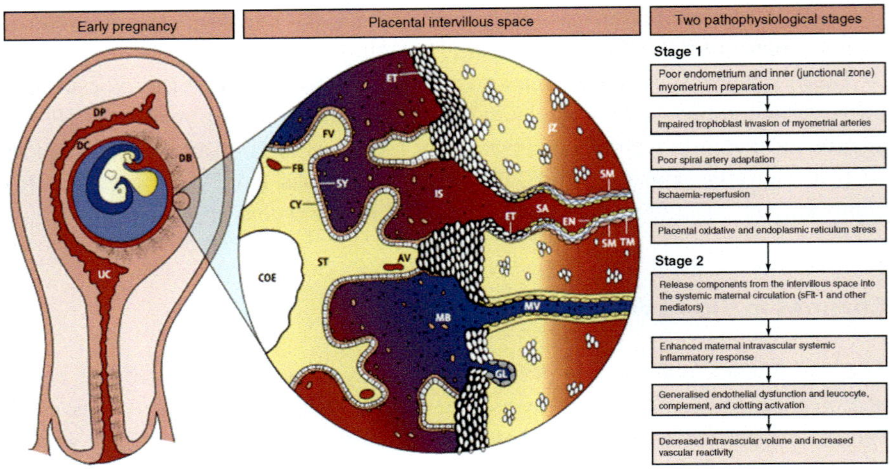

Fig. 15.2 Possible pathophysiological processes in pre-eclampsia. (Figure adapted from Steegers et al., with permission from Elsevier [21]). AV anchoring villus, COE coelomic cavity, CY cytotrophoblast, DB decidua basalis, DC decidua capsularis, DP decidua parietalis, EN endothelium, ET extravillous trophoblast, FB fetal blood vessel, FV floating villus, GL gland, IS intervillous space, JZ junctional zone myometrium, MB maternal blood, leaving the intervillous space with various components such as anti-angiogenic factors. MV maternal vein, SA spiral artery, SM smooth muscle, ST stroma, SY syncytiotrophoblast, TM tunica media, UC uterine cavity, sFlt-1 soluble form of the vascular endothelial growth factor receptor

the entire picture, and perhaps, this has hampered the ability to predict and prevent the outcomes of these complex disease processes.

More recently the role of the maternal circulation in the pathogenesis of FGR has received greater attention. While there are some differences between studies, a common finding is that in comparison to normal pregnancies, FGR is associated with a less dramatic rise in maternal heart rate, stroke volume and cardiac output. Furthermore, women whose pregnancies are complicated by FGR display higher mean arterial pressures and total vascular resistance and an element of both systolic and diastolic dysfunction. These markers of cardiovascular function have been examined in both the preclinical and clinical phases of FGR.

Cardiac Output, Stroke Volume and Heart Rate

Various studies have shown a lower heart rate, stroke volume and cardiac output in pregnancies complicated by FGR when compared to uncomplicated pregnancies [22–24]. Interestingly, the lower stroke volume and cardiac output appear to correlate with a smaller end-diastolic volume and left atrial diameter [25]. This suggests that this relatively smaller rise in stroke volume and cardiac output is a result of inadequate plasma volume expansion and thus a lower preload [25, 26]. Supporting this hypothesis are the findings of lower renin, angiotensin and aldosterone (RAAS) levels in women with PE and FGR [27, 28]. These hormones play a key role in regulation of plasma volume and blood pressure. Furthermore, studies have reported these disparities in cardiovascular adaptation as early as 5–8 weeks' gestation, suggesting that such haemodynamic maladaptation precedes the clinical manifestations of FGR [29, 30]. As a result, cardiovascular markers have shown some promise as screening tools, particularly in the high-risk population [30, 31]. However, further research into the predictive value of these cardiac indices is required.

Mean Arterial Pressures and Total Vascular Resistance

Studies have consistently shown that maternal total vascular resistance (TVR) and mean arterial pressures are higher in pregnancies complicated by FGR [1, 25, 32]. The rise in systolic and diastolic blood pressures, and TVR is not only independent of concomitant hypertension or PE but also appears to precede the clinical phase [18, 32]. This suggests at least some element of causality. In fact, TVR can be used as a predictive marker for "placental syndromes of pregnancy" [18]. Vasapollo et al. showed that, in high-risk pregnancies, TVR >1400 dynes at 24 weeks' gestation has a 89% sensitivity, 94% specificity, 77% positive predictive value (PPV) and 97% negative predictive value (NPV) for predicting the likelihood of a pregnancy complicated by a "placental syndrome". In this particular study, TVR performed better than the standard uterine artery Doppler indices currently used for predicting pregnancy complications [18]. However, further research is required to confirm the value of TVR as a screening tool in the general obstetric population.

Cardiac Morphology and Remodelling

The findings of abnormal cardiac remodelling in FGR pregnancies have been reported some decades ago. Scandinavian studies from the 1960s have shown that women with smaller heart volumes are at a higher risk of delivering small for gestational age infants [33]. More recent echocardiographic studies have shown that FGR pregnancies are characterized by smaller left atrial diameters, left ventricular outflow tracts and left ventricular diastolic dimensions [25, 29, 34, 35]. Pregnancies complicated by "placental syndromes" have also been associated with a depressed left atrial function and altered concentric hypertrophy of the left ventricle, in contrast to the eccentric hypertrophy that normally takes place [18]. The underlying causes of this maladaptation may be attributed to a number of factors. Firstly, the smaller left atrial diameters and diastolic volumes are suggestive of decreased preload [25]. This may be a result of inadequate compensation to the vasodilation and decreased intravascular volume seen in early pregnancy [26]. Secondly, the concentric left ventricular hypertrophy is likely a reflection of the pressure overload that is characteristic of "placental syndromes" of pregnancy [36]. This is in contrast to the volume increase seen in physiologically normal pregnancies accompanied by eccentric left ventricular hypertrophy.

Diastolic Dysfunction

There is significant disparity between studies with regard to diastolic dysfunction in the "placental syndromes" of pregnancy. Some echocardiographic studies have suggested an element of diastolic dysfunction in pregnancies complicated by FGR and PE, demonstrating a decreased E/A ratio and longer isovolumetric relaxation time [22, 34, 35]. This suggests mild diastolic dysfunction and impaired relaxation of the left ventricle [22, 34, 35]. However, this has been contradicted in other studies [25] where no difference has been identified in diastolic function between FGR and normal pregnancy population groups. Further research with larger sample cohorts is required to clarify these findings.

Vascular Dysfunction

The association between vascular dysfunction and "placental syndromes" of pregnancy has received somewhat less attention than the heart. The few studies within this area have mainly focused on PE rather than FGR and have shown a positive correlation between PE and arterial stiffness (increased central BP, PWV and AIx) [37, 38]. Such vascular remodelling is evident in the carotid artery, which has proven to be a well-established marker for cardiovascular morbidity and mortality [38]. These changes in arterial function appear to precede the clinical phase of the disease. When used in the first trimester, in addition to maternal history in the screening for PE, these indices improve the detection rate significantly from 33% to 43% at a 5% FPR [37]. However, the overall low detection rate renders the changes in arterial function a poor predictive tool. There is a paucity of research examining vascular remodelling in FGR with these studies showing conflicting results [39, 40].

The relationship between "placental syndromes" and vascular dysfunction has also been examined through assessment of cerebral vasculature. The ophthalmic and middle cerebral artery Doppler studies are thought to reflect hyperperfusion of the central nervous system (CNS) as a result of endothelial dysfunction. Supporting the CNS hyperperfusion hypothesis are various studies, which have shown that FGR and PE patients exhibit lower ophthalmic artery resistance, that is, an increase in vascular flow [41–43]. While these findings again predate the clinical phase of the disease, the predictive value of the ophthalmic artery Doppler requires further evaluation [42, 44, 45].

Issues with the Cardiac Hypothesis

Inconsistent Study Results

The discrepancy between studies examining maternal cardiovascular changes in FGR pregnancies can be attributed to two main reasons:

1. Definition of the population group: studies that include small for gestational age fetuses and neonates as a marker of FGR tend to show less dramatic differences between cases and controls. However, when FGR is defined by fetal weight, abdominal circumference and abnormal umbilical artery Doppler indices, there are more drastic differences between population groups. The latter method is more representative of the pathological process of FGR, while fetuses that are constitutionally small confound the former.
2. Sample size: the majority of studies in this research area have a small sample size and are likely underpowered to detect a difference between population groups. Larger prospective studies and meta-analyses are required in order to better identify the trends in cardiovascular function in FGR and PE.

The Uncertainties Around Cause Versus Effect, and Early Versus Late FGR

It is unclear whether cardiovascular maladaptation causes or is the result of uteroplacental dysfunction. Pregnancy is a physiological stress test. Cardiovascular maladaptation may therefore be a reflection of failing this stress test, and the resultant impaired fetal perfusion and fetal growth restriction are just symptoms of underlying cardiovascular dysfunction. Alternatively, it is also plausible that cardiovascular maladaptation is itself a symptom of a poorly functioning uteroplacental unit and abnormal placentation. Lastly, it may be the failure of both processes that manifests in "placental syndromes". Defective placentation results in a high-resistance placental bed, which causes changes in the maternal cardiovascular system. However, not everyone with abnormal placentation develops PE or FGR. One way to explain this contradiction would be to surmise that the clinical syndrome develops only in those unable to undergo the necessary cardiovascular adaptations in response to defective placentation. All three of these hypotheses currently remain conjecture, and hopefully longitudinal studies including the pre-pregnancy period will clarify this issue.

It has also been proposed that early- and late-onset FGR represent separate pathological processes, and perhaps cardiovascular maladaptation may explain the differing pathologies [46]. There is a strong consensus that early-onset FGR is a result of true placental insufficiency. Supporting this, the current screening methods of low PAPP-A and raised uterine artery Dopplers can reliably predict early-onset disease. However, 70–80% of cases of FGR are defined as late onset, and within this population group, these placental markers are of modest value [47]. It has thus been proposed that such late-onset disease is not a result of true placental insufficiency but rather the inability of the maternal cardiovascular system to meet the increasing demands of pregnancy [46]. There is certainly evidence that placental histology is different between early- and late-onset FGR, with the former reflecting abnormal placentation and ischaemia and the latter reflecting more heterogeneous changes [48]. Supporting these findings is also evidence of lower cardiac output and higher TVR in pregnancies complicated by late-onset FGR [24].

The single largest risk factor for stillbirth is undiagnosed fetal growth restriction [49]. Perhaps, through a better understanding of the role of maternal haemodynamics in the pathogenesis of early- and late-onset FGR, we will be able to better predict and monitor the population groups at risk of what is essentially a preventable adverse outcome.

Long-Term Cardiovascular Implications of Fetal Growth Restriction to the Mother

Placental syndromes of pregnancy are associated with long-term maternal cardiovascular sequelae. Studies have shown that mothers with FGR infants have a twofold increased risk of cardiovascular disease and cardiovascular disease-related deaths [50, 51]. These findings have also been replicated in the pre-eclamptic population [52, 53]. Mothers of FGR infants have also been shown to have higher rates of glucose impairment, abnormal lipids, persistent endothelial dysfunction and evidence of subclinical atherosclerosis [54, 55]. It is unclear whether this vascular impairment is a result of PE and FGR causing a permanent vascular insult, or a reflection of underlying cardiovascular dysfunction in this population group in the first place. Nonetheless, it does appear that these women could benefit from closer long-term follow-up and risk modifications for prevention of cardiovascular disease.

Key Points

- Adequate cardiovascular adaptation is essential to meeting the metabolic demands of the mother, fetus and uteroplacental unit. Cardiovascular changes in pregnancy include a drop in total vascular resistance; a rise in stroke volume, heart rate and cardiac output; a significant expansion of blood volume; and temporary eccentric remodelling of the heart.
- Evidence suggests that pregnancies complicated by FGR are associated with cardiovascular maladaptation. Mothers of FGR fetuses have been shown to have a higher systemic vascular resistance and a lower stroke volume and cardiac output in comparison to normal pregnancies.
- It is unclear whether such maladaptation is the cause or the result of abnormal placentation or whether it is a combination of both pathological processes that results in the clinical phenotype of FGR.
- The cardiovascular maladaptation associated with FGR appears to predate the clinical phase of the disease, and as such, cardiovascular indices may have a role in predicting early- and late-onset FGR. Further research is required to explore and validate the use of these markers in predictive models.

References

1. Prefumo F, Muiesan ML, Perini R, Paini A, Bonzi B, Lojacono A, et al. Maternal cardiovascular function in pregnancies complicated by intrauterine growth restriction. Ultrasound Obstet Gynecol. 2008;31:65–71.
2. Beltramo F, Menteer J, Razavi A, Khemani RG, Szmuszkovicz J, Newth CJ, et al. Validation of an ultrasound cardiac output monitor as a bedside tool for pediatric patients. Pediatr Cardiol. 2016;37:177–83.
3. van Lelyveld-Haas LE, van Zanten AR, Borm GF, Tjan DH. Clinical validation of the non-invasive cardiac output monitor USCOM-1A in critically ill patients. Eur J Anaesthesiol. 2008;25:917–24.
4. Vinayagam D, Patey O, Thilaganathan B, Khalil A. Cardiac output assessment in pregnancy: comparison of two automated monitors with echocardiography. Ultrasound Obstet Gynecol. 2017;49:32–8.
5. McNamara H, Barclay P, Sharma V. Accuracy and precision of the ultrasound cardiac output monitor (USCOM 1A) in pregnancy: comparison with three-dimensional transthoracic echocardiography. Br J Anaesth. 2014;1:669–76.
6. Roman MJ, Devereux RB, Kizer JR, Lee ET, Galloway JM, Ali T, et al. Central pressure more strongly relates to vascular disease and outcome than does brachial pressure: the Strong Heart Study. Hypertension. 2007;50:197–203.
7. Iacobaeus C, Andolf E, Thorsell M, Bremme K, Jörneskog G, Östlund E, et al. Longitudinal study of vascular structure and function during normal pregnancy. Ultrasound Obstet Gynecol. 2017;49:46–53.
8. Franz MB, Burgmann M, Neubauer A, Zeisler H, Sanani R, Gottsauner-Wolf M, et al. Augmentation index and pulse wave velocity in normotensive and pre-eclamptic pregnancies. Acta Obstet Gynecol Scand. 2013;92:960–6.
9. Townsend RR, Black HR, Chirinos JA, Feig PU, Ferdinand KC, Germain M, et al. Clinical use of pulse wave analysis: proceedings from a symposium sponsored by North American Artery. J Clin Hypertens. 2015;17:503–13.
10. Pereira T, Correia C, Cardoso J. Novel methods for pulse wave velocity measurement. J Med Biol Eng. 2015;35:555–65.
11. Mancia G, Fagard R, Narkiewicz K, Redón J, Zanchetti A, Böhm M, et al. 2013 ESH/ESC Guidelines for the management of arterial hypertension: the task force for the management of arterial hypertension of the European Society of Hypertension (ESH) and of the European Society of Cardiology (ESC). J Hypertens. 2013;31:1281–357.
12. Cornette J, Roos-Hesselink JW. Normal cardiovascular adaptation to pregnancy. In: Stergiopoulos K, Brown D, editors. Evidence-based cardiology consult. London: Springer; 2014.
13. Hunter S, Robson SC. Adaptation of the maternal heart in pregnancy. Br Heart J. 1992;68:540–3.
14. Robson SC, Hunter S, Boys RJ, Dunlop W. Serial study of factors influencing changes in cardiac output during human pregnancy. Am J Phys. 1989;256:H1060–5.
15. Savu O, Jurcut R, Giusca S, van Mieghem T, Gussi I, Popescu BA, et al. Morphological and functional adaptation of the maternal heart during pregnancy. Circ Cardiovasc Imaging. 2012;5:289–97.
16. Sanghavi M, Rutherford JD. Cardiovascular physiology of pregnancy. Circulation. 2014;130:1003–8.
17. Grindheim G, Estensen ME, Langesaeter E, Rosseland LA, Toska K. Changes in blood pressure during healthy pregnancy: a longitudinal cohort study. J Hypertens. 2012;30:342–50.
18. Vasapollo B, Novelli GP, Valensise H. Total vascular resistance and left ventricular morphology as screening tools for complications in pregnancy. Hypertension. 2008;51:1020–6.
19. Pritchard JA. Changes in the blood volume during pregnancy and delivery. Anesthesiology. 1965;26:393–9.

20. Khalil A, Maiz N, Garcia-Mandujano R, Penco JM, Nicolaides KH. Longitudinal changes in maternal serum placental growth factor and soluble fms-like tyrosine kinase-1 in women at increased risk of pre-eclampsia. Ultrasound Obstet Gynecol. 2016;47:324–31.
21. Steegers EA, von Dadelszen P, Duvekot JJ, Pijnenborg R. Pre-eclampsia. Lancet. 2010;376:631–44.
22. Vasapollo B, Valensise H, Novelli GP, Larciprete G, Di Pierro G, Altomare F, et al. Abnormal maternal cardiac function and morphology in pregnancies complicated by intrauterine fetal growth restriction. Ultrasound Obstet Gynecol. 2002;20:452–7.
23. Mahendru AA, Foo FL, McEniery CM, Everett TR, Wilkinson IB, Lees CC. Change in maternal cardiac output from preconception to midpregnancy is associated with birth weight in healthy pregnancies. Ultrasound Obstet Gynecol. 2017;49:78–84.
24. Guy GP, Ling HZ, Machuca M, Poon LC, Nicolaides KH. Maternal cardiac function at 35–37 weeks' gestation: relationship with birth weight. Ultrasound Obstet Gynecol. 2017;49:67–72.
25. Bamfo JE, Kametas NA, Chambers JB, Nicolaides KH. Maternal cardiac function in fetal growth-restricted and non-growth-restricted small-forgestational age pregnancies. Ultrasound Obstet Gynecol. 2007;29:51–7.
26. de Haas S, Ghossein-Doha C, van Kuijk SM, van Drongelen J, Spaanderman ME. Physiological adaptation of maternal plasma volume during pregnancy: a systematic review and meta-analysis. Ultrasound Obstet Gynecol. 2017;49:177–87.
27. Salas SP, Rosso P, Espinoza R, Robert JA, Valdes G, Donoso E. Maternal plasma volume expansion and hormonal changes in women with idiopathic fetal growth retardation. Obstet Gynecol. 1993;81:1029–33.
28. Laskowska M, Leszczynska-Gorzelak B, Laskowska K, Oleszczuk J. Evaluation of the renin-angiotensin-aldosterone system in pregnancy complicated by preeclampsia with and without intrauterine growth retardation. Ann Univ Mariae Curie Sklodowska Med. 2004;59:451–6.
29. Duvekot JJ, Cheriex EC, Pieters FA, Peeters LL. Severely impaired fetal growth is preceded by maternal hemodynamic maladaptation in very early pregnancy. Acta Obstet Gynecol Scand. 1995;74:693–7.
30. De Paco C, Kametas N, Rencoret G, Strobl I, Nicolaides KH. Maternal cardiac output between 11 and 13 weeks of gestation in the prediction of preeclampsia and small for gestational age. Obstet Gynecol. 2008;111:292–300.
31. Stott D, Bolten M, Salman M, Paraschiv D, Clark K, Kametas NA. Maternal demographics and hemodynamics for the prediction of fetal growth restriction at booking, in pregnancies at high risk for placental insufficiency. Acta Obstet Gynecol Scand. 2016;95:329–38.
32. Bamfo JE, Kametas NA, Chambers JB, Nicolaides KH. Maternal cardiac function in normotensive and pre-eclamptic intrauterine growth restriction. Ultrasound Obstet Gynecol. 2008;32:682–6.
33. Hedberg E, Radberg C. Maternal heart volume and prematurity. Acta Obstet Gynecol Scand. 1962;41:48–56.
34. Valensise H, Vasapollo B, Novelli GP, Larciprete G, Romanini ME, Arduini D, et al. Maternal diastolic function in asymptomatic pregnant women with bilateral notching of the uterine artery waveform at 24 weeks' gestation: a pilot study. Ultrasound Obstet Gynecol. 2001;18:450–5.
35. Vasapollo B, Valensise H, Novelli GP, Altomare F, Galante A, Arduini D. Abnormal maternal cardiac function precedes the clinical manifestation of fetal growth restriction. Ultrasound Obstet Gynecol. 2004;24:23–9.
36. Ghossein-Doha C, Khalil A, Lees CC. Maternal hemodynamics: a 2017 update. Ultrasound Obstet Gynecol. 2017;49:10–4.
37. Khalil A, Akolekar R, Syngelaki A, Elkhouli M, Nicolaides KH. Maternal hemodynamics at 11-13 weeks' gestation and risk of pre-eclampsia. Ultrasound Obstet Gynecol. 2012;40:28–34.
38. Yuan LJ, Xue D, Duan YY, Cao TS, Yang HG, Zhou N. Carotid arterial intima-media thickness and arterial stiffness in pre-eclampsia: analysis with a radiofrequency ultrasound technique. Ultrasound Obstet Gynecol. 2013;42:644–52.

39. Khalil A, Sodre D, Syngelaki A, Akolekar R, Nicolaides KH. Maternal hemodynamics at 11-13 weeks of gestation in pregnancies delivering small for gestational age neonates. Fetal Diagn Ther. 2012;32:231–8.
40. Stergiotou I, Bijnens B, Cruz-Lemini M, Figueras F, Gratacos E, Crispi F. Maternal subclinical vascular changes in fetal growth restriction with and without pre-eclampsia. Ultrasound Obstet Gynecol. 2015;46:706–12.
41. Melo NA, Araujo Junior E, Helfer TM, Caetano AC, Zamarian AC, Moron AF, et al. Assessment of maternal Doppler parameters of ophthalmic artery in fetuses with growth restriction in the third trimester of pregnancy: a case-control study. J Obstet Gynaecol Res. 2015;41:1330–6.
42. Gurgel Alves JA, Maia e Holanda Moura SB, Araujo Junior E, Tonni G, Martins WP, Da Silva Costa F. Predicting small for gestational age in the first trimester of pregnancy using maternal ophthalmic artery Doppler indices. J Matern Fetal Neonatal Med. 2016;29:1190–4.
43. Diniz AL, Moron AF, dos Santos MC, Sass N, Pires CR, Debs CL. Ophthalmic artery Doppler as a measure of severe pre-eclampsia. Int J Gynaecol Obstet. 2008;100:216–20.
44. Gurgel Alves JA, Praciano de Sousa PC, Maia e Holanda Moura SB, Kane SC, da Silva Costa F. First-trimester maternal ophthalmic artery Doppler analysis for prediction of pre-eclampsia. Ultrasound Obstet Gynecol. 2014;44:411–8.
45. Kalafat E, Laoreti A, Khalil A, Da Silva CF, Thilaganathan B. Ophthalmic artery Doppler prediction of preeclampsia: a systematic review and meta-analysis. Ultrasound Obstet Gynecol. 2018;51:731–7.
46. Thilaganathan B. Placental syndromes: getting to the heart of the matter. Ultrasound Obstet Gynecol. 2017;49:7–9.
47. Crovetto F, Crispi F, Scazzocchio E, et al. First-trimester screening for early and late small-for-gestational-age neonates using maternal serum biochemistry, blood pressure and uterine artery Doppler. Ultrasound Obstet Gynecol. 2014;43:34–40.
48. Mifsud W, Sebire NJ. Placental pathology in early-onset and late-onset fetal growth restriction. Fetal Diagn Ther. 2014;36:117–28.
49. Gardosi J, Madurasinghe V, Williams M, Malik A, Francis A. Maternal and fetal risk factors for stillbirth: population based study. BMJ. 2013;346:f108.
50. Smith GC, Pell JP, Walsh D. Pregnancy complications and maternal risk of ischaemic heart disease: a retrospective cohort study of 129,290 births. Lancet. 2001;357:2002–6.
51. Pariente G, Sheiner E, Kessous R, Michael S, Shoham-Vardi I. Association between delivery of a small-for-gestational-age neonate and longterm maternal cardiovascular morbidity. Int J Gynaecol Obstet. 2013;123:68–71.
52. Grand'Maison S, Pilote L, Okano M, Landry T, Dayan N. Markers of vascular dysfunction after hypertensive disorders of pregnancy: a systematic review and meta-analysis. Hypertension. 2016;68:1447–58.
53. Wu P, Haththotuwa R, Kwok CS, et al. Preeclampsia and future cardiovascular health: a systematic review and meta-analysis. Circ Cardiovasc Qual Outcomes. 2017;10:e003497.
54. Hillman SL, Kubba T, Williams DJ. Delivery of small-for-gestational-age neonate and association with early-onset impaired maternal endothelial function. Ultrasound Obstet Gynecol. 2017;49:150–4.
55. Kanagalingam MG, Nelson SM, Freeman DJ, et al. Vascular dysfunction and alteration of novel and classic cardiovascular risk factors in mothers of growth restricted offspring. Atherosclerosis. 2009;205:244–50.

Index

L. M. M. Nardozza et al. (eds.), *Fetal Growth Restriction*,
https://doi.org/10.1007/978-3-030-00051-6

Printed by Printforce, the Netherlands